50 LANDMARK PAPERS

every

Breast Surgeon Should Know

There has been an exponential increase in the volume and quality of published research relating to breast disease over the past decades. This book identifies the 50 key scientific articles in the field of breast disease and breast surgery and examines their importance to and impact on current clinical care.

Among thousands of articles, a small fraction are truly 'game changing'. Such studies form the foundations of breast surgery today, and the selection of papers within this book provide the 50 landmark papers every 21st-century breast surgeon needs to know. A commentary to each carefully selected paper explains why these papers are so important, thus providing every surgeon with the foundation stones of knowledge in this fast-moving area.

This is a valuable reference not only to the established surgeon, but also to breast surgery residents and trainees, as well as to more experienced surgeons as they continue to learn new techniques and approaches and to improve their knowledge of breast disease and treatments. The papers provide an evidence-based resource for those surgeons preparing for professional exams and may inspire clinicians to produce new research.

50 Landmark Papers Series

50 Landmark Papers every Spine Surgeon Should Know
Alexander R Vaccaro, Charles G Fisher and Jefferson R Wilson

50 Landmark Papers every Trauma Surgeon Should Know
Stephen M Cohn and Ara J Feinstein

50 Landmark Papers every Acute Care Surgeon Should Know
Stephen M Cohn and Peter Rhee

50 Landmark Papers every Vascular and Endovascular Surgeon Should Know
Juan Carlos Jimenez and Samuel Eric Wilson

50 Landmark Papers every Oral and Maxillofacial Surgeon Should Know
Niall MH McLeod and Peter A Brennan

50 Landmark Papers every Intensivist Should Know
Stephen M Cohn, Alan Lisbon and Stephen Heard

50 Landmark Papers every Thyroid and Parathyroid Surgeon Should Know
Sam Wiseman and Sebastian Aspinall

50 Landmark Papers every Pediatric Surgeon Should Know
Mark Davenport, Bashar Aldeiri and Joseph Davidson

50 Landmark Papers every Breast Surgeon Should Know
Lynda Wyld, Ramsey Cutress and Jenna Morgan

For more information about this series, please visit www.routledge.com/50-Landmark-Papers/book-series/50LP

50 LANDMARK PAPERS

every

Breast Surgeon Should Know

EDITED BY

Lynda Wyld
Ramsey Cutress
Jenna Morgan

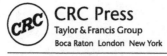

CRC Press
Taylor & Francis Group
Boca Raton London New York

CRC Press is an imprint of the
Taylor & Francis Group, an **informa** business

First edition published 2024
by CRC Press
4 Park Square, Milton Park, Abingdon, Oxon, OX14 4RN

and by CRC Press
2385 NW Executive Center Drive, Suite 320, Boca Raton, FL 33431

CRC Press is an imprint of Informa UK Limited

British Library Cataloguing-in-Publication Data
A catalogue record for this book is available from the British Library

ISBN: 9781032522388 (hbk)
ISBN: 9781032471273 (pbk)
ISBN: 9781003405696 (ebk)

DOI: 10.1201/b23352

Typeset in Times New Roman
by KnowledgeWorks Global Ltd.

We dedicate this book to the pioneering researchers who led these seminal works, the teams of research-active doctors, nurses, scientists and administrators who conducted this research and all the patients who have given up their time/blood/tissue, and often endured gruelling new treatment and follow-up schedules, to take part in these studies over the years.

Lynda Wyld, Ramsey Cutress and Jenna Morgan

Contents

FOREWORD XIX
PREFACE XXI
EDITORS XXIII
CONTRIBUTORS XXV

Section One   Epidemiology

1 TYPE AND TIMING OF MENOPAUSAL HORMONE THERAPY AND BREAST
CANCER RISK: INDIVIDUAL PARTICIPANT META-ANALYSIS OF THE
WORLDWIDE EPIDEMIOLOGICAL EVIDENCE   1
Collaborative Group on Hormonal Factors in Breast Cancer.
Lancet 394(10204):1159–1168, 2019

Expert Commentary by Toral Gathani and Isobel Barnes

2 MODERATE ALCOHOL INTAKE AND CANCER INCIDENCE
IN WOMEN   7
Allen N, Beral V, Cassabone D, Kan SW, Reeves GK, Brown A,
Green J on behalf of the Million Women Study Collaborators.
J Natl Cancer Inst 101(5):296–305, 2009

Expert Commentary by Toral Gathani and Isobel Barnes

Section Two   Screening and Prevention

3 TAMOXIFEN FOR PREVENTION OF BREAST CANCER: REPORT
OF THE NATIONAL SURGICAL ADJUVANT BREAST AND BOWEL
PROJECT P-1 STUDY (NSABP P-1)   13
Fisher B, Costantino J, Wickerman D, et al.
J Natl Cancer Inst 97(22):1652–1662, 2005

Expert Commentary by Andrew Kilshaw and Lynda Wyld

4 THE SWEDISH TWO-COUNTY TRIAL OF MAMMOGRAPHIC SCREENING
FOR BREAST CANCER: RECENT RESULTS AND CALCULATION OF
BENEFIT   19
Tabar L, Fagerberg G, Duffy SW, et al.

J Epidemiol Community Health 43:107–114, 1989

Expert Commentary by Alasdair Findlay and Lynda Wyld

5 THE BENEFITS AND HARMS OF BREAST CANCER SCREENING:
AN INDEPENDENT REVIEW   25
*Marmot MG, Altman DG, Cameron DA, Dewar JA, Thompson SG,
Wilcox M.*

Br J Cancer 108(11):2205–2240, 2013

Expert Commentary by Colin McIlmunn and Stuart McIntosh

Section Three   Diagnostic Imaging

6 DIAGNOSTIC PERFORMANCE OF DIGITAL VERSUS FILM MAMMOGRAPHY
FOR BREAST-CANCER SCREENING   31
*Pisano ED, Gatsonis C, Hendrick E, Yaffe M, Baum JK, Acharyya S,
Conant EF, Fajardo LL, Bassett L, D'Orsi C, Jong R, Rebner M.*

N Engl J Med 353(17):1773–1783, 2005

Expert Commentary by Jonathan James, Mariana Matias and Nisha Sharma

7 SCREENING WITH MAGNETIC RESONANCE IMAGING AND
MAMMOGRAPHY OF A UK POPULATION AT HIGH FAMILIAL RISK
OF BREAST CANCER: A PROSPECTIVE MULTICENTRE COHORT STUDY
(MARIBS)   39
Leach MO, Boggis CRM, Dixon AK, Easton DF, et al.

Lancet 365(9473):1769–1778, 2005

Expert Commentary by Jonathan James, Mariana Matias and Nisha Sharma

8 COMPARATIVE EFFECTIVENESS OF MRI IN BREAST CANCER
(COMICE) TRIAL: A RANDOMISED CONTROLLED TRIAL   45
Turnbull L, Brown S, Harvey I, Olivier C, Drew P, Napp V, Hanby A, Brown J.

Lancet 375:563–571, 2010

Expert Commentary by Jonathan James, Mariana Matias and Nisha Sharma

Section Four   Surgery: Mastectomy versus Conservation

9 TWENTY-YEAR FOLLOW-UP OF A RANDOMIZED TRIAL COMPARING TOTAL MASTECTOMY, LUMPECTOMY, AND LUMPECTOMY PLUS IRRADIATION FOR THE TREATMENT OF INVASIVE BREAST CANCER   51
Fisher B, Anderson S, Bryant J, Margolese RG, Deutsch M, Fisher ER, Jeong JH, Wolmark N.
N Engl J Med 347(16):1233–1241, 2002
Expert Commentary by Bahar Mirshekar-Syahkal and John Benson

10 THE ASSOCIATION OF SURGICAL MARGINS AND LOCAL RECURRENCE IN WOMEN WITH EARLY-STAGE INVASIVE BREAST CANCER TREATED WITH BREAST-CONSERVING THERAPY: A META-ANALYSIS   57
Houssami N, Macaskill P, Marinovich ML, Morrow M.
Ann Surg Oncol 21(3):717–730, 2014
Expert Commentary by Leah Kim and Mehra Golshan

11 TEN YEAR SURVIVAL AFTER BREAST-CONSERVING SURGERY PLUS RADIOTHERAPY COMPARED WITH MASTECTOMY IN EARLY BREAST CANCER IN THE NETHERLANDS: A POPULATION-BASED STUDY   61
van Maaren MC, de Munck L, de Back GH, Jobsen J, van Dalen T, Poortmans P, Strobbe LC, Siesling S.
Lancet Oncol 17:1258–1270, 2016
Expert Commentary by Ismail Jatoi and John Benson

Section Five   De-Escalation of Axillary Surgery

12 TWENTY-FIVE-YEAR FOLLOW-UP OF A RANDOMIZED TRIAL COMPARING RADICAL MASTECTOMY, TOTAL MASTECTOMY, AND TOTAL MASTECTOMY FOLLOWED BY IRRADIATION   67
Fisher B, Jeong JH, Anderson S, Bryant J, Fisher ER, Wolmark N.
N Engl J Med 347(8):567–575, 2002
Expert Commentary by Eilidh Bruce and Beatrix Elsberger

13 EFFECT OF AXILLARY DISSECTION VS NO AXILLARY DISSECTION ON
10-YEAR OVERALL SURVIVAL AMONG WOMEN WITH INVASIVE BREAST
CANCER AND SENTINEL NODE METASTASIS: THE ACOSOG Z0011
(ALLIANCE) RANDOMIZED CLINICAL TRIAL   73
Giuliano AE, Ballman KV, McCall L, et al.
JAMA 318(10):918–926, 2017
Expert Commentary by Eilidh Bruce and Beatrix Elsberger

14 RADIOTHERAPY OR SURGERY OF THE AXILLA AFTER A POSITIVE
SENTINEL NODE IN BREAST CANCER (EORTC 10981-22023
AMAROS): A RANDOMISED, MULTICENTRE, OPEN-LABEL,
PHASE 3 NON-INFERIORITY TRIAL   77
Donker M, van Tienhoven G, Straver ME, et al.
Lancet Oncol 15(12):1303–1310, 2014
Expert Commentary by Eilidh Bruce and Beatrix Elsberger

15 SENTINEL LYMPH NODE SURGERY AFTER NEOADJUVANT
CHEMOTHERAPY IN PATIENTS WITH NODE-POSITIVE BREAST
CANCER: THE ACOSOG Z1071 (ALLIANCE) CLINICAL TRIAL   81
Boughey JC, Suman VJ, Mittendorf EA, et al.
JAMA 310(14):1455–1461, 2013
Expert Commentary by Eilidh Bruce and Beatrix Elsberger

Section Six   Oncoplastic Breast Surgery/Breast Reconstruction

16 PLANNING AND USE OF THERAPEUTIC MAMMAPLASTY: THE
NOTTINGHAM APPROACH   87
McCulley SJ, Macmillan RD.
Br J Plast Surg 58(7):889–901, 2005
Expert Commentary by Danielle Banfield and Shelley Potter

17 ONCOPLASTIC BREAST-CONSERVING SURGERY FOR WOMEN
WITH PRIMARY BREAST CANCER   91
Nanda A, Hu J, Hodgkinson S, Ali S, Rainsbury R, Roy PG.
Cochrane Database Syst Rev (10):CD013658, 2021
Expert Commentary by Katherine Fairhurst and Shelley Potter

18 SHORT-TERM SAFETY OUTCOMES OF MASTECTOMY AND
    IMMEDIATE IMPLANT-BASED BREAST RECONSTRUCTION WITH
    AND WITHOUT MESH (iBRA): A MULTICENTRE, PROSPECTIVE
    COHORT STUDY   95
    Potter S, Conroy EJ, Cutress RI, et al.

    Lancet Oncol 20:254–266, 2019

    Expert Commentary by Danielle Banfield and Shelley Potter

19 IMPROVING BREAST CANCER SURGERY: A CLASSIFICATION
    AND QUADRANT PER QUADRANT ATLAS FOR ONCOPLASTIC
    SURGERY   101
    Clough KB, Kaufman GJ, Nos C, Buccimazza I, Sarfati IM.

    Ann Surg Oncol 17:1375–1391, 2010

    Expert Commentary by David Stark and Shelley Potter

Section Seven   Breast Cancer Genomics and Prognostic Tools

20 GENE EXPRESSION PATTERNS OF BREAST CARCINOMAS
    DISTINGUISH TUMOR SUBCLASSES WITH CLINICAL
    IMPLICATIONS   107
    Sørlie T, Perou CM, Tibshirani R, Aas T, Geisler S, Johnsen H, et al.

    Proc Natl Acad Sci 98(19):10869–10874, 2001

    Expert Commentary by Cliona Kirwan and Rachel Foster

21 COMPREHENSIVE MOLECULAR PORTRAITS OF HUMAN BREAST
    TUMOURS   111
    The Cancer Genome Atlas Network.

    Nature 490:61–70, 2012

    Expert Commentary by Rachel Foster and Cliona Kirwan

22 70-GENE SIGNATURE AS AN AID TO TREATMENT DECISIONS
    IN EARLY-STAGE BREAST CANCER   117
    Cardoso F, van't Veer LJ, Bogaerts J, et al. for the MINDACT Investigators.

    N Engl J Med 375(8):717–729, 2016

    Expert Commentary by Cliona Kirwan and Rachel Foster

23 21-GENE ASSAY TO INFORM CHEMOTHERAPY BENEFIT IN NODE-POSITIVE BREAST CANCER (RxPONDER)   123
    Kalinsky K, Barlow WE, Gralow JR, et al.

    New Engl J Med 385:2336–2347, 2021

    Expert Commentary by Cliona Kirwan and Rachel Foster

24 PREDICT: A NEW UK PROGNOSTIC MODEL THAT PREDICTS SURVIVAL FOLLOWING SURGERY FOR INVASIVE BREAST CANCER   129
    Wishart GC, Azzato EM, Greenberg DC, et al.

    Breast Cancer Res 12:R1–R10, 2010

    Expert Commentary by Rachel Foster and Cliona Kirwan

Section Eight   Ductal Carcinoma *In Situ*

25 GENOMIC ANALYSIS DEFINES CLONAL RELATIONSHIPS OF DUCTAL CARCINOMA *IN SITU* AND RECURRENT INVASIVE BREAST CANCER   135
    Lips EH, Kumar T, Megalios A, Visser LL, Sheinman M, Fortunato A, et al.

    Grand Challenge PRECISION Consortium. Nature Genet 54:850–860, 2022

    Expert Commentary by Thomas Seddon, Pavneet S. Kohli and Tim Rattay

26 PATHOLOGICAL FEATURES OF 11,337 PATIENTS WITH PRIMARY DUCTAL CARCINOMA *IN SITU* (DCIS) AND SUBSEQUENT EVENTS: RESULTS FROM THE UK SLOANE PROJECT   141
    Shaaban AM, Hilton B, Clements K, Provenzano E, Cheung S, Wallis MG, et al.

    Br J Cancer 2021 Mar;124(5):1009–1017

    Expert Commentary by Stacey Carter, Elizabeth Bonefas, Karen Clements and Alastair Thompson

27 EFFECT OF TAMOXIFEN AND RADIOTHERAPY IN WOMEN WITH LOCALLY EXCISED DUCTAL CARCINOMA *IN SITU*: LONG-TERM RESULTS FROM THE UK/ANZ DCIS TRIAL   147
    Cuzick J, Sestak I, Pinder SE, Ellis IO, Forsyth S, Bundred NJ, et al.

    Lancet Oncol 12(1):21–29, 2011

    Expert Commentary by Nicole James and Gurdeep Mannu

28 A Prognostic Index for Ductal Carcinoma *In Situ* of the
    Breast   153
    Silverstein MJ, Lagios MD, Craig PH, et al.

    Cancer 77(11):2267–2274, 1996

    Expert Commentary by Amit Agrawal and Mahmoud Soliman

Section Nine   Adjuvant Chemotherapy

29 Comparisons between Different Polychemotherapy Regimens
    for Early Breast Cancer: Meta-Analyses of Long-Term
    Outcome among 100,000 Women in 123 Randomised Trials   159
    Peto R, Davies C, Godwin J, Gray, R, Pan, HC, Clarke, M, et al.

    Lancet 379(9814):432–444, 2012

    Expert Commentary by Jessica Banks, Lynda Wyld and Janet Brown

30 Adjuvant Capecitabine for Breast Cancer after Preoperative
    Chemotherapy: CREATE-X   165
    Masuda N, Lee S-J, Ohtani S, Im Y-H, Lee E-S, Yokota I, et al.

    N Engl J Med 376:2147–2159, 2017

    Expert Commentary by Soudamini Nayak, Lynda Wyld and Janet Brown

Section Ten   Adjuvant Endocrine Therapy

31 Relevance of Breast Cancer Hormone Receptors and Other
    Factors to the Efficacy of Adjuvant Tamoxifen: Patient-Level
    Meta-Analysis of Randomised Trials   171
    Early Breast Cancer Trialists' Collaborative Group (EBCTCG).

    Lancet 378:771–784, 2011

    Expert Commentary by Fiona James and Tom Hubbard

32 Long-Term Effects of Continuing Adjuvant Tamoxifen to
    10 Years versus Stopping at 5 Years after Diagnosis
    of Oestrogen Receptor–Positive Breast Cancer:
    ATLAS, a Randomised Trial   177
    Davies C, Pan H, Godwin J, et al.

    Lancet 9869:805–816, 2013

    Expert Commentary by Fiona James and Tom Hubbard

33 TAILORING ADJUVANT ENDOCRINE THERAPY FOR PREMENOPAUSAL
    BREAST CANCER   183
    Francis PA, Pagani O, Fleming GF, et al.

    N Engl J Med 379:122–137, 2018

    Expert Commentary by Fiona James and Douglas Ferguson

34 ANASTROZOLE ALONE OR IN COMBINATION WITH TAMOXIFEN VERSUS
    TAMOXIFEN ALONE FOR ADJUVANT TREATMENT OF POSTMENOPAUSAL
    WOMEN WITH EARLY BREAST CANCER: FIRST RESULTS OF THE ATAC
    RANDOMISED TRIAL   187
    Arimidex, Tamoxifen, Alone or in Combination; ATAC Trialists' Group.

    Lancet 359(9324):2131–2139, 2002

    Expert Commentary by Alex Humphreys and Douglas Ferguson

Section Eleven   Immunotherapy/Systemic Therapy

35 11 YEARS' FOLLOW-UP OF TRASTUZUMAB AFTER ADJUVANT
    CHEMOTHERAPY IN *HER2*-POSITIVE EARLY BREAST CANCER:
    FINAL ANALYSIS OF THE HERCEPTIN ADJUVANT (HERA)
    TRIAL   193
    *Cameron D, Piccart-Gebhart MJ, Gelber RD, Procter M, Goldhirsch A,
    de Azambuja E, et al. and Herceptin Adjuvant (HERA) Trial Study Team.*

    Lancet 389(10075):1195–1205, 2017

    Expert Commentary by Wilson Cheah Pui Fui and Ellen Copson

36 ADJUVANT OLAPARIB FOR PATIENTS WITH *BRCA1-* OR *BRCA2-*
    MUTATED BREAST CANCER   199
    Tutt ANJ, Garber JE, Kaufman B, et al.

    N Engl J Med 384(25):2394–2405, 2021

    Expert Commentary by Anthony Mark Monaghan and Ellen Copson

37 PEMBROLIZUMAB FOR EARLY TRIPLE-NEGATIVE BREAST
    CANCER   205
    Schmid P, Cortes J, Dent R, et al.

    New Engl J Med 386(6):556–567, 2022

    Expert Commentary by Constantinos Savva and Ellen Copson

38 TRASTUZUMAB EMTANSINE FOR RESIDUAL INVASIVE
    HER2-POSITIVE BREAST CANCER   211
    von Minckwitz G, Huang C-S, Mano MS, et al. for the KATHERINE
    Investigators.

    N Engl J Med 380:617–628, 2019

    Expert Commentary by Maclyn Augustine and Ellen Copson

Section Twelve   Adjuvant Radiotherapy

39 BREAST-CONSERVING SURGERY WITH OR WITHOUT
    IRRADIATION IN EARLY BREAST CANCER
    (PRIME II)   217
    Kunkler IH, Williams LJ, Jack WJL, Cameron DA, Dixon JM
    Breast-conserving surgery with or without irradiation
    in early breast cancer.

    New England Journal of Medicine. 16;388(7):585–94, 2023

    Expert Commentary by Puteri Abdul Haris and David Dodwell

40 EFFECT OF RADIOTHERAPY AFTER BREAST-CONSERVING
    SURGERY ON 10-YEAR RECURRENCE AND 15-YEAR
    BREAST CANCER DEATH: META-ANALYSIS OF INDIVIDUAL
    PATIENT DATA FOR 10,801 WOMEN IN 17 RANDOMISED
    TRIALS   221
    Early Breast Cancer Trialists' Collaborative Group (EBCTCG)
    Darby S, McGale P, Correa C, et al.

    Lancet 378(9804):1707–1716, 2011

    Expert Commentary by Puteri Abdul Haris and David Dodwell

41 WHOLE-BREAST IRRADIATION WITH OR WITHOUT A BOOST FOR
    PATIENTS TREATED WITH BREAST-CONSERVING SURGERY FOR EARLY
    BREAST CANCER: 20-YEAR FOLLOW-UP OF A RANDOMISED PHASE 3
    TRIAL   225
    Bartelink H, Maingon P, Poortmans P, et al. On behalf of the European
    Organisation for Research and Treatment of Cancer Radiation Oncology
    and Breast Cancer Groups.

    Lancet 16:47–56, 2015

    Expert Commentary by Puteri Abdul Haris and David Dodwell

42 EFFECT OF RADIOTHERAPY AFTER MASTECTOMY AND AXILLARY
    SURGERY ON 10-YEAR RECURRENCE AND 20-YEAR BREAST CANCER
    MORTALITY: META-ANALYSIS OF INDIVIDUAL PATIENT DATA FOR 8135
    WOMEN IN 22 RANDOMISED TRIALS   229
    Early Breast Cancer Trialists' Collaborative Group.

    Lancet 383(9935):2127–2135, 2014

    Expert Commentary by Puteri Abdul Haris and David Dodwell

43 HYPOFRACTIONATED BREAST RADIOTHERAPY FOR 1 WEEK VERSUS
    3 WEEKS (FAST-FORWARD): 5-YEAR EFFICACY AND LATE NORMAL
    TISSUE EFFECTS; RESULTS FROM A MULTICENTRE, NON-INFERIORITY,
    RANDOMISED, PHASE 3 TRIAL   233
    *Brunt AM, Haviland JS, Wheatley DA, et al., on behalf of the
    FAST-Forward Trial Management Group.*

    Lancet 395(10237):1613–1626, 2020

    Expert Commentary by Puteri Abdul Haris and David Dodwell

Section Thirteen   Bisphosphonates

44 ADJUVANT ZOLEDRONIC ACID IN PATIENTS WITH EARLY BREAST
    CANCER: FINAL EFFICACY ANALYSIS OF THE AZURE (BIG 01/04)
    RANDOMISED OPEN-LABEL PHASE 3 TRIAL   237
    *Coleman R, Cameron D, Dodwell D, et al., on behalf of the AZURE
    Investigators.*

    Lancet Oncol 15(9):997–1006, 2014

    Expert Commentary by Steven Wood, Emma Green and Janet Brown

45 LONG-TERM EFFECTS OF ANASTROZOLE ON BONE MINERAL DENSITY:
    7-YEAR RESULTS FROM THE ATAC TRIAL   243
    *Eastell R, Adams J, Clack G, Howell A, Cuzick J, Mackey J, et al.
    Annals Oncol 22(4):857–862, 2011*

    Expert Commentary by Sophie Trotter and Janet Brown

Section Fourteen   Surgery for Metastatic Disease

46 LOCOREGIONAL TREATMENT VERSUS NO TREATMENT OF THE
    PRIMARY TUMOUR IN METASTATIC BREAST CANCER: AN OPEN-LABEL
    RANDOMISED CONTROLLED TRIAL   249
    Badwe R, Hawaldar R, Nair N, Kaushik R, Parmar V, Siddique S, et al.

    Lancet Oncol 16:1380–1388, 2015

    Expert Commentary by Urvashi Jain, Ashutosh Kothari and Rajendra Badwe

Section Fifteen   Breast Cancer in Pregnancy/ Prophylactic Surgery for Family History

47 TREATMENT OF BREAST CANCER DURING PREGNANCY: AN OBSERVATIONAL STUDY   255
Loibl S, Han SN, Minckwitz GV, Bontenbal M, Ring A, Giermek J, et al.

Lancet Oncol 13:887–896, 2012

Expert Commentary by Lydia Newman, Chris Coyle, Avi Agrawal and Edward R. St John

48 GERMLINE *BRCA* MUTATION AND OUTCOME IN YOUNG-ONSET BREAST CANCER (POSH): A PROSPECTIVE COHORT STUDY   261
Copson ER, Maishman TC, Tapper WJ, Cutress RI, Greville-Heygate S, Altman DG, et al.

Lancet Oncol 19(2):169–180, 2018

Expert Commentary by Wilson Cheah Pui Fui, Camellia Richards, Constantinos Savva and Ramsey Cutress

49 EFFICACY OF BILATERAL PROPHYLACTIC MASTECTOMY IN WOMEN WITH A FAMILY HISTORY OF BREAST CANCER   269
Hartmann L, Schaid D, Woods J, Crotty T, Myers J, Arnold P, et al.

N Engl J Med 340(2):77–84, 1999

Expert Commentary by Hamza Ikram and Lynda Wyld

50 WIRE- AND MAGNETIC-SEED-GUIDED LOCALIZATION OF IMPALPABLE BREAST LESIONS: iBRA-NET LOCALISATION STUDY (ARM 1)   275
Dave RV, Barrett E, Morgan J, et al., on behalf of the iBRA-NET Localisation Study Collaborative.

Br J Surg 109:274–282, 2022

Expert Commentary by Iram Hassan, Samantha Chen, Masooma Zaidi, Peter A Barry and Edward R. St John

INDEX   281

Foreword

As President of the Association of Breast Surgery (ABS) of Great Britain and Northern Ireland, it is a privilege and honour to be invited to write this foreword. The association has a thriving and extremely active academic and research committee, and all three editors and most of the chapter authors are members of the association. Despite being busy clinicians, they are academics and leaders in the field and understand the pressures to keep up to date with research findings.

Breast cancer is the commonest cancer worldwide, and probably the most written about cancer in literature. I remember studying for my final fellowship examination years ago and pondering over what I would consider to be the most significant landmark papers. How I wish there had been a book like this available at that time.

With so much literature available, Cutress, Morgan and Wyld have done a fantastic job of not only picking 50 landmark papers but presenting them in a manner that enables the book to cover topics as opposed to isolated papers.

The simple layout covering the salient features of the paper, followed by the expert commentary and easy-to-grasp style of presentation, makes this an ideal book for everyone—students, trainees, busy clinicians wanting to check facts and lecturers and professors preparing their talks.

I would also like to congratulate all the chapter authors. This is a wonderful book, extremely useful, and gives a solid foundation for understanding the rationale behind clinical practice and current research. I feel every breast unit should have a copy, as a useful resource for members of their team.

Leena S Chagla, MS, FRCS
President, Association of Breast Surgery, UK (2023–2025)

Preface

Breast cancer outcomes have improved massively in the past 50 years, from 50% 5-year survival in the 1970s to over 80% today, and this progress has been driven by high-quality research. Breast oncology (surgical, medical and radiation) has led the way in embracing evidence-based practice and adopting new management paradigms to keep pace with the research data. Pioneering researchers over the past 50 years have often faced criticism for challenging the status quo. Prime examples include Bernard Fisher and Umberto Veronesi for their practice-changing trials into breast conservation surgery, leading to millions of women being spared mastectomy for their breast cancer. At the time they were derided as heretics by the mainstream surgical establishment, but time, and their excellent, rigorous trial data, proved them right. We have therefore moved from monodisciplinary breast care (surgery) to multidisciplinary care, with integrated teams of experts contributing to improve outcomes whilst simultaneously improving long-term quality of life.

The role of research cannot be overstated, but sadly these key works are often distilled into a reference number in a guideline, and many practitioners are not familiar with the actual study (warts and all) that changed practice.

Understanding these works, their context and the impact they have made is essential for a modern breast practitioner (of whatever discipline). Acquiring the skills to critically evaluate new research is also an essential skill for all clinicians so they may continue the trend of improving evidence-based practice, so that in another 50 years, breast cancer survival rates have moved from 80% to 95% and a cure is in sight.

Lynda Wyld
Ramsey Cutress
Jenna Morgan

Editors

Lynda Wyld is Professor of Surgical Oncology at the University of Sheffield and a Consultant Oncoplastic Surgeon at Doncaster and Bassetlaw Teaching Hospitals. She is the Past President of the British Association of Surgical Oncology (BASO) and Past Chair of the European Society of Surgical Oncology (ESSO) Education Committee and is a Trustee of the Association of Breast Surgery (ABS).

Ramsey Cutress is Professor of Breast Surgery at University of Southampton and a Consultant Surgeon at University Hospital Southampton. He is Chair of the Association of Breast Surgery (ABS) Academic and Research Committee, Course Director for the ABS Advanced Skills in Breast Disease Management course, Head of the School for Clinical Academic Training at the Wessex Deanery and breast disease subspecialty editor for the *Annals of the Royal College of Surgeons of England*, demonstrating his interests in research and teaching.

Jenna Morgan is an NIHR Advanced Fellow Breast Surgery at the University of Sheffield and a Consultant Oncoplastic Surgeon at the Jasmine Breast Unit in Doncaster, UK. She is Past Chair of the Mammary Fold Academic Committee of the ABS. She is a clinical academic with an interest in mixed-methods research, geriatric oncology and the psychology of ageing in healthcare settings.

Contributors

Puteri Abdul Haris
Oxford University Hospitals
  NHS Trust
Oxford, UK

Amit Agrawal
Cambridge University Hospitals
  NHS Trust
Cambridge, UK

Avi Agrawal
Portsmouth Hospitals University
  NHS Trust
Portsmouth, UK

Maclyn Augustine
University of Southampton
Southampton, UK

Rajendra Badwe
Tata Memorial Centre
Maharashtra, Mumbai, India

Danielle Banfield
North Bristol NHS Trust
Bristol, UK

Jessica Banks
University of Sheffield
Sheffield, UK

Isobel Barnes
University of Oxford
Oxford, UK

Peter A Barry
The Royal Marsden Hospital
  NHS Foundation Trust
London, UK

John Benson
Cambridge University Hospitals
  NHS Foundation Trust
University of Cambridge
Cambridge, UK
and
School of Medicine
Anglia Ruskin University
Cambridge and Chelmsford, UK

Elizabeth Bonefas
Women's Health Surgeons
Houston, Texas, USA

Janet Brown
Weston Park Hospital
University of Sheffield
Sheffield, UK

Eilidh Bruce
Aberdeen Royal Infirmary, NHS
  Grampian
Aberdeen, Scotland, UK

Stacey Carter
Baylor College of Medicine
Houston, Texas, USA

Wilson Cheah Pui Fui
University of Southampton and University
  Hospital Southampton
Southampton, UK

Samantha Chen
The Royal Marsden Hospital
London, UK

Karen Clements
NHS England
Birmingham, UK

Ellen Copson
University Hospital Southampton
Southampton, UK

Chris Coyle
Queen Alexandra Hospital
Portsmouth, UK

David Dodwell
University of Oxford
Oxford, UK

Beatrix Elsberger
Aberdeen Royal Infirmary, NHS
    Grampian
Aberdeen, Scotland, UK

Katherine Fairhurst
University of Bristol
Bristol, UK

Douglas Ferguson
Royal Devon University Healthcare
    Trust NHS Foundation Trust
University of Exeter
Exeter, UK

Alasdair Findlay
Doncaster Royal Infirmary (Doncaster
    and Bassetlaw Teaching Hospitals
    NHS Trust)
Doncaster, UK

Rachel Foster
Manchester Foundation Trust
Manchester, UK

Toral Gathani
University of Oxford
Oxford, UK

Mehra Golshan
Yale School of Medicine
New Haven, Connecticut, USA

Emma Green
University of Sheffield
Sheffield, UK

Iram Hassan
University Hospital Southampton
    NHS Foundation Trust
Southampton, UK

Tom Hubbard
University of Exeter
Exeter, UK

Alex Humphreys
Northumbria Healthcare NHS
    Foundation Trust
Newcastle, England, UK

Hamza Ikram
Barnsley Hospital NHS Foundation Trust
Yorkshire, UK

Urvashi Jain
Royal Marsden NHS Foundation Trust
London, UK

Fiona James
Leeds Teaching Hospitals NHS Trust
University of Leeds
Leeds, UK

Jonathan James
Nottingham Breast Institute
Nottingham University Hospital
Nottingham, UK

Nicole James
Royal Berkshire NHS Foundation Trust
Berkshire, UK

Ismail Jatoi
University of Texas Health Science Center
    at San Antonio
San Antonio, Texas, USA

Andrew Kilshaw
Doncaster and Bassetlaw Hospitals
    NHS Trust
Doncaster, UK

Leah Kim
Yale School of Medicine
New Haven, Connecticut, USA

Cliona Kirwan
The University of Manchester and
    Manchester University NHS
    Foundation Trust
Manchester, UK

Pavneet S. Kohli
Glenfield Hospital
University Hospital of Leicester
Leicester, UK

Ashutosh Kothari
Guy's and St Thomas' NHS Foundation
    Trust
London, UK

Gurdeep Mannu
University of Oxford
Oxford, UK

Mariana Matias
Leeds Teaching Hospital
    NHS Trust
Leeds, UK

Colin McIlmunn
Altnagelvin Area Hospital
Derry, Northern Ireland, UK

Stuart McIntosh
Patrick G Johnson Centre for Cancer
    Research
Queen's University Belfast
Belfast, Northern Ireland, UK

Bahar Mirshekar-Syahkal
Cambridge University Hospitals
Cambridge, UK

Anthony Mark Monaghan
University Hospital Southampton
    NHS Foundation Trust
Southampton, UK

Soudamini Nayak
University of Leicester
Leicester, UK

Lydia Newman
University Hospitals Southampton
    NHS Trust
Southampton, UK

Shelley Potter
Bristol Medical School and North Bristol
    NHS Trust
Bristol, UK

Tim Rattay
Leicester Cancer Research Centre,
    University of Leicester
Leicester, UK

Camellia Richards
University of Southampton
Southampton, UK

Constantinos Savva
University of Southampton
Southampton, UK

Thomas Seddon
Glenfield Hospital
Leicester, UK

Nisha Sharma
St James Hospital
Leeds Teaching Hospital NHS Trust
Leeds, UK

Mahmoud Soliman
Manchester University Hospitals
    NHS Foundation Trust
Manchester, UK
and
Mansoura University
Mansoura, Egypt

David Stark
North Bristol NHS Trust
Bristol, UK

Edward R St John
Portsmouth Hospitals University
    NHS Trust
University of Portsmouth
Portsmouth, UK

Alastair Thompson
Baylor College of Medicine
Houston, Texas, USA

Sophie Trotter
Weston Park Hospital
Sheffield Teaching Hospitals Trust
University of Sheffield
Sheffield, UK

Steven Wood
University of Sheffield
Sheffield, UK

Masooma Zaidi
University Hospital Southampton
  NHS Foundation Trust
Southampton, UK

CHAPTER 1

Type and Timing of Menopausal Hormone Therapy and Breast Cancer Risk: Individual Participant Meta-Analysis of the Worldwide Epidemiological Evidence

Collaborative Group on Hormonal Factors in Breast Cancer.
Lancet 394(10204):1159–1168, 2019

The benefits and risks of the use of menopausal hormone therapy (MHT, also known as hormone replacement therapy [HRT]) comprise an area of considerable debate. The widespread use of MHT began in the 1960s with initial preparations containing only oestrogen. Subsequent observations that these preparations led to endometrial disorders in postmenopausal women with an intact uterus resulted in the addition of progestogens to MHT preparations to confer protection to the endometrial lining in these women. As the use of MHT became more widespread, concerns began to be raised about breast cancer risk related to the use of these preparations. Broadly, modern MHT preparations may include oestrogen and progestogen, in which the progestogen component is given continuously or intermittently (for women with an intact uterus), or they may be oestrogen-only preparations (for women without an intact uterus). The different types of MHT are usually administered orally or transdermally (as creams or patches). Topical vaginal preparations are used only to treat local vaginal symptoms and are minimally absorbed systemically.

Epidemiological studies try to establish causal associations between risk factors or exposures and defined outcomes of interest. The two main study designs are prospective cohort studies and retrospective case–control studies. Historically, case–control studies were easier to design and implement but were subject to particular biases, such as recall bias of exposures and difficulties in recruiting suitable controls. With the ability to conduct large-scale prospective studies with data linkage, cohort studies are a reliable way to examine aetiological factors in disease. In this study design, recording of the main exposure of interest occurs prior to the main outcome of interest, and as such minimises risks such as recall bias.

The Collaborative Group on Hormonal Factors in Breast Cancer (CGHFBC) was set up in 1992 and is led by epidemiologists at the University of Oxford. The

DOI: 10.1201/b23352-1

1

aim of the CGHFBC is to bring together worldwide observational studies to conduct pooled analyses of participant-level data and generate the most robust epidemiological evidence on the associations of particular risk factors with breast cancer risk. To date, the CGHFBC has published on the associations of alcohol and tobacco,[1] breastfeeding,[2] abortion,[3] family history,[4] menarche and menopause[5] and oral contraceptives[6] with risk of breast cancer.

The CGHFBC published initial findings on the use of MHT and risk of breast cancer in 1997[7] and showed that current and recent users of MHT were at increased risk of breast cancer. Little information was available about the effects of different types of MHT and the longer-term risks after MHT use had stopped. In 2019, the CGHFBC published updated analyses[8] on the associations of MHT and breast cancer risk which we will present and discuss in this chapter.

PAPER DESCRIPTION

- **Objective/Research Question**: Examine the associations of MHT and breast cancer risk.

- **Design**: Pooled analyses of participant-level data from published obser-vational studies. A nested case–control study design was used, with four controls for every case. Logistic regression models were used to calculate adjusted risk ratios (RRs) comparing particular groups of MHT users versus never users, and to examine in detail the effects of different types and different durations of use of MHT.

- **Sample Size**: The main analyses in the 2019 CGHFBC paper included participant-level information from 24 prospective studies and included 108,647 postmenopausal women who had developed breast cancer at a mean age of 65 years, among whom 51% had ever used MHT.

- **Results**: The key findings of this paper were:
  1. Every MHT type, except vaginal oestrogens, was associated with an increased risk of breast cancer, which increased steadily with increased duration of use.
  2. The increased risks of breast cancer were greater for users of combined oestrogen–progestogen compared with oestrogen-only preparations.
  3. The increased risks of breast cancer were greater in current rather than past users, but persist for up to a decade after MHT use ceased.
  4. There was little excess risk associated with short duration of MHT use (< 1 year) but definite increased risks with use of 1–4 years, and risks increased with increasing duration of use.
  5. For a given duration of use, the excess risk of breast cancer among cur-rent users of MHT was greater for oestrogen receptor–positive disease compared to oestrogen receptor–negative disease.

The absolute risks of developing breast cancer by age 70 associated with starting different types of MHT at age 50 and continuing for 5 or 10 years were also estimated. The absolute risks assumed that 6.3% of never users of average weight would develop breast cancer during the 20-year age range of 50–69 years. With 5 years of MHT use, followed by 15 years of past use, the 20-year risk for oestrogen plus daily progestogen combined MHT would become about 8.3%, an absolute increase of 2.0 per every 100 women (one in every 50 users). For oestrogen plus intermittent progestogen combined MHT, the 20-year risk would become about 7.7%, an absolute increase of 1.4 per 100 women (one in every 70 users). For oestrogen-only MHT preparations, the risk would become about 6.8%, an absolute increase of 0.5 per 100 women (one in every 200 users). Importantly, about half the excess risk would be during the first 5 years of current MHT use, and about half the excess risk would be during the next 15 years of past use. These absolute risks would be approximately double with 10 years of use from the age of 50 compared to 5 years of use.

EXPERT COMMENTARY BY TORAL GATHANI AND ISOBEL BARNES

Paper significance

The main strengths of the CGHFBC are the large number of women included in the analyses and restriction of the main analyses to prospective studies only. In addition, detailed information was available on the type and duration of MHT use with long periods of follow-up, allowing for reliable estimation of longer-term risks.

The dominant risk factor for breast cancer is age, with over 80% of all cases diagnosed in women aged over 50 years, and a third in women aged over 70 years. There are few modifiable risk factors for breast cancer, but arguably these include body mass index (BMI), alcohol consumption (discussed in Chapter 2) and use of MHT, and knowledge of the effects of these factors at an age when absolute risks of breast cancer are increasing is important. The findings of the CGHFBC reliably show that current users of MHT are at increased risk of breast cancer compared to never users, that the risks are increased with increasing duration of use and with combined rather than oestrogen-alone preparations and that these risks persist after usage stops. The effect of MHT to increase mammographic density means that users of MHT are less likely to be diagnosed with cancers at screening, but are more likely to present in the interval between screenings, and these cancers are known to have a more aggressive tumour characteristic profile.

In context of the relevant current literature

Other important large studies that have examined the risk of breast cancer associated with MHT use include the UK Million Women Study (MWS)[9] and the US Women's Health Initiative (WHI) trial.[10] The MWS is a large prospective cohort study which recruited 1.3 million UK women aged 50–64 years during 1996–2001 via the breast-screening units participating in the National Health Service Breast Screening Programme. The first results on the associations of MHT and breast cancer risk were published in 2003 and showed similar findings to those described in the CGHFBC. Unlike the present study and the MWS, the WHI trial was a formal randomised trial with women randomised to either combined oestrogen–progestogen MHT or oestrogen-only MHT. The trial was stopped early due to safety issues in the combined MHT treatment arm, with an excess number of women diagnosed with breast cancer and cardiovascular events such as heart disease and stroke. This study also reported increased mammographic density in women on MHT, which will have an impact on screening sensitivity and is another risk of MHT use that women who are eligible for population-based screening need to be aware of.

Conclusions

Women should be able to make informed choices about their own health, and reliable evidence on the risks and benefits of treatments helps to inform these choices. The use of MHT declined sharply following publication of the MWS and the WHI trial, but rates of MHT use are increasing again with recent campaigns to raise awareness of the menopause and the benefits of treatments in the mainstream media. However, it should be noted that the advice from the UK government on the use of MHT remains unchanged, that women should be prescribed MHT to alleviate acute symptoms of the menopause taking into account the risks and benefits and that the lowest effective dose should be prescribed and for the shortest time.

REFERENCES

1. Collaborative Group on Hormonal Factors in Breast Cancer. Alcohol, tobacco and breast cancer—collaborative reanalysis of individual data from 53 epidemiological studies, including 58,515 women with breast cancer and 95,067 women without the disease. *Br J Cancer*. 2002;87(11):1234–45.
2. Collaborative Group on Hormonal Factors in Breast Cancer. Breast cancer and breastfeeding: Collaborative reanalysis of individual data from 47 epidemiological studies in 30 countries, including 50302 women with breast cancer and 96973 women without the disease. *Lancet*. 2002;360(9328):187–95.
3. Beral V, Bull D, Doll R, Peto R, Reeves G, Collaborative Group on Hormonal Factors in Breast Cancer. Breast cancer and abortion: Collaborative reanalysis of data from 53 epidemiological studies, including 83000 women with breast cancer from 16 countries. *Lancet*. 2004;363(9414):1007–16.
4. Collaborative Group on Hormonal Factors in Breast Cancer. Familial breast cancer: Collaborative reanalysis of individual data from 52 epidemiological studies including 58,209 women with breast cancer and 101,986 women without the disease. *Lancet*. 2001;358(9291):1389–99.
5. Collaborative Group on Hormonal Factors in Breast Cancer. Menarche, menopause and breast cancer risk: individual participant meta-analysis including 118964 women with breast cancer from 117 epidemiological studies. *Lancet Oncol*. 2012;13:1141–51.

6. Collaborative Group on Hormonal Factors in Breast Cancer. Breast cancer and hormonal contraceptives: collaborative reanalysis of individual data on 53 297 women with breast cancer and 100 239 women without breast cancer from 54 epidemiological studies. *Lancet.* 1996;347(9017):1713–27.

7. Collaborative Group on Hormonal Factors in Breast Cancer. Breast cancer and hormone replacement therapy: Collaborative reanalysis of data from 51 epidemiological studies of 52,705 women with breast cancer and 108,411 women without breast cancer. *Lancet.* 1997;350(9084):1047–59.

8. Collaborative Group on Hormonal Factors in Breast Cancer. Type and timing of menopausal hormone therapy and breast cancer risk: Individual participant meta-analysis of the worldwide epidemiological evidence. *Lancet.* 2019;394(10204):1159–68.

9. Million Women Study Collaborators. Breast cancer and hormone replacement therapy in the Million Women Study. *Lancet.* 2003;362:419–27.

10. Chlebowski RT, Hendrix SL, Langer RD. Influence of estrogen plus progestin on breast cancer and mammogrophy in healthy postmenopausal women. The Women's Health Initiative Randomized Trial. *J AMA.* 2003;289(24):3243–53.

Moderate Alcohol Intake and Cancer Incidence in Women

*Allen N, Beral V, Cassabone D, Kan SW, Reeves GK, Brown A,
Green J on behalf of the Million Women Study Collaborators.*
J Natl Cancer Inst 101(5):296–305, 2009

This chapter discusses a paper examining the associations of moderate alcohol
intake with cancer incidence in women who were participants of the UK Million
Women Study (MWS), a landmark prospective cohort study.[1]

PAPER DESCRIPTION

- **Objective/Research Question**: Although the primary aim of the MWS
  was to investigate the associations of menopausal hormone therapy
  (MHT, otherwise known as hormone replacement therapy [HRT]) with
  the risk of breast cancer, a clear strength of large-scale cohort studies is
  to be able to reliably assess the effects of many different exposures with
  many different outcomes. In this study, the effects of different types of
  alcohol consumption and the associations with 21 different cancer sites
  could be examined reliably, to provide important information on the
  risks of this common lifestyle factor.
  The study examined cancer risk overall and at 21 different sites, including breast.

- **Design**: Women aged 50–64 years were recruited into the study via the
  breast-screening units of the National Health Service Breast Screening
  Programme. At recruitment, participants completed a questionnaire
  about sociodemographic, lifestyle and reproductive factors and were
  resurveyed at roughly 3-year intervals. All participants are electroni-
  cally linked to central National Health Service databases, and the study
  investigators are routinely notified of any deaths and incident cancer
  registrations.

- **Sample Size**: Between 1996 and 2001, 1.38 million women aged
  50–64 years were recruited into the study, which represented one in four
  women of that age group in the UK at that time.

- **Results**: During an average of 7.2 years of follow-up per woman, 68,775 incident cancers (of which 28,380 were breast cancers) were registered in the cohort. Cox regression models were used to estimate relative risks (RRs) with various measures of alcohol intake, using attained age as the underlying time variable. Analyses were stratified by region, and adjusted for deprivation, cigarette consumption, body mass index, physical activity, use of oral contraceptives and use of MHT. All variables were derived from information reported at recruitment. The association of alcohol intake and cancer incidence was summarised in the form of a log-linear trend in risk per 10 g alcohol/day (broadly equivalent to an increase of one unit per day) among drinkers.

  Among the participants of the MWS, a quarter of women reported drinking no alcohol. Among those women who consumed alcohol, average consumption was a drink per day. Women who drank alcohol tended to be younger, leaner, more affluent and more likely to engage in strenuous exercise compared to non-drinkers. Among drinkers of alcohol, the proportion of current smokers increased with increasing alcohol intake. Approximately 30% of the drinkers consumed wine exclusively. Overall, 93% of the women who reported not consuming alcohol at recruitment also reported at the 3-year resurvey that they drank no alcohol or less than one drink per week. Among the 7% who reported being non-drinkers at recruitment but reported 3 years later drinking some alcohol, 58% reported drinking only one or two drinks per week.

  Increased risks of cancer were observed for low and moderate alcohol consumption for several cancer sites, including oral cavity and pharynx, oesophagus, larynx, rectum, liver and breast. For breast cancer, the increase in risk was 12% per drink per day (95% confidence interval [CI] = 9%–14%). The increase in the overall risk of cancer was 6% per drink per day (95% CI = 4%–7%). The observed effects were similar in women who drank wine exclusively and other consumers of alcohol. There was evidence of a reduced risk of thyroid cancer, non-Hodgkin lymphoma and renal cell carcinoma with increasing alcohol consumption. It is important to note that increased risks of oral cavity and pharynx, oesophagus and liver cancer were also observed in non-drinkers, as this category also included women who had consumed alcohol previously. To allow for the effect of past alcohol consumption, analyses of trends were restricted to current drinkers.

  Applying the estimated RRs to the cumulative incidence rates of cancer, the excess incidence of cancer up to age 75 years associated with a drink per day increase in alcohol consumption was 11 per 1,000 women for breast cancer, and 15 per 1,000 women for all cancers combined. Further calculations showed that in the UK, alcohol accounts for about 11% of all breast cancer cases (5,000 extra cancers annually).

EXPERT COMMENTARY BY TORAL GATHANI AND ISOBEL BARNES

Paper significance

Although alcohol is known to be a risk factor for many cancers, most of the evidence has come from studies in men with high levels of consumption, and relatively little was known about the effects of moderate alcohol consumption in women. The associations of alcohol, tobacco and breast cancer risk have been investigated by the Collaborative Group on Hormonal Factors in Breast Cancer (CGHFBC). The group conducted participant-level pooled analyses from 53 epidemiological studies which included 58,515 women with breast cancer and 95,067 women without the disease and published findings in 2002.[2]

Alcohol and tobacco consumption are closely correlated, and previous studies had not all reliably assessed the effect of confounding between these two exposures. In the CGHFBC analysis, average alcohol consumption among the controls in developed countries was roughly three drinks per week, and was higher in ever smokers compared to never smokers. The risk of breast cancer was higher among women who consumed alcohol compared to those who did not, and the risks increased by 7.1% per extra drink consumed daily. The increased risks were the same in ever smokers and never smokers. Importantly, the effect of smoking on breast cancer risk was confounded by alcohol consumption. When analyses were restricted to women who never consumed alcohol, there was no increased risk of breast cancer in those who smoked. If the observed relationship was causal, then it was estimated that about 4% of breast cancers diagnosed in women in the developed world are attributable to alcohol.

The main strengths of the study are the prospectively collected exposure data and complete follow-up for incident cancers. The size of the study also allowed for detailed examination of the effects of alcohol by number of drinks and the type of alcohol consumed on different cancer sites. The resurveying of participants provided repeat measurements of alcohol consumption which is important to minimise the effects of measurement error. The findings clearly show that low and moderate levels of alcohol consumption are associated with increased risks of certain cancers, and provide reliable evidence to inform public health messaging and the choices women make about their own health.

In context of the relevant current literature

The MWS has provided important evidence about other potentially modifiable risk factors for breast cancer, most notably on MHT as discussed in Chapter 1.[3] An analysis investigating the associations of adiposity and risk of breast cancer[4] showed that greater adiposity in childhood and, to a lesser extent, early adulthood was associated with a reduced risk of breast cancer. However, greater BMI at age 60 was associated with an increased risk of breast cancer

(RR per 7 kg/m^2 = 1.20). Important work has been done, including data from the MWS, to investigate the effects of shift work patterns and sleep duration on breast cancer risk, which have been hypothesised to increase breast cancer risk through suppression of melatonin production leading to increased oestrogen production. Night shift work, including long-term shift work, has little or no effect on breast cancer incidence,[5] and no significant associations with duration of sleep and breast cancer risk are observed.[6] The study has also been able to examine ethnic differences in breast cancer incidence, taking into account known risk factors for the disease, and has shown the lower incidence of breast cancer observed in women from ethnic minority backgrounds is largely, if not wholly, explained by differences in known risk factors.[7]

Well-designed large-scale epidemiological studies provide important evidence to help understand the drivers of disease incidence, and where public health interventions may be of benefit. The UK is uniquely placed to host such studies like the MWS and UK Biobank,[8] as linkage to routinely collected national datasets within the National Health Service is possible and provides the most detailed and reliable follow-up information on disease incidence and deaths. There is an increasing focus on the importance of cancer as a public health concern, and the increased incidence is largely due to an ageing population. However, evidence from epidemiological studies shows that common personal and lifestyle characteristics collectively have a significant impact on cancer incidence and there is much individuals can do to modify their own cancer risk. In 2015, almost 4 out of 10 cancers overall were attributable to known risk factors,[9] of which smoking was the most significant but also included alcohol consumption, obesity and exposure to ultraviolet (UV) radiation.

Conclusions

For breast cancer, women in midlife when the absolute risks of breast cancer are increasing should aim to moderate their alcohol intake, maintain a healthy weight and be cognisant of the risks and benefits of using MHT.

REFERENCES

1. Green J, Reeves GK, Floud S, et al. Cohort Profile: The Million Women Study. *Int J Epidemiol.* 2019;48(1):28–9e.
2. Collaborative Group on Hormonal Factors in Breast Cancer. Alcohol, tobacco and breast cancer—collaborative reanalysis of individual data from 53 epidemiological studies, including 58,515 women with breast cancer and 95,067 women without the disease. *Br J Cancer.* 2002;87(11):1234–45.
3. The Million Women Study Collaborators. Breast cancer and hormone replacement therapy in the Million Women Study. *Lancet.* 2003;362:419–27.
4. Yang TO, Cairns BJ, Pirie K, et al. Body size in early life and the risk of postmenopausal breast cancer. *BMC Cancer.* 2022;22(1):232.

5. Travis RC, Balkwill A, Fensom GK, et al. Night shift work and breast cancer incidence: three prospective studies and meta-analysis of published studies. *J Natl Cancer Inst.* 2016;108(12).

6. Wong ATY, Heath AK, Tong TYN, et al. Sleep duration and breast cancer incidence: Results from the Million Women Study and meta-analysis of published prospective studies. *Sleep.* 2021;44(2).

7. Gathani T, Ali R, Balkwill A, et al. Ethnic differences in breast cancer incidence in England are due to differences in known risk factors for the disease: Prospective study *Br J Cancer.* 2014;7(110(1)):224–9.

8. Sudlow C, Gallacher J, Allen N, et al. UK biobank: An open access resource for identifying the causes of a wide range of complex diseases of middle and old age. *PLoS Med.* 2015;12(3):e1001779.

9. Brown KF, Rumgay H, Dunlop C, et al. The fraction of cancer attributable to modifiable risk factors in England, Wales, Scotland, Northern Ireland, and the United Kingdom in 2015. *Br J Cancer.* 2018;118(8):1130–41.

CHAPTER 3

Tamoxifen for Prevention of Breast Cancer: Report of the National Surgical Adjuvant Breast and Bowel Project P-1 Study (NSABP P-1)

Fisher B, Costantino J, Wickerman D, et al.

J Natl Cancer Inst 97(22):1652–1662, 2005

The adage 'Prevention is better than cure' has been adopted as a fundamental principle in modern health care worldwide, and is inherent in strategies to reduce disease burden. The National Surgical Adjuvant Breast and Bowel Project (NSABP) proposed, in its inception, that there was a need to evaluate medicines that were potentially capable of altering, or even preventing, the initiation or promotion of non–clinically detectable cancers.[1]

Oestrogen has long been known as a contributory factor in breast cancer development. The marked reduction in the rate of new contralateral breast cancers in patients treated with tamoxifen for their ipsilateral carcinoma led to the drug being considered in cancer prevention.[2] With this in mind, the NSABP implemented a trial to appraise its use in preventing breast cancer in high-risk patients.[3]

PAPER DESCRIPTION

- **Objective/Research Question**: The primary aim of the NSABP Breast Cancer Prevention Trial was to determine whether tamoxifen, administered for 5 years, prevented invasive breast cancer in women at higher risk. Secondary aims were to determine whether tamoxifen would lower the incidence of fatal and non-fatal myocardial infarctions and reduce the incidence of bone fractures.

- **Design**: The study was a multicentre, double-blind, randomised placebo-controlled trial. Importantly the study included formal interim monitoring by a third party and allowed for early cessation if the primary end point of the trial had been reached.

- **Sample Size**: A total of 13,388 women were recruited, of whom 6,681 were given tamoxifen while 6,707 were given placebo across 131 centres in the USA and Canada from June 1992 until September 1997.

- **Inclusion Criteria**:
  1. One of the following:
     a. Age ≥ 60
     b. Age 35–59 with a Gail model 5-year risk of breast cancer ≥ 1.66%
     c. Age 35–59 with a history of lobular carcinoma *in situ* (LCIS)
  2. Life expectancy greater than 10 years
  3. No evidence of breast cancer by clinical breast exam or mammogram within the previous 180 days

- **Exclusion Criteria**:
  1. Those on oestrogen/progesterone replacement therapy, the oral contraceptive pill or androgens within the previous 3 months
  2. Patients with a history of deep vein thrombosis (DVT) or pulmonary embolism (PE)
  3. Abnormal white blood cells, platelet counts or liver or renal function
  4. Pregnant or planning to become pregnant during the study period

- **Intervention or Treatment Received**: Randomisation of participants was performed centrally by the NSABP Biostatistical Centre. Participants were stratified by age, race, history of LCIS and breast cancer relative risk. The 13,388 participants were randomised to either tamoxifen (20 mg per day) or placebo for 5 years.

- **Results**: Excluding 212 participants lost to follow-up (108 in the placebo group and 104 in the tamoxifen group), and one patient removed as had in fact developed breast cancer and not a non invasive lesion, a total of 13,175 women at increased risk were analysed. Mean follow-up was 47.7 months, with the final date of follow-up in March 1998 due to the study being unblinded. This was 7 months after the final participant was recruited and due to an independent monitoring committee determining that the findings were strong enough to justify disclosure of the results: Tamoxifen had significantly reduced the risk of breast cancer development.

  Tamoxifen reduced the risk of invasive breast cancers by 49% ($p < 0.00001$) and non-invasive breast cancers by 50%, with the decrease being greatest in those patients over the age of 60 (55%). The risk was reduced in women with LCIS (56%) and more so in women with atypical ductal hyperplasia (86%.) It reduced the occurrence of cancer in oestrogen receptor (ER)-positive tumours (69%) but did not reduce the incidence of ER-negative tumours.

  With regard to the study's secondary aims, tamoxifen did not alter the annual rate of ischaemic heart disease but did reduce the rates of hip, distal radius and spinal fractures.

  Importantly, the rates of endometrial cancer, DVT, PE and stroke were increased in the tamoxifen group and predominantly affected those participants over the age of 50.

EXPERT COMMENTARY BY ANDREW KILSHAW AND LYNDA WYLD

Paper significance

Tamoxifen's use in the risk reduction setting was first suggested following numerous significant studies implicating its significance in overall survival and reduction of contralateral cancers in the adjuvant setting. The NSABP Breast Cancer Prevention Trial (NSABP P-1) was the first randomised trial to demonstrate tamoxifen's effectiveness in the primary prevention of breast cancer among women at higher risk. Overall it was very well received, although some critics proclaimed that the participants should not have been informed of the marked benefit achieved with tamoxifen until a survival benefit was demonstrated.[1] The authors understandably believed this failed to take into account the ethical considerations under which medical research is conducted. By unblinding the study and publishing the results, those participants in the placebo arm were given the opportunity to commence tamoxifen, thus diluting any final benefit.

To date, the NSABP P-1 is the largest double-blind placebo-controlled trial exploring tamoxifen as a chemopreventative. This as well as other, smaller studies have informed guidance on chemoprevention by medical institutions in the UK and further afield. The National Institute for Health and Care Excellence (NICE) in the UK recommend that, for higher risk women (if lifetime risk is 30% or greater), chemopreventative therapy should be offered; and, for those at medium risk (lifetime risk of 17%–30%), it should be considered, taking into account its lack of effect on mortality and its significant side effects.[4] The US Food and Drug Administration (FDA) has approved tamoxifen in a chemopreventative setting in those patients with a Gail 5-year risk of 1.67% or higher.[5]

Paper limitations

Of the 13,175 participants included in the study, 96.4% were white, 3.4% were black, while 3.8% were of other races. The authors note this in their discussion, suggesting that they had made every effort to recruit non-white participants, albeit unsuccessfully. They do, however, acknowledge that the results of the study may not be generalisable to the non-white population.

There was no overall survival benefit from taking tamoxifen. Although not initially specified, the follow-up study[1] did state that any significant findings in this regard would likely take 15–20 years of follow-up. As the study was unblinded, over 30% of the placebo cohort were commenced on tamoxifen; thus, significant long-term comparisons could not be obtained.

In context of the relevant current literature

Further studies have confirmed this finding, including the UK IBIS-I trial. A meta-analysis comparing different selective ER modulators (SERMs) in the prevention of breast cancer showed tamoxifen to have an overall reduction in risk of 33%.[6] This is somewhat less than that reported in the NSAPB P-1 trial; however, some of the trials' entry criteria accepted patients with a low risk of developing breast cancer, while others were trialling the use of SERMs to reduce the risk of developing osteoporosis. In a head-to-head randomisation between tamoxifen and another SERM, raloxifene, in postmenopausal women, the Study of Tamoxifen and Raloxifene (STAR) trial demonstrated that tamoxifen was equally effective at reducing invasive breast cancers but more effective in non-invasive types. However, it did have more side effects, including thromboembolic events.[7] Hence, raloxifene is recommended in postmenopausal women in the USA.[5]

In regard to postmenopausal women, the Mammary Prevention 3 (MAP.3) trial showed a risk reduction after 2.5 years of 60% with the use of exemestane,[8] while the IBIS-II trial comparing anastrozole with placebo demonstrated a 50% reduction in risk after 3.5 years.[9] Similarly, neither of these studies showed a statistically significant risk reduction in ER-negative cancers. Importantly, neither study showed an increased risk of thromboembolic events or endometrial cancers, unlike in the tamoxifen studies.

With this in mind, NHS England, through their medicines-repurposing pro-gramme, are pushing for anastrozole to be licenced as a chemopreventative in postmenopausal women. Using it in this way will save the National Health Service (NHS) an estimated £14.7 million by allowing 79,000 people to receive the drug and preventing around 2,257 cases of breast cancer and its subsequent treatment.[10]

Conclusions

A large percentage of breast cancers express the ER, and the progression of these cancers is dependent on intact ER signalling. The NSABP P-1 trial clearly demonstrated tamoxifen's positive effect in reducing ER+ breast cancer devel-opment in high-risk patients. This has been demonstrated in further studies of both SERMs and aromatase inhibitors. None of these studies to date have demonstrated a survival advantage, and compliance and uptake of these drugs are generally poor. Consequently, despite their huge potential impact, very few women have benefitted from these drugs in the primary prevention setting.

REFERENCES

1. Fisher B, Costantino JP, Wickerham DL, Redmond CK, Kavanah M, Cronin WM, et al. Tamoxifen for the prevention of breast cancer: current status of the National Surgical Adjuvant Breast and Bowel Project P-1 study. *J Natl Cancer Inst*. 2005;97(22):1652–62. doi:10.1093/jnci/dji372
2. Fisher B, Redmond C. New perspective on cancer of the contralateral breast: a marker for assessing tamoxifen as a preventive agent. *J Natl Cancer Inst*. 1991;83(18):1278–80. doi:10.1093/jnci/83.18.1278

3. Fisher B, Costantino JP, Wickerham DL, et al. Tamoxifen for prevention of breast cancer: report of the National Surgical Adjuvant Breast and Bowel Project P-1 Study. *J Natl Cancer Inst.* 1998;90(18):1371–88. doi:10.1093/jnci/90.18.1371

4. *Familial breast cancer: classification, care and managing breast cancer and related risks in people with a family history of breast cancer.* London: National Institute for Health and Care Excellence (NICE); November 2019.

5. The U.S Food and Drug Administration. Nolvadex (Tamoxifen Citrate) Tablets [Internet]. United States of America 2004 [cited 2023 Aug 10]. Available from: https://www.access-data.fda.gov/drugsatfda_docs/label/2005/17970s053lbl.pdf

6. Cuzick J, Sestak I, Bonanni B, et al. Selective oestrogen receptor modulators in prevention of breast cancer: an updated meta-analysis of individual participant data. *Lancet.* 2013;381(9880):1827–34. doi:10.1016/S0140-6736(13)60140-3

7. Vogel VG, Costantino JP, Wickerham DL, et al. Effects of tamoxifen vs raloxifene on the risk of developing invasive breast cancer and other disease outcomes: the NSABP Study of Tamoxifen and Raloxifene (STAR) P-2 trial [published correction appears in JAMA. 2006 Dec 27;296(24):2926] [published correction appears in JAMA. 2007 Sep 5;298(9):973]. *JAMA.* 2006;295(23):2727–41. doi:10.1001/jama.295.23.joc60074

8. Goss PE, Ingle JN, Alés-Martínez JE, et al. Exemestane for breast-cancer prevention in postmenopausal women [published correction appears in N Engl J Med. 2011 Oct 6;365(14):1361]. *N Engl J Med.* 2011; 364(25): 2381–91. doi:10.1056/NEJMoa1103507

9. Cuzick J, Sestak I, Forbes JF, et al. Use of anastrozole for breast cancer prevention (IBIS-II): Long-term results of a randomised controlled trial [published correction appears in Lancet. 2020 Feb 15;395(10223):496] [published correction appears in Lancet. 2021 Feb 27;397(10276):796]. *Lancet.* 2020; 395(10218): 117–22. doi:10.1016/S0140-6736(19)32955-1

10. NHS England. Teaching old drugs new tricks: preventing breast cancer with a repurposed medicine. [Internet] England. 2022 [cited 2023 Aug 25]. Available from https://www.england.nhs.uk/blog/teaching-old-drugs-new-tricks-preventing-breast-cancer-with-a-repurposed-medicine/

The Swedish Two-County Trial of Mammographic Screening for Breast Cancer: Recent Results and Calculation of Benefit

Tabar L, Fagerberg G, Duffy SW, et al.
J Epidemiol Community Health 43:107–114, 1989

The National Health Service Breast Screening Programme (NHSBSP) was introduced in 1988, inviting all women aged between 50 and 70 years for mammographic screening. In 2021–2022, the screening programme in England screened 2.2 million women and identified 20,152 cancers (9.2 per 1,000 screened).[1] Breast screening is effective at reducing mortality by 20%–30% based on a number of randomised controlled trials (RCTs), the earliest being the Health Insurance Plan (HIP) study carried out in New York in 1963.[2] One of the largest, most notable and influential studies, prior to implementation of the NHSBSP, was the 1985 'Swedish Two-County Trial'. Its findings were key in a 1986 report to the health ministers of the UK recommending breast screening (the Forrest Report).[3] Conducted by the Swedish National Board of Health and Welfare, this trial randomised patients from the counties of Kopparberg (renamed Dalarna in 1997) and Östergötland. Initially published in 1985, it was criticised for presenting overall mortality which did not differentiate deaths from breast cancer from other illnesses, for not assessing mortality in separate age groups and for a lack of comparison between the two counties. The present paper was published several years after the original report, elaborates on the initial publication with additional follow-up and addresses some of the observed shortcomings.

PAPER DESCRIPTION

- **Objective/Research Question**: To what extent does single-view mammographic screening reduce mortality from breast cancer?

- **Design**: Randomised controlled trial.

- **Sample Size**: One hundred and thirty-four thousand eight hundred and sixty-seven women from both counties in Sweden who responded to invitations for screening were entered into the trial.

- **Trial Setup**: Between 1977 and 1980, all women aged 40 years or older from Kopparberg and Östergötland in Sweden, who had not previously had surgery for breast cancer, were invited to take part in screening. A total of 162,981 women responded. However, due to less than 50% compliance in women older than 74 years, the age range was set at 40–74, reducing the sample size to 134,867. Women aged 40–49 were invited to screening every 24 months, and those aged 50 and older every 33 months. Screening was in the form of single medial-lateral oblique (MLO) mammogram views only.

  Randomisation was carried out at a community level, the aim being to provide socioeconomic homogeneity. Each county was divided into 19 blocks; in Östergötland, each block was then subdivided into two units and randomly allocated into an active surveillance programme (ASP; $n = 38,491$) or a passive surveillance programme (PSP; $n = 37,403$). In Kopparberg, the 19 blocks were divided into three units, two randomly allocated screening ($n = 38,589$) and one as the control ($n = 18,582$).

  The primary outcome was death due to breast cancer, decided at the consensus of local project groups after review of clinical records. After 7 years, the trial was closed, and those on PSP were invited to attend screening.

- **Results**: Annual follow-up data were presented for 1984–1986 in Kopparberg and 1984–1987 in Östergötland, respectively; the additional year achieved an equivalent average follow-up duration of 7.9 years for both counties. Results were presented as the relative risk (RR) of mortality from breast cancer. At the study end point, the RR was 0.64 (95% confidence interval [CI] = 0.41–0.9, $p = 0.008$) in Kopparberg and 0.7 (95% CI = 0.55–0.87, $p = 0.001$) in Östergötland. Age-based analysis showed nonsignificance in 40–49 year-olds (with a RR of 0.92, 95% CI = 0.52–1.6, $p = 0.8$) and 70–74 year-olds (RR = 0.77, 95% CI = 0.47–1.27, $p = 0.3$). There was a significant benefit in 50–59 year-olds (RR = 0.6, 95% CI = 0.4–0.9, $p = 0.01$) and 60–69 year-olds (RR = 0.65, 95% CI = 0.44–0.95, $p = 0.03$).

  In a comparison of ASP to PSP, there was a 31% reduction in the mortality rate in those allocated to screening. This is one death prevention per year per 9,600 women screened. The cohort with maximum benefit were the 50–59 year-olds in years 4–9, who had one death prevented per year per 4,000 women screened.

EXPERT COMMENTARY BY ALASDAIR FINDLAY AND LYNDA WYLD

Paper significance

This study is one of the largest RCTs for breast cancer screening and was groundbreaking, as it demonstrated a reduction in mortality of 31% with mammographic screening only. It built on evidence from the New York HIP trial, which also showed a reduction in mortality, although the HIP trial evaluated a combined clinical examination and mammographic screening intervention. The Two-County Trial demonstrated similar reductions in mortality with mammography only and an interval between screening of nearly three times as long as that of the HIP trial. It is the second largest RCT for breast cancer screening ever carried out, surpassed only by the UK Age trial, and has the largest age range (40–74 years old) of any RCT to date.

Paper limitations

The initial study, published in 1985, did come under a large amount of scrutiny, and its original publication was criticised for: presenting overall mortality which did not differentiate causes of death, not assessing mortality in separate age groups, lack of comparison between the two counties, the randomisation process and bias.

The present paper, published in 1989, presented data on the patients with an additional 2 years of follow-up. They also addressed some of the criticism by removing patients who had already had breast cancer from the study, analysing patients in age categories and between the two counties and finally differentiating breast cancer mortality from unrelated causes. Whilst again demonstrating reduced mortality in the screening cohort, they concluded there was no difference between the counties. Notably, statistical significance was not achieved until 1986 in Kopparberg and 1987 in Östergötland, suggesting that the longer the duration of follow-up, the greater the benefit to reduction in mortality. There was variation between age categories, suggesting that patients aged 50–69 demonstrated the greatest benefit in screening.

Further criticism was levelled at the study for nonblinding of the ascertainment of death in addition to inconsistencies between the assessed cause of death recorded by the authors and that recorded on the Swedish Cause of Death Register. A further study, by the same authors, in 2003 addressed criticism of the cluster randomisation process and alleged bias in the classifications of causes of death, concluding these criticisms to be baseless.[4] In 2011, the authors published a 29-year follow-up of the original study. They assessed case status and cause of death determined by a local end point committee and also an independent external one. Once again, they demonstrated a significant reduction in breast cancer mortality for the women randomised to screening.[5]

In context of the relevant current literature

The study was included as part of a Cochrane systematic review of screening for breast cancer in 2013 by Gøtzsche and Jørgensen, which assessed the variation in estimation of screening benefits.[6] They evaluated eight RCTs comprising 650,000 women. With regard to the Swedish Two-County Trial, they highlighted issues around the randomisation process, particularly the different randomisation ratios between counties and even speculation that the process involved the rudimentary tossing of a coin in Östergötland.[7] The review criticised the Two-County Trial in several ways: Breast cancer mortality in Kopparberg was almost double that in Östergötland ($p = 0.02$), something not highlighted in the original 1985 paper. In Kopparberg there was an apparent imbalance of exclusion, with a greater number of the PSP being excluded ($p = 0.03$), especially in the 60–69 year-olds ($p = 0.007$). Finally, the quoted sample sizes across publications varied, with at least 12 different figures quoted. The review concluded that the trial was suboptimally randomised and likely biased.

Only three of the eight assessed trials were found to be adequately randomised: the Malmö Mammographic Screening Trial (1986), the Canadian National Breast Screening Study (1980) and the UK Age trial.

Meta-analysis in this Cochrane Review showed no statistically significant reduction in mortality at 7 years or 13 years in the three studies deemed to have appropriate randomisation, whereas there was significant reduction shown in those with inadequate randomisation. Overall, the study questioned the benefit of screening programmes, suggesting that they led to overtreatment and exposure of patients to harm. Trials consistently used breast cancer mortality as the primary measured outcome which the authors believed exaggerated benefit. This controversial review prompted a number of countries to re-evaluate and review in detail the potential benefits and harms of breast cancer screening.

In the UK, an independent review was commissioned. This was carried out in 2012, chaired by Professor Sir Michael Marmot. The panel concluded that breast screening did indeed extend lives, with an estimated 20% reduction in mortality. They concluded that the current UK screening programme would prevent around 1,300 breast cancer deaths per year, with an estimated 1% overdiagnosis rate.[8]

The Two-County Trial is a landmark study, in that it pioneered the use of mammography-only breast screening, demonstrating a reduction in mortality from breast cancer especially in those aged 50–69. Whilst the trial design and interpretation have undergone persistent scrutiny and criticism, it is one of the largest clinical trials for breast cancer screening ever carried out. It heavily influenced UK healthcare policy in the recommended introduction of the NHSBSP.

Conclusions

Mammographic breast screening is both domestically and internationally[9] recognised to reduce mortality from breast cancer. There are still variation and discrepancy between countries regarding the age range and screening interval used.

For example, the UK screens 40–70 year-olds every 3 years, whereas the USA annually screens 45–54 year-olds, increasing to biennially from 55. In Canada and Australia, regular screening occurs every 2 years for 50–74 year-olds.

The future of breast screening does not lie in asking *if* screening should be carried out, but *how*. Research is ongoing in the UK into the optimum age range (the AgeX trial) or with the introduction of novel techniques such as digital breast tomosynthesis screening currently being trialled in Alabama and Arizona. Risk-stratified screening is also being actively studied. This is the legacy of the Two-County Trial: It has provided the foundation from which to build and improve breast cancer care.

REFERENCES

1. NHS Breast Screening Programme, England 2021–2022 [Internet]. England; 2023 Feb. Available from: https://digital.nhs.uk/data-and-information/publications/statistical/breast-screening-programme/england—2021-22
2. Shapiro S. Periodic screening for breast cancer: the HIP randomized controlled trial. health insurance plan. *J Natl Cancer Inst Monogr.* 1997;(22):27–30.
3. Forrest, Patrick, Sir. Breast cancer screening: Report to the Health Ministers of England, Wales, Scotland & Northern Ireland by a working group chaired by Sir Patrick Forrest. London H.M.S.O; 1986.
4. Duffy SW, Tabar L, Vitak B, Yen MF, Warwick J, Smith RA, et al. The Swedish Two-County Trial of mammographic screening: cluster randomisation and end point evaluation. *Ann Oncol.* 2003;14(8):1196–8.
5. Tabár L, Vitak B, Chen THH, Yen AMF, Cohen A, Tot T, et al. Swedish Two-County trial: Impact of mammographic screening on breast cancer mortality during 3 decades. *Radiology.* 2011;260(3):658–63.
6. Gøtzsche PC, Jørgensen KJ. Screening for breast cancer with mammography. *Cochrane Database Syst Rev.* 2013(6):CD001877.
7. Nyström, Lennarth. Assessment of population screening. The case of mammography. [Faculty of Medicine]: Umeå University; 2000.
8. Marmot MG, Altman DG, Cameron DA, Dewar JA, Thompson SG, Wilcox M. The benefits and harms of breast cancer screening: an independent review. *Br J Cancer.* 2013;108(11):2205–40.
9. Lauby-Secretan B, Scoccianti C, Loomis D, Benbrahim-Tallaa L, Bouvard V, Bianchini F, et al. Breast-Cancer screening — Viewpoint of the IARC Working Group. *N Engl J Med.* 2015;372(24):2353–8.

The Benefits and Harms of Breast Cancer Screening: An Independent Review

Marmot MG, Altman DG, Cameron DA, Dewar JA, Thompson SG, Wilcox M.
Br J Cancer 108(11):2205–2240, 2013

Breast screening was introduced to the UK in 1989–1990 following publication of the Forrest Report. This had recommended breast screening based on data from a number of large randomised trials such as the Health Insurance Plan (HIP) trial of New York and the Swedish Two-County Trial. A Cochrane Review of screening in 2011 raised concerns about the methodological quality of many of these trials, suggesting that they were subject to bias, the benefits of screening were less than initially thought and the risks of overdiagnosis and overtreatment were greater. This review caused controversy and ultimately led to several countries commissioning formal reviews of the evidence base for screening. The Marmot Review was the UK review triggered by this controversy.

PAPER DESCRIPTION

- **Objective/Research Question**: Review the relative and absolute mortality benefits of the breast-screening programme, weighed against the risk of overdiagnosis.

- **Design**: Systematic review of randomised clinical trials comparing breast screening with no screening. This was conducted by an independent panel review, commissioned by Cancer Research UK and the Department of Health (England) in 2012.

- **Sample Size**: Ten studies comprising 673,573 women included in the review of mortality, and three trials including 132,413 women in the review of overdiagnosis.

- **Inclusion Criteria**: Reported randomised trials of mammographic breast screening, as previously identified in the Cochrane Review.

- **Intervention or Treatment Received**: Review of studies comparing groups of women undergoing mammographic screening with women not undergoing mammographic screening.

DOI: 10.1201/b23352-5

- **Results**: The Independent UK Panel on Breast Cancer Screening's estimate of the relative risk (RR) of breast cancer mortality in the mammographically screened patient population was 0.80 (95% confidence interval [CI] = 0.72–0.89). This was based on data reported in the Cochrane Review and is in keeping with other estimates of a RR reduction in breast cancer mortality of 20% (US Preventive Services Task Force,[1] Canadian Task Force on Preventive Health Care[2] and Duffy review[3]). The Panel thus confirmed that invitation to mammographic screening did indeed result in a reduction in the risk of dying from breast cancer.

  The Panel calculated absolute reduction in breast cancer mortality risk using this 20% RR reduction, and estimated that for every 235 women first invited for screening at age 50 years, one breast cancer death would be prevented, which would equate to 43 breast cancer deaths prevented per 10,000 women invited for screening.

  The Panel also examined the harms of breast screening—principally 'overdiagnosis', which can be defined as the detection by screening of cancers that would never have become clinically apparent in a patient's lifetime. This results in treatment of these cancers with surgery, radiotherapy and endocrine therapy, with attendant morbidity. The Panel made estimates of overdiagnosis from meta-analyses of the randomised trials, concluding that the best estimate of overdiagnosis for a population invited to be screened is 11%. The Panel also estimated that for an individual invited to screening who is diagnosed with breast cancer during the screening period, the likelihood of overdiagnosis is 19%. The application of this estimate of overdiagnosis risk to UK women aged 55–69 suggests that one in 77 women aged 50 who is invited to screening for 20 years will have an overdiagnosed cancer. This is a rate of 129 overdiagnosed cancers per 10,000 women invited to screening.

  Regarding radiotherapy, the Malmö Breast Tomosynthesis Screening Trial's RR of 1.24 (95% CI = 1.04–1.49) and the Swedish Two-County Trial's Kopparberg County RR of 1.40 (95% CI = 1.17–1.69) reported higher radiotherapy rates in screened populations.[4,5]

EXPERT COMMENTARY BY COLIN McILMUNN AND STUART McINTOSH

Paper significance

This review of the benefits and harms of breast screening has directly informed UK policy, supporting ongoing population-based mammographic breast screening. It provided best estimates for the benefits of screening in terms of preventing breast cancer death, and of overdiagnosis within the UK's National Health Service Breast Screening Programme (NHSBSP). It led to review of how information is communicated to women attending for breast screening, and a redesign of information leaflets for the NHSBSP.

Paper limitations

The Panel noted that there remained significant uncertainties in the published results of randomised trials. Reasons for this included variability between studies in terms of randomisation approaches, ages of the women involved, mammographic approach, screening intervals, follow-up time, number of screening visits, use of physical examination or self-examination and the adjudication of breast cancer deaths. In view of these uncertainties, the Panel noted that the figures cited give a false impression of accuracy, and that these are only estimates of the benefits and harms of screening.

In context of the relevant current literature

The Cochrane Review which triggered this report was published by Gøtzsche and Nielsen in 2011.[6] They used a similar methodology and reviewed eight randomised clinical trials, but only included three as being adequately randomised (the Canadian National Breast Screening Study, Malmö and the UK Age trial); four were considered to be suboptimally randomised (the Gothenburg Breast Screening Trial [Göteborg], the HIP trial, the Stockholm Mammographic Screening Trial and the Swedish Two-County Trial; Malmö II, an extension of Malmö, was also suboptimally randomised), and one was inadequately randomised (the Edinburgh Randomized Trial of Breast Cancer Screening). The Edinburgh trial used cluster randomisation leading to baseline differences between the control and study groups, resulting in selection bias, which was considered to preclude provision of reliable data.

The results for the adequately randomised and the suboptimally randomised trials were reported separately, whilst the inadequately randomised trial was reported for completeness only. Of the adequately randomised trials, breast cancer mortality was *not* significantly different between groups at 7 years (a RR of breast cancer death of 0.93, 95% CI = 0.79–1.09) or at 13 years (an RR of 0.90, 95% CI = 0.79–1.02). In the suboptimally randomised trials, a significant benefit was noted at 7 years (RR = 0.71, 95% CI = 0.61–0.83) and at 13 years (RR = 0.75, 95% CI = 0.67–0.83). Taken together, the seven trials noted a RR of 0.81 (95% CI = 0.72–0.90) at 7 years and an RR of 0.81 (95% CI = 0.74–0.87) at 13 years, which is similar to the result found by Marmot. The Cochrane Group also noted that significantly more breast surgery was performed on the screening-group participants than the non-screening participants: an RR of 1.31 (95% CI = 1.22–1.42) for the two adequately randomised trials reporting surgery rates and an RR of 1.42 (95% CI = 1.26–1.61) for the suboptimally randomised trials. This difference persisted when observing mastectomy-only rates between the groups: an RR of 1.20 (95% CI = 1.08–1.32) for the adequately randomised trials and an RR of 1.21 (95% CI = 1.06–1.38) for the suboptimally randomised trials.

As a result, the Cochrane Review concluded that existing trials had significant methodological limitations, and whilst it did conclude that breast screening reduced breast cancer mortality, this was at a cost of significant harm. It highlighted the issue of 'overdiagnosis', and estimated this level to be around 30% in optimally randomised trials, and higher in suboptimally randomised trials. This review sparked the debate around the harms and benefits of breast screening, which led to the commissioning of the Marmot UK Independent Panel on Breast Screening. This acknowledged that overdiagnosis was a significant issue but reinforced the benefits of screening, leading to a more balanced appreciation of the role of screening and how the risks and benefits should be communicated to women.

Conclusions

The Panel concluded that breast screening extends lives, but at the cost of overdiagnosis. For every 10,000 women invited to screening from age 50 for 20 years, it was estimated that around 681 cancers will be diagnosed; of these, 129 will represent an overdiagnosis, and 43 breast cancer deaths will be prevented.

Relevant additional studies

Updated US Task Force recommendations: Effectiveness of Breast Cancer Screening: Systematic Review and Meta-analysis to Update the 2009 U.S. Preventive Services Task Force Recommendation. HD Nelson et al. *Ann Intern Med.* 2016 Feb 16;164(4):244–255. doi: 10.7326/M15-0969.

Current recommendations for screening women with dense breast tissue: Breast cancer screening in women with extremely dense breasts recommendations of the European Society of Breast Imaging (EUSOBI). RM Mann et al. *Eur Radiol.* 2022 Jun;32(6):4036-4045. doi: 10.1007/s00330-022-08617-6.

Results of the UK AgeX trial for breast screening in women aged 40–50 years: Effect of mammographic screening from age 40 years on breast cancer mortality (UK Age trial): final results of a randomised, controlled trial. SW Duffy et al. *Lancet Oncol.* 2020 Sep;21(9):1165–1172.

Review of the role of artificial intelligence (AI) in breast screening and mammographic diagnosis of breast cancer: Artificial intelligence for breast cancer detection in mammography and digital breast tomosynthesis: State of the art. I Sechopoulos et al. *Semin Cancer Biol.* 2021 Jul;72:214–225. doi: 10.1016/j. semcancer.2020.06.002.

A review of the evidence around risk-stratified screening: The current status of risk-stratified breast screening. A Kieran Clift et al. *Br J Cancer.* 2022 Mar;126(4):533–550. doi: 10.1038/s41416-021-01550-3.

Meta-analysis comparing tomosynthesis with digital mammography in the screening setting: An individual participant data meta-analysis of breast cancer detection and recall rates for digital breast tomosynthesis versus digital mammography population screening. S Libesman et al. *Clin Breast Cancer.* 2022 Jul;22(5):e647–e654. doi: 10.1016/j.clbc.2022.02.005.

Evaluation of magnetic resonance imaging (MRI) for screening of patients at high risk of breast cancer: MRI versus mammography for breast cancer screening in women with familial risk (FaMRIsc): a multicentre, randomised, controlled trial. S Saadatmand et al. *Lancet Oncol.* 2019 Aug;20(8):1136–1147.

REFERENCES

1. Woolf SH. The 2009 Breast Cancer screening recommendations of the US Preventive Services Task Force. *JAMA*. 2010;303:162–3.
2. Canadian Task Force on Preventive Health Care. Recommendations on screening for breast cancer in average-risk women aged 40–74 years. *CMAJ*. 2011;183:1991–2001.
3. Duffy SW, Ming-Fan Yen A, Hsui-His Chen T, Li-Sheng Chen S, Yeuh-Hsia Chiu S, Jean-Yu Fan J, et al. Long-term benefits of breast screening. *Breast Cancer Manag*. 2021;1:31–8.
4. Nyström L, Andersson I, Bjurstam N, Frisell J, Nordenskjold B, Rutqvist LE. Long-term effects of mammography screening: Updated overview of the Swedish randomised trials. *Lancet*. 2002;359:909–19.
5. Tabar L, Vitak B, Hsiu-Hsi Chen T, Ming-Fang Yen A, Cohen A, Tot T, et al. Swedish Two-County Trial: Impact of mammographic screening on breast cancer mortality during 3 decades. *Radiology*. 2011;260:658–63.
6. Gøtzsche PC, Nielsen M. Screening for breast cancer with mammography. *Cochrane Database Syst Rev*. 2011;(1)CD001877.

CHAPTER 6

Diagnostic Performance of Digital versus Film Mammography for Breast-Cancer Screening

Pisano ED, Gatsonis C, Hendrick E, Yaffe M, Baum JK, Acharyya S, Conant EF, Fajardo LL, Bassett L, D'Orsi C, Jong R, Rebner M.

N Engl J Med 353(17):1773–1783, 2005

PAPER DESCRIPTION

- **Objective/Research Question**: The Digital Mammographic Imaging Screening Trial (DMIST) was conducted to compare the diagnostic accuracy of film and digital mammography for breast cancer screening.

- **Design**: Prospective, multicentre, paired group trial involving 33 recruiting sites across the USA and Canada, during a 25.5-month period.

- **Sample Size**: A total of 49,528 asymptomatic women were initially recruited.

    On further analysis, 195 women did not meet the study's eligibility criteria, 194 women withdrew their consent from the study and 1,489 women were excluded as the study protocol was not accurately followed. With imaging rereporting, an extra 39 women were excluded as both their mammograms were read by the same radiologist or the radiologist knew the results of the other examination whilst doing their interpretation. In addition, 12 women were also excluded because their examinations were considered technically inadequate. A further 4,339 women were excluded due to missing data, and 500 women were excluded because their cancer status was considered indeterminate.

    Therefore, the final data of 42,760 women (86.7% of those eligible) were used for primary analysis.

- **Inclusion Criteria**: Women eligible for screening mammography.

- **Exclusion Criteria**:
    1. Symptomatic women
    2. Women with breast implants

DOI: 10.1201/b23352-6

3. Women thought to be pregnant
4. Women who had undergone mammography within the previous 11 months
5. Women with a previous history of breast cancer treated with breast-conserving surgery and radiotherapy

- **Intervention Received**: All asymptomatic women screened for breast cancer at the 33 sites included in this trial underwent both film and digital mammography in random order.

   The screen-film and digital mammograms of each woman were independently interpreted by two radiologists and rated according to a seven-point malignancy scale, with 1 indicating a definitely non-malignant score and 7 a definitely malignant score. The mammograms were also classified according to the Breast Imaging Reporting and Data System (BIRADS) score from 0 (incomplete data) to 5 (highly suggestive of cancer). Additionally, mammograms were reported in terms of breast density according to the standard BIRADS scale (extremely dense, heterogeneously dense, scattered fibroglandular densities and almost completely fat).

   If findings of either examination were interpreted as abnormal, subsequent workup, including biopsy or aspiration of suspicious-looking lesions, occurred according to the recommendations of the interpreting reader. Breast cancer status was determined as positive or negative based on biopsy results or follow-up mammography within 455 days after study entry. Indeterminate status was assigned for women with indeterminate biopsy results; with a follow-up mammogram with a BIRADS score of 3, 4 or 5; or who passed away during the study with a formal breast cancer diagnosis.

   Receiver operating characteristic (ROC) analysis was used to assess and compare the results.

- **Primary and secondary end points**: The primary aim of the DMIST trial was the measurement of diagnostic accuracy of asymptomatic breast cancer by digital mammography in comparison with film mammography.

   Secondary end points of DMIST included the evaluation of subgroups for age (< 50 years versus > 50 years), menopausal status, breast density, ethnicity, lifetime risk of breast cancer and four manufactures of digital mammographic equipment used. Subgroup comparison included a Bonferroni analysis (to adjust for multiple tests), and a $p = < 0.003$ was set to indicate statistical significance.

- **Results**: The DMIST trial results were presented considering:
   1. **Image interpretation**: To facilitate results comparation, the scores of the seven-point malignancy scale were dichotomised as negative

(scores of 1–3) and positive (scores of 4–7). The BIRADS scores were also dichotomised as negative (scores of 1–3) and positive (scores of 0, 4 or 5).

Based on the above criteria, and considering the dichotomised seven-point malignancy scale, 223 women were reported as positive on both digital and film mammograms, 947 women had only positive digital mammograms while 832 women had only positive film mammograms. A total of 40,553 women were reported as negative on both examinations. For the remaining 205 women, interpretations for either film or digital studies were missing.

According to the dichotomised BIRADS scale, the authors reported 1,249 women as positive on both digital and film mammograms, 2,399 women had positive digital mammograms and 2,416 women had positive film mammograms. A total of 36,696 women were reported as negative on both film and digital mammograms.

2. **Number of breast cancers**: During the DMIST trial, a total of 335 breast cancers were diagnosed, with similar detection findings for both film and digital mammography based on the histology and the stage of the breast cancers identified.

3. **Diagnostic performance of digital and film mammography**: Considering the paired test design of the trial, the areas under the curve (AUCs) were compared with the use of a bivariate, binormal model.

   Primary analysis showed similar diagnostic accuracy between digital and film mammography, with a mean AUC of 0.78±0.02 for digital mammography and of 0.74±0.02 for film mammography (difference in AUC = 0.03, 95% confidence interval [CI] = −0.02 to 0.08, $p = 0.18$).

   Further analysis showed that the AUC for digital mammography also did not vary significantly from that for film mammography according to race, the risk of breast cancer or the type of digital machine used. However, on subgroup analysis, digital mammography demonstrated better performance among women aged 50 years or younger (AUC for digital mammography = 0.84±0.03, AUC for film mammography = 0.69±0.05, difference = 0.15, 95% CI = 0.05–0.25, $p = 0.002$), among women considered to have heterogeneously or extremely dense breast by the readers (AUC for digital mammography = 0.78±0.03, AUC for film mammography = 0.68±0.03, difference = 0.11, 95% CI = 0.04–0.18, $p = 0.003$) and among pre- or perimenopausal women (AUC for digital mammography = 0.82±0.03, AUC for film mammography = 0.67±0.05, difference = 0.15, 95% CI = 0.05–0.24, $p = 0.002$).

   There were no statistically significant differences between digital and film mammogram AUCs among women aged 50 years or older, women with fatty breasts and postmenopausal women.

EXPERT COMMENTARY BY JONATHAN JAMES, MARIANA MATIAS AND NISHA SHARMA

Paper significance

While showing similar detection rates of breast cancer, the DMIST trial highlighted the power of digital mammography over film mammography in the diagnosis of breast cancer among young women, pre- or perimenopausal women and those with dense breast tissue. Digital mammography was also non-inferior both overall and in other groups.

Digital mammography also offers several other advantages, including easier transmission, access and storage of images and computer-assisted diagnosis and, most importantly, the use of a lower average radiation dose without compromising diagnostic accuracy.

Paper limitations

The DMIST trial did not measure mortality end points, as authors assumed that screening mammography using either film or digital systems reduces the death rate from breast cancer.

In comparison to previous studies, the sensitivities of both film and digital mammography assessed by the DMIST trial were generally lower than anticipated. The authors suggest this was the result of a different concept of sensitivity and the use of an unconventional follow-up period of 455 days.

The DMIST trial was the first time that the seven-point malignancy scale was used in a large study. Therefore, comparing these trial results with previous published studies can be challenging.

The recall rate (14%) of this study was relatively high, as women underwent two screening tests.

In context of the relevant current literature

The DMIST trial results were supported by the findings of Vinnicombe and colleagues,[1] who conducted a similar study within the UK's National Health Service Breast Screening Programme. This group compared retrospectively the performance between digital and film mammography in one screening centre between January 2006 and June 2007, including 8,478 digital and 31,720 film mammograms. Within this period of time, 263 breast cancers were diagnosed, with a similar detection rate per 100 screening mammograms (0.68 [95% CI = 0.47–0.89] for digital vs. 0.72 [95% CI = 0.58–0.85] for film, $p = 0.74$), and similar recall rates (3.2% [95% CI = 2.8–3.6] for digital vs. 3.4% [95% CI = 3.1–3.6] for film, $p = 0.44$).

The authors also conducted a systematic review of eight studies, reporting a higher detection rate of asymptomatic breast cancer for digital mammography, particularly at 60 years of age or younger (pooled digital and film mammography difference: 0.11 [95% CI = 0.04–0.18] per 100 screening mammograms), but no obvious modality differences in recall rates.

Breast Cancer Surveillance Consortium data for 2003–2011 was published in 2015 by Henderson and colleagues.[2] This study included 3,021,515 screening mammograms and assessed if histology findings of screen-detected and interval cancers differ for digital versus film mammography. A total of 15,729 breast cancers were identified, from which 85.3% were screen-detected and 14.7% were interval cancers. Digital and film mammography showed similar detection rates of both screen-detected cancers (4.47 vs. 4.42 per 1,000 mammograms) and interval cancers (0.73 vs. 0.79 per 1,000 mammograms). Regarding pathology findings, interval cancers diagnosed after digital mammography were less likely to have more aggressive features when compared with those detected on film mammography, although with very small absolute differences.

A similar study was published in 2016 by Munck and colleagues,[3] comparing digital and film mammography to evaluate screen-detected and interval breast cancer performance indicators and histology characteristics. The study was conducted between 2004 and 2010 and included a total of 902,868 examinations. Their results showed similar detection rates of both screen-detected and interval cancers for digital versus film mammography. Recall rates were 2.1% (film mammography) and 3.0% (digital; $p < 0.001$), and the positive predictive values were 25.6% (film mammography) and 19.9% (digital; $p = 0.002$). Regarding tumour characteristics, similar percentages of low-grade ductal carcinoma *in situ* (DCIS) were found for film and digital mammography. Invasive cancers diagnosed after subsequent screens with digital were more often of high-grade ($p = 0.024$) and ductal type ($p = 0.030$). More recently, Dabbous and colleagues[4] published their data comparing digital and film mammography performance characteristics, including 297,629 digital and 416,791 film mammograms. They reported a similar sensitivity between modalities, with a higher specificity (1%–2% higher) for digital across age and breast density categories. The authors also mentioned a lower recall rate for digital that could account for performance differences between digital and film mammography.

The DMIST trial and these other studies have demonstrated the clear advantages of digital over film mammography. However, digital mammography still has some limitations as a screening tool, such as low sensitivity in women with dense breasts and reduced specificity when possible breast masses are simulated by the summation of normal glandular breast tissue. The development of digital technology has enabled the development of digital breast tomosynthesis (DBT). This advanced mammographic technique generates pseudo-3D imaging by constructing thin slices through the breast from multiple low-dose digital projections, potentially increasing the sensitivity and specificity of screening mammography. Studies, including a meta-analysis by Marinovich and colleagues,[5] have demonstrated the potential of DBT to improve cancer detection rates and lower recall rates, particularly in high-recall environments. Consequently, breast cancer screening with DBT has been widely adopted in North America, but there is as yet little evidence that the increase in cancer detection seen with DBT translates into a reduction in the interval cancer rate, which is an important measure of the effectiveness of any screening modality. There is concern that the extra breast cancers detected with DBT may represent overdiagnosis, and so the adoption of DBT as the routine screening modality in European population-based screening programmes is more limited. Research into the cost-effectiveness of this advanced digital mammographic technique is ongoing, including the Tomosynthesis Mammographic Imaging Screening Trial (TMIST) led by the researchers responsible for the original DMIST study.

Conclusions

The publication of the results of the DMIST trial in 2005, demonstrating no difference in performance between traditional film-based and digital mammograms for the whole screening population and improved diagnostic accuracy in some subgroups such as younger women, pre- and perimenopausal women and those with dense breasts, precipitated the widespread replacement of traditional film mammography systems. Screening programmes worldwide quickly benefited from the more efficient image acquisition, storage and display that digital images offered. Digital mammography has led to the development of more advanced mammographic techniques such as DBT that are now being investigated and implemented as screening tools in their own right.

REFERENCES

1. Vinnicombe S, Pereira SMP, McCormack VA, Shield S, Perry N, Silva IMS. Full-field digital versus screen-film mammography: Comparison within the UK breast screening program and systematic review of published data. *Radiology*. 2009;251(2):347–58.
2. Henderson LM, Miglioretti DL, Kerlikowske K, Wernli KJ, Sprague BL, Lehman CD. Breast Cancer Characteristics Associated with Digital vs Film-screen Mammography for Screen-detected and Interval Cancers. *AJR Am J Roentgenol*. 2015;206(3):676–84.
3. Munck L, Bock GH, Otter R, Reiding D, Broeders MJ, Willemse PH, Siesling S. Digital vs screen-film mammography in population-based breast cancer screening: Performance indicators and tumour characteristics of screen-detected and interval cancers. *Br J Cancer*. 2016;115(5):517–24.
4. Dabbous F, Dolecek TA, Friedewald SM, Tossas-Milligan KY, Macarol T, Summerfelt WT, Rauscher GH. Performance characteristics of digital vs film screen mammography in community practice. *Breast J*. 2018;24(3):369–72.

5. Marinovich ML, Hunter KE, Macaskill P, Houssami N. Breast cancer screening using tomosynthesis or mammography: A meta-analysis of cancer detection and recall. *J Natl Cancer Inst.* 2018;110:942–9.
6. Pisano ED, Gatsonis CA, Yaffe MJ, et al. The American College of Radiology Imaging Network Digital Mammographic Imaging Screening Trial: Objectives and methodology. *Radiology.* 2005;236:404–12.

CHAPTER 7

Screening with Magnetic Resonance Imaging and Mammography of a UK Population at High Familial Risk of Breast Cancer: A Prospective Multicentre Cohort Study (MARIBS)

Leach MO, Boggis CRM, Dixon AK, Easton DF, et al.
Lancet 365(9473):1769–1778, 2005

PAPER DESCRIPTION

- **Objective/Research Question**: The Magnetic Resonance Imaging for Breast Screening (MARIBS) study was designed to assess the diagnostic accuracy of contrast-enhanced magnetic resonance imaging (CE MRI) in women at high risk of breast cancer as a result of either a known pathogenic gene mutation or a strong family history. These women are at elevated breast cancer risk, and standard screening with mammography is less effective in younger women due to increased breast density. CE MRI was proposed as a surveillance modality as it has enhanced sensitivity in younger women, on whom this study focussed.

- **Design**: Prospective multicentre cohort study (non randomised) including 22 screening centres in the UK.

- **Sample Size**: The study was conducted between August 1997 and May 2004, and 838 women were originally recruited. From those, 106 women were excluded due to logistic problems.
  According to the study profile, 732 women were initially screened with CE MRI (2,065 examinations) and mammography (1,973 examinations). On further analysis, 83 of these women were excluded as they were screened with only one of the two modalities. Therefore, a total of 649 women were included for the final analysis, corresponding to 1,881 screens.

- **Inclusion Criteria**: The MARIBS study included women aged 35–49 years and one of the following:
  1. Known to have a *BRCA1*, *BRCA2* or *TP53* mutation (*TP53* carriers were screened from age 25 years)

DOI: 10.1201/b23352-7

   2. First-degree relative of someone with a *BRCA1*, *BRCA2* or *TP53*
      mutation
   3. Strong family history of breast or ovarian cancer, or both
   4. Family history of Li–Fraumeni syndrome

• **Exclusion Criteria**:
   1. Women with a history of previous breast cancer
   2. Women diagnosed with other types of cancer and an expected prog-
      nosis of less than 5 years
   3. Women who underwent genetic testing during the study and whose
      results were negative

• **Intervention Received**: Based on the above inclusion and exclusion
  criteria, women at high risk of breast cancer enrolled in the MARIBS
  study were screened annually with CE MRI and film mammography for
  2–7 years. All studies were independently double-reported by radiologists unaware of the findings of the other modality.

• **Primary and Secondary End Points**: The MARIBS study primarily compared the diagnostic sensitivity and specificity for breast cancer of CE
  MRI with mammography amongst asymptomatic women at high risk of
  developing breast cancer during their lifetime.
     The diagnostic accuracy of CE MRI examinations was subanalysed,
  including the assessment of 100 symptomatic cases.

• **Results**: Screening with CE MRI alone showed a greater sensitivity (77%,
  95% confidence interval [CI] = 60–90) when compared with mammography alone (40%, 95% CI = 24–58, $p = 0.01$), although CE MRI alone was
  less specific (81% for CE MRI vs. 93% for mammography, $p < 0.0001$).
  The combination of CE MRI and mammography presented higher sensitivity (94%, 95% CI = 81–99) than either modality independently, but
  lower specificity (77%). The positive predictive values (PPVs) of CE MRI
  and mammography were 7.3% (95% CI = 4.9–10) and 10% (95%
  CI = 5.8–17), respectively. The negative predictive value (NPV) was 99%
  for both (95% CI = 99–100 for CE MRI, and 98–99 for mammography).
     Further subanalyses were conducted considering:

   1. *Prevalence screen*: CE MRI sensitivity of 75% and mammography
      sensitivity of 40% ($p = 0.12$), and specificity of 82% and 93%, respec-
      tively ($p < 0.0001$).
   2. *Cancer diagnosis*: During the study, a total of 35 breast cancers were
      diagnosed; of those, 2 were interval cancers, 19 were identified by CE
      MRI, 6 by mammography and 8 by both modalities.
   3. *Carriers of a BRCA1 mutation or with a relative known to have the
      BRCA1 mutation*: Within this group (13 breast cancers), the sensitiv-
      ity of CE MRI was greater than that of mammography ($p = 0.004$)

and the specificity was lower, but both modalities were comparable with the results for the whole cohort. The PPV for CE MRI was 14% and for mammography was 9.1%. Both tests together had a sensitivity of 92% and a specificity of 72%. If excluding the ductal carcinoma *in situ* (DCIS)-only case, the sensitivity of the CE MRI increased to 100% and decreased to 25% for mammography.

4. *Carriers of a BRCA2 mutation or with a relative known to have the BRCA2 mutation:* Amongst this group, eight breast cancers were diagnosed. CE MRI sensitivity was similar to that of mammography ($p = 1.0$). Excluding the three DCIS-only cases, CE MRI sensitivity increased to 67% and mammography sensitivity decreased to 33%, although due to the small numbers considered, the differences between CE MRI and mammography were nonsignificant ($p = 0.45$).

The authors reported a cancer detection rate of 26.9 per 1,000 women in the prevalent screen and 12.8 per 1,000 women at subsequent screens (incident).

Regarding recall rates, 3.9% of the whole cohort were recalled based on mammographic findings and 10.7% based on the CE MRI reading. When combining both modalities, the recall rate increased to 12.7%.

A total of 124 women withdrew from the study, with the five most common reasons being: negative predictive genetic test ($n = 30$), the development of breast cancer ($n = 35$) (trial participation discontinued after a breast cancer diagnosis), personal reasons including stress ($n = 19$), claustrophobia ($n = 12$) and undergoing a risk-reducing mastectomy ($n = 28$).

EXPERT COMMENTARY BY JONATHAN JAMES, MARIANA MATIAS AND NISHA SHARMA

Paper significance

Despite some differences in terms of study design and population, the MARIBS results proved to be concordant with the results of two major prospective screening studies, one from Canada[1] and the Dutch MRI Screening (MRISC) Study.[2] Overall, these studies highlighted the benefit of CE MRI as part of the screening program of women known to be *BRCA* mutation carriers. Kriedge and colleagues demonstrated a cancer detection rate of 26.2 per 1,000 women screened, compared to 5.4 per 1,000 in high-risk nonmutation carriers.[2] When considering the whole high-risk cohort studied, the combination of CE MRI and mammography offers the most effective screening regimen.

In context of the relevant current literature

Following the MARIBS trial, multiple other studies were published comparing CE MRI with mammography as a potential screening modality for women at high risk of developing breast cancer.

In 2019, Saadatmand and colleagues published the results of a multicentre, randomised controlled trial of Dutch women aged 30–55 years with a cumulative lifetime breast cancer risk of at least 20% due to their familial history, but who were *BRCA1, BRCA2* and *TP53* negative.[3] Women taking part in this study were randomised (1:1) to receive either an annual MRI and clinical breast examination plus biennial mammography or an annual mammography and clinical breast examination. Between January 2011 and December 2017, 1,355 women were enrolled in this study, and the results demonstrated a higher cancer detection rate in the MRI group (40 cancers vs. 15 cancers in the mammography group, $p = 0.0017$). Invasive cancers diagnosed in the MRI group (24 cancers) were smaller than in the mammography group (median size 9 mm vs. 17 mm, $p = 0.010$) and less frequently node-positive (4 of 24 vs. 5 of 8, $p = 0.023$). The authors also highlighted the role of MRI in the detection of cancers at an earlier stage (12 of 25 in the MRI group vs. 1 of 15 in the mammography group were stage T1, and 1 of 25 vs. 2 of 15, respectively, were stage T2 or higher; $p = 0.035$). More recently, Whitaker and colleagues[4] published a review of the role of MRI for risk-stratified screening in *BRCA* mutation carriers or those with a high familial risk of breast cancer. Similarly, they concluded that breast MRI screening allows earlier detection of breast cancer with potential beneficial impact on overall survival.

There is good evidence for MRI screening for women at the highest risk of developing breast cancer. In recent years, there has been considerable interest in the use of MRI in women with intermediate risk factors, particularly those with dense breast tissue. As well as having an increased breast cancer risk, women with dense breasts are more prone to false-negative mammographic interpretations due to dense glandular breast tissue masking tumours. The Dutch Dense Tissue and Early Breast Neoplasm Screening (DENSE) trial showed that supplemental screening with breast MRI led to a cancer detection rate of 16.5 per 1,000 women screened.[5] Interval cancer rates are an important predictor of the effectiveness of a screening modality, and importantly, the DENSE trial was able to demonstrate a fall in interval cancer rates from 5.0 per 1,000 in the mammography-only group to 2.5 per 1,000 in the MRI invitation cohort. On the downside, MRI is associated with false-positive findings. In the DENSE trial, the recall rate was 9.5%, with a false-positive rate of 8%. In the MARIBS study, MRI was associated with a recall rate of 10.7%. In intermediate-risk groups, a better understanding of the effectiveness of supplemental screening with MRI is still required. For instance, does the tumour biology of the extra cancers detected justify the greater number of false positives, the risk of overdiagnosis and the increased expenditure? To reduce costs, abbreviated MRI protocols with shorter acquisition and interpretation times are also under investigation.

Conclusions

The MARIBS study led the way in demonstrating that amongst high-risk groups, breast MRI is a highly sensitive breast cancer screening tool when compared with conventional mammography. Multiple studies have now shown that MRI can identify breast cancer at an earlier stage and that the combination of MRI and mammography is associated with improved survival. Consequently, for the highest risk women, particularly genetic mutation carriers, the use of MRI screening has become the standard of care in many countries including the UK.

REFERENCES

1. Warner E, Plewes DB, Hill KA, et al. Surveillance of BRCA 1 and BRCA 2 mutation carriers with magnetic resonance imaging, ultrasound, mammography, and clinical breast examination. *JAMA*. 2004;292:1317–25.
2. Kriedge M, Brekelmans CT, Boetes C, et al. Efficacy of MRI and mammography for breast-cancer screening in women with a familial or genetic predisposition. *N Engl J Med*. 2004;351:427–37.
3. Saadatmand S, Geuzinge HA, Rutgers EJT, et al. MRI versus mammography for breast cancer screening in women with familial risk (FaMRIsc): A multicentre, randomised, controlled trial. *Lancet Oncol*. 2019;20(8):1136–47.
4. Whitaker KD, Sheth D, Olopade OI. Dynamic contrast-enhanced magnetic resonance imaging for risk-stratified screening in women with BRCA mutations or high familial risk for breast cancer: Are we there yet? *Breast Cancer Res Treat*. 2020;183(2):243–50.
5. Bakker MF, De Lange SV, Pijnappel RM, et al. Supplemental MRI screening for women with extremely dense breast tissue. *N Engl J Med*. 2019;381:2091–102.

Comparative Effectiveness of MRI in Breast Cancer (COMICE) Trial: A Randomised Controlled Trial

Turnbull L, Brown S, Harvey I, Olivier C, Drew P, Napp V, Hanby A, Brown J.
Lancet 375:563–571, 2010

PAPER DESCRIPTION

- **Objective/Research Question**: The Comparative Effectiveness of MRI in Breast Cancer (COMICE) trial was conducted to evaluate the clinical efficacy and cost-effectiveness of contrast-enhanced magnetic resonance imaging (MRI) in decreasing reoperation rates in women with primary breast cancer who were deemed suitable for breast-conserving surgery (BCS) in comparison with standard triple assessment (imaging with mammography and ultrasound alone).

- **Design**: Multicentre, randomised, controlled, open-label, parallel group trial involving 107 consultant breast surgeons and radiologists from 45 UK centres.

- **Sample Size**: According to the trial profile, 5,496 patients were initially assessed for eligibility, of whom 3,871 were excluded (1,360 patients did not meet the inclusion criteria, 1,173 patients refused to participate and 1,338 patients were excluded for other reasons).

    A total of 1,625 patients were randomised, with 817 patients assigned to receive MRI in addition to triple assessment, and 808 assigned to triple assessment only. One patient from each group was further excluded due to lack of consent.

    During the trial, four patients from the intervention group and six patients from the control group were lost to follow-up. Therefore, a total of 816 patients who received MRI plus triple assessment and 807 patients who received triple assessment alone were analysed for the primary end point.

- **Inclusion Criteria**:
    1. Female patients aged over 18 years with biopsy-proven primary breast cancer who were considered for wide local excision after triple assessment

DOI: 10.1201/b23352-8

- **Exclusion Criteria**:
  1. Contraindications to MRI
  2. Allergy to paramagnetic contrast agents
  3. Renal dialysis
  4. Patients who had undergone chemotherapy or hormonal therapy for cancer for the contralateral breast in the previous 12 months
  5. Planned neoadjuvant chemotherapy
  6. Previous recent breast surgery within the past 4 months
  7. Pregnant or breastfeeding patients

- **Intervention Received**: After triple assessment, patients were randomised to receive either additional MRI or no MRI on a 1:1 basis.

- **Primary and Secondary End Points**: The primary end point was the proportion of participants needing further surgery (re-excision of margins or completion mastectomy within 6 months of randomisation, or a mastectomy considered pathologically avoidable at initial surgery).

  Pathologically avoidable mastectomy was defined by the Data Monitoring Ethics Committee (DMEC) as: multifocal disease detected on MRI resulting in mastectomy, with histopathology showing only localised malignant disease; or index lesion size overestimated by MRI resulting in mastectomy, but histopathology reporting an index lesion and ductal carcinoma *in situ* (DCIS) diameter of 30 mm or less.

  A health economic analysis was also performed.

  The secondary end points of the COMICE trial included:

  1. Change in clinical management
  2. Quality of life as assessed by the functional assessment of cancer therapy at 8 weeks after initial surgery
  3. Local recurrence
  4. Imaging technique effectiveness

- **Results**: Between February 2002 and January 2007, 1,623 patients were randomised (816 to MRI and 807 to the control group), slightly less than needed to meet the study's predefined power calculation.

  Considering the study's primary end point, 309 patients (19%) underwent either a repeat operation or mastectomy within 6 months of initial randomisation or a pathologically avoidable mastectomy at initial surgery, with a difference between the two groups of 0.58% (95% confidence interval [CI] = 3.24%–4.40%), with this being statistically non-significant (OR = 0.96, 95% CI = 0.75–1.24, $p = 0.77$). The authors also report no association between the minimisation factors of breast density ($p = 0.51$) and surgeon effect ($p = 0.34$) and reoperation rates. Patients aged over 50 years were less likely to undergo further surgery (OR = 0.64, 95% CI = 0.47–0.86, $p = 0.0029$).

When analysing the reoperation rates, the authors also highlight the lack of a significant relationship between the type of breast cancer (lobular carcinoma vs. all other types) and the addition of MRI to conventional triple assessment ($\chi^2 = 0.13$, $p = 0.72$), or age plus MRI ($\chi^2 = 0.16$, $p = 0.69$).

The health economic end point, assessed by the EQ-5D quality-of-life/quality-adjusted life year metric, showed no statistically significant difference between the two groups ($p = 0.075$).

Considering the study's secondary end points, 55 patients in the MRI group had a change in clinical management based on MRI findings, such as additional disease found in 91% of these patients. On further analysis, 30% of these patients were found to have undergone a pathologically avoidable mastectomy.

Tumour staging using MRI data was compared with histopathology results showing that all imaging modalities offer minimal agreement with pathology when considering the size of the index lesion (κ values: ultrasound = 0.46, 95% CI = 0.41–0.50; X-ray mammography = 0.45, 95% CI = 0.41–0.49; and MRI = 0.45, 95% CI = 0.39–0.50). Similar analysis including DCIS showed poor agreement with ultrasound and MRI (κ values: ultrasound = 0.38, 95% CI = 0.34–0.42; X-ray mammography = 0.41, 95% CI = 0.37–0.46; and MRI = 0.48, 95% CI = 0.42–0.53).

No radiologist effect was reported to be associated with differences in the extent of disease.

The authors reported comparable quality-of-life scores between the MRI and non-MRI groups, decreasing slightly within the first 8 weeks following randomisation, then recovering between 6 and 12 months after initial surgery.

EXPERT COMMENTARY BY JONATHAN JAMES, MARIANA MATIAS AND NISHA SHARMA

Paper significance

The COMICE study was the first large pragmatic prospective multicentre trial showing that the addition of MRI to the traditional triple assessment of patients with breast cancer, whilst increasing service and patients' burden, had no clinical benefit on decreasing the reoperation rate or any health-related quality-of-life benefits in both groups of patients following initial surgery.

The authors suggest that the trial results can be generalised to clinical practice as well as be globally adopted by all healthcare providers. The trial outcomes support previously published systematic reviews and meta-analyses with similar outcomes.

Study limitations

The final sample size (1,623 patients) was smaller than the sample size (1,840 patients) needed for a 90% power relating to the primary end point.

The variability of radiologists' experience with MRI reporting and differences between patients may also introduce some heterogeneity.

In context of the relevant current literature

Despite the many studies published so far, the benefit of preoperative MRI in the context of breast cancer staging and surgical planning, management and outcomes remains controversial.

Fancellu and colleagues[1] conducted a systematic review examining the association between preoperative MRI and surgical management of DCIS. They concluded that having a preoperative MRI led to an increased odds of having a mastectomy (OR = 1.72, p = 0.012; adjusted OR = 1.76, p = 0.010), although there were no significant differences in the proportion of women with positive margins following BCS in the MRI and non-MRI groups (OR = 0.80, p = 0.059; adjusted OR = 1.10, p = 0.716), nor in the necessity of reoperation for positive margins after BCS (OR = 1.06, p = 0.759; adjusted OR = 1.04, p = 0.844). Overall mastectomy rates did not vary significantly regardless of whether a preoperative MRI was considered or not (OR = 1.23, p = 0.340; adjusted OR = 0.97, p = 0.881).

A similar systematic analysis by Houssami and colleagues[2] considered all types of invasive breast cancer. Their primary analysis included 85,975 subjects and highlighted that preoperative MRI increases the odds of patients having a mastectomy (OR = 1.39, 95% CI = 1.23–1.57, p < 0.001) as part of their surgical management, as well as a contralateral prophylactic mastectomy (OR = 1.91, 95% CI = 1.25–2.91, p = 0.003). A subgroup analysis of patients diagnosed with invasive lobular carcinoma (ILC) did not show any association between MRI and the odds of receiving mastectomy (OR = 1.00, 95% CI = 0.75–1.33, p = 0.988) or the odds of re-excision (OR = 0.65, 95% CI = 0.35–1.24, p = 0.192). Their review, therefore, supports previous studies suggesting that the use of preoperative MRI is not associated with improvement in surgical outcomes.

A more recent review published by Li and colleagues[3] supports the Houssami result. Their review included 19 studies showing that preoperative MRI significantly increases mastectomy rates (OR = 1.36, p = 0.001), although it reduces reoperation rates (OR = 0.77, p = 0.02). On a subanalysis of patients with ILC, preoperative MRI did not significantly affect the rate of secondary mastectomy (OR = 0.77, p = 0.02), the rate of positive margins (OR = 1.08, p = 0.66), the mastectomy rate (OR = 1.00, p < 0.05) or the reoperation rate (OR = 0.65, p = 0.19).

Alaref and colleagues[4] in a review reiterated the power of MRI in the detection of early small breast cancers due to its superior sensitivity and specificity when compared with conventional imaging, including mammography and ultrasound. MRI plays a particularly important role in the detection of multifocal, multicentric and contralateral lesions. However, the authors concluded that MRI should only be used when clinically relevant.

Overall, although many individual published studies report conflicting results, recent meta-analyses suggest that preoperative MRI may be potentially overutilised with very minimal to no benefit to patients. Therefore, further high-quality prospective multicentre studies are needed to fully determine the justification for MRI use in the context of breast cancer diagnosis and surgical management. The current UK guidelines[5] advocate MRI in the following circumstances:

> Tumour size uncertainty (conventional imaging discordancy), lobular breast cancer being considered for conservation, mammographically occult cancer, malignant axillary nodes with an occult primary and Paget's disease being considered for conservation.

Conclusions

The COMICE study concluded that the addition of MRI to the diagnostic pathway for women with a recent breast cancer diagnosis had few or no benefits. Over 10 years later, routine preoperative staging of primary breast cancer with breast MRI is still controversial. Breast MRI demonstrates more disease, but there is little evidence that this translates into an improvement in patient outcomes.

REFERENCES

1. Fancellu A, Turner RM, Dixon JM, Pinna A, Cottu P, Houssami N. Meta-analysis of the effect of preoperative breast MRI on the surgical management of ductal carcinoma *in situ*. *Br J Surg*. 2015;102(8):883–93.
2. Houssami N, Turner RM, Morrow M. Meta-analysis of pre-operative magnetic resonance imaging (MRI) and surgical treatment for breast cancer. *Breast Cancer Res Treat*. 2017;165(2):273–83.
3. Li L, Zhang Q, Qian C, Lin H. Impact of preoperative magnetic resonance imaging on surgical outcomes in women with invasive breast cancer: A systematic review and meta-analysis. *Int J Clin Pract*. 2022;2022:6440952.
4. Alaref A, Hassan A, Kandel RS, Mishra R, Gautam J, Jahan N. Magnetic resonance imaging features in different types of invasive breast cancer: A systematic review of the literature. *Cureus*. 2021;13(3):e13854.
5. Royal College of Radiologists, RCR, 2019.

CHAPTER 9

Twenty-Year Follow-Up of a Randomized Trial Comparing Total Mastectomy, Lumpectomy, and Lumpectomy plus Irradiation for the Treatment of Invasive Breast Cancer

Fisher B, Anderson S, Bryant J, Margolese RG, Deutsch M, Fisher ER, Jeong JH, Wolmark N.
N Engl J Med 347(16):1233–1241, 2002

PAPER DESCRIPTION

- **Background**: The National Surgical Adjuvant Breast and Bowel Project (NSABP) B-06 trial was designed to determine whether resection of breast cancer with a margin of surrounding breast tissue and tumour-free resection margins (lumpectomy, hereafter referred to as wide local excision [WLE]) with or without radiotherapy is as effective as total mastectomy for treatment of invasive breast cancer.

- **Objective/Research Question**: The trial aimed specifically to examine the impact of radiotherapy on ipsilateral breast tumour recurrence (IBTR) and whether WLE increased the risk of distant disease and death.

- **Design**: Multicentre randomised controlled trial.

- **Sample Size**: The trial originally enrolled 2,163 patients, with 1,851 included in an analysis of comparisons between total mastectomy versus WLE alone or combined with radiotherapy.

- **Inclusion Criteria**: Patients with invasive breast cancer (stages I and II) and tumours measuring up to 4 cm amenable to WLE with attainment of acceptable cosmetic results based on size and location were eligible.

- **Exclusion Criteria**: Patients with tumours >4 cm and/or skin involvement, non-invasive pathology only, unknown nodal status or previous/concomitant cancers were excluded.

DOI: 10.1201/b23352-9

- **Intervention or Treatment Received**: Patients were randomly allocated to one of three treatment arms: (1) total mastectomy with removal of the entire breast and pectoral fascia, (2) WLE and breast radiotherapy (50 Gy, 25 fractions) and (3) WLE alone. All patients underwent level II axillary lymph node dissection (ALND), and those with positive nodes received adjuvant chemotherapy.

- **Results**: Analysis of trial data at 20 years confirmed findings at 5 years[1] with no significant differences in disease-free survival, distant-disease-free survival or overall survival between the three treatment arms. Hazard ratios for risk of death were 1.05 (95% CI = 0.9–1.23, $p = 0.51$) for comparison of total mastectomy with WLE alone and 0.97 (95% CI = 0.83–1.14, $p = 0.74$) for comparison of total mastectomy with WLE with radiotherapy, with overall survival rates of 47% for total mastectomy and 46% for WLE irrespective of radiotherapy. The cumulative incidence of ipsilateral breast tumour recurrence (IBTR) was notably reduced when breast radiotherapy followed WLE (39.2% vs. 14.3%, $p < 0.001$). Furthermore, amongst women undergoing WLE with tumour-free resection margins, the mortality ratio was similar for the irradiated and non-irradiated groups (0.91, 95% CI = 0.77–1.06, $p = 0.23$).

EXPERT COMMENTARY BY BAHAR MIRSHEKAR-SYAHKAL AND JOHN BENSON

Paper significance

William Halsted (1852–1922) is accredited with the first formal description of an operation for breast cancer that involved en bloc removal of the breast, pectoral muscles and axillary lymph nodes (level III).[2] This 'radical mastectomy' was predicated on the observation that many patients developed local recurrence before manifestation of any distant metastasis or death from breast cancer. Halsted believed that breast cancer is a locoregional disease that spreads in a progressive centrifugal manner through local tissues within the breast, then spreads to regional nodes and thereafter accesses the bloodstream via lymphatico-venous communications within axillary lymph nodes. A basic tenet of this paradigm was that nodal involvement always preceded haematogenous dissemination, with nodal metastases being determinants of distant disease and survival. The radical mastectomy reduced rates of local recurrence from 60% to 6%, but no improvement in overall survival ensued from this mutilating surgery that was associated with poor functional and cosmetic outcomes.

The so-called Halstedian paradigm was increasingly challenged by the concept of biological predeterminism proposed by Bernard Fisher (1918–2019).[3] In contrast to Halstedian principles, a breast tumour is considered to be a local manifestation of a systemic disease with complex interactions between the host, the primary tumour and distant micro-metastases. According to this model, surgery can only achieve local control of disease, and systemic treatment is necessary to improve survival outcomes by targeting distant micro-metastases that pre-exist at the time of presentation and determine a patient's clinical outcome.

During the 1970s, Fisher initiated the NSABP B-04 trial[4] in the United States, and the Cancer Research Campaign conducted the Kings/Cambridge trial[5] in the United Kingdom. A key aspect of these trials was randomisation of patients to ALND or radiotherapy that was either performed at the time of mastectomy or delayed until there was recurrent disease in the axilla. Overall survival was not adversely affected in the delayed axillary treatment arms, and hence foci of tumour within axillary nodes did not appear to act as a regional disease focus for dissemination of micro-metastases to distant sites. Although it was considered surgical heresy to suggest anything less than full mastectomy for treatment of breast cancer, results of the NSABP B-04 and Kings/Cambridge trials alluded to the possibility of less radical surgical intervention for breast cancer without any survival detriment.

The NSABP B-06 trial was the largest of several seminal trials demonstrating the survival equivalence of breast-conserving therapy (BCT) compared with radical or modified radical mastectomy. This trial had a profound influence on surgical practice and led to widespread acceptance of WLE combined with breast radiotherapy as the standard and preferred treatment for early-stage breast cancer.[6] This in turn has spurred the development of oncoplastic techniques that have advanced the limits of breast conservation, although BCT trials did not include tumours exceeding 5 cm in maximum size. Follow-up of NSABP B-06 at 20 years has confirmed that radiotherapy halves the risk of IBTR after breast-conserving surgery, with similar distant-disease-free and overall survival rates for modified radical mastectomy, WLE and radiotherapy or WLE alone. Hence, permutations of breast surgery have no impact on breast cancer–specific mortality, and this has justified trends for less extensive breast surgical procedures. Residual cancer cells are a determinant of local failure, with IBTR being a marker of propensity for development of distant micro-metastases. Despite finite rates of IBTR with BCT, these are very low in contemporary practice (<1% per annum) with multimodality treatments and increased stringency with surgical margins. A corollary of Fisher's alternative hypothesis is the necessity for systemic therapies to obliterate distant micro-metastases and thereby reduce mortality; systemic treatments not only improve breast cancer–specific survival but also reduce locoregional recurrence by approximately one-third overall and by up to one-half when targeting tumour biology with anti-*HER2* therapies.

In context of the relevant current literature

Umberto Veronesi (1925–2016) initiated the Milan I trial[7] just prior to NSABP B-06 and followed a personal campaign for a trial of BCT that had previously been rejected by the World Health Organisation in 1968. This trial randomised 701 women with clinically node-negative cancers of smaller average size than in NSABP B-06 (≤2 cm) to either radical mastectomy or quadrant resection (quadrantectomy) with breast radiotherapy. Both groups received ALND, and long-term follow-up at 20 years confirmed earlier reports of no significant differences in rates of distant metastases, breast cancer–associated deaths and all-cause mortality. Twenty-year follow-up of both the Milan I and NSABP B-06 trials were published simultaneously in the *New England Journal of Medicine*, with initial results of the former appearing on the front page of the *New York Times* in 1981. Similar conclusions on survival outcomes for comparisons of modified radical mastectomy and BCT were reached in the European Organisation for Research and Treatment of Cancer (EORTC) 10801 trial[8] that also reported improved body image and patient satisfaction without undue fear of local recurrence within the conserved breast. Interestingly, there were higher rates of IBTR in the breast-conserving arms of these trials, and only NSABP B-06 mandated microscopically negative resection margins defined as no tumour on ink (other trials refer to 'gross' excision of tumours). The Early Breast Cancer Trialists' Collaborative Group meta-analysis[9] reinforced the link between local control and survival and showed that more substantial differences in local relapse (>10%) translated into modest reductions in survival at 15 years. This emphasized the importance of adequate locoregional treatments with elimination of residual foci of disease in the breast and axilla that might otherwise act as a source or determinant of distant metastatic disease. This accords with the Halstedian concept, whereas biological predeterminism, expounded by Fisher, implies that the extent of locoregional treatments has a minimal effect on survival. A spectrum paradigm now prevails with recognition that some tumours have a propensity to spread locoregionally, whereas others disseminate early on by haematogenous spread. Genetic profiling of tumours has now revealed a dichotomy, with luminal tumours behaving in a more Halstedian fashion and triple-negative/*HER2*-positive tumours being intrinsically more aggressive with increased likelihood of early spread into the bloodstream. In theory, a relatively high proportion of smaller (namely, screen-detected) invasive cancers are luminal types and will be cured by surgery either alone or combined with breast radiotherapy—these tumours have an excellent prognosis and do not have pre-existing micro-metastases at the time of diagnosis.

Conclusions

NSABP B-06 is the largest of six randomised controlled trials and confirmed that with prolonged follow-up, BCT is equivalent to either radical or modified radical mastectomy in terms of survival outcomes for patients with stage I or II breast cancer measuring up to 4 cm (NSABP B-06) or 5 cm (EORTC) in size. More recently, it has been suggested that BCT may be associated with a survival advantage over mastectomy[10] based on meta-analysis of a large number of patients in largely nonrandomised, observational studies but with heterogeneity of study design. Non-randomised cohort studies are subject to bias from unmeasured confounders, and currently WLE combined with radiotherapy remains standard treatment for the majority of early-stage breast cancer cases. However, patients should not be dissuaded from undergoing mastectomy if it is their personal choice.

REFERENCES

1. Fisher B, Bauer M, Margolese R, Poisson R, Pilch Y, Redmond C, et al. Five-year results of a randomized clinical trial comparing total mastectomy and segmental mastectomy with or without radiation in the treatment of breast cancer. *N Engl J Med*. 1985;312(11):665–73.
2. Halsted WS. I. The results of operations for the cure of cancer of the breast performed at the Johns Hopkins Hospital from June, 1889, to January, 1894. *Ann Surg*. 1894;20(5):497–555.
3. Fisher B. The surgical dilemma in the primary therapy of invasive breast cancer: a critical appraisal. *Curr Probl Surg*. 1970;1–53.
4. Fisher B, Jeong JH, Anderson S, Bryant J, Fisher ER, Wolmark N. Twenty-five-year follow-up of a randomized trial comparing radical mastectomy, total mastectomy, and total mastectomy followed by irradiation. *N Engl J Med*. 2002;347(8):567–75.
5. Cancer Research Campaign (King's/Cambridge) trial for early breast cancer. A detailed update at the tenth year. Cancer Research Campaign Working Party. *Lancet*. 1980;2(8185):55–60.
6. NIH consensus conference. Treatment of early-stage breast cancer. *JAMA*. 1991;265(3):391–5.
7. Veronesi U, Cascinelli N, Mariani L, Greco M, Saccozzi R, Luini A, et al. Twenty-year follow-up of a randomized study comparing breast-conserving surgery with radical mastectomy for early breast cancer. *N Engl J Med*. 2002;347(16):1227–32.
8. Litière S, Werutsky G, Fentiman IS, Rutgers E, Christiaens M, Van Limbergen E, et al. Breast conserving therapy versus mastectomy for stage I–II breast cancer: 20 year follow-up of the EORTC 10801 phase 3 randomised trial. *Lancet Oncol*. 2012;13(4):412–9.
9. Clarke M, Collins R, Darby S, Davies C, Elphinstone P, Evans V, et al. Effects of radiotherapy and of differences in the extent of surgery for early breast cancer on local recurrence and 15-year survival: an overview of the randomised trials. *Lancet*. 2005;366(9503):2087–106.
10. De la Cruz Ku G, Karamchandani M, Chambergo-Michilot D, Narvaez-Rojas AR, Jonczyk M, Príncipe-Meneses FS, et al. Does breast-conserving surgery with radiotherapy have a better survival than mastectomy? A meta-analysis of more than 1,500,000 patients. *Ann Surg Oncol*. 2022;29(10):6163–88.

The Association of Surgical Margins and Local Recurrence in Women with Early-Stage Invasive Breast Cancer Treated with Breast-Conserving Therapy: A Meta-Analysis

Houssami N, Macaskill P, Marinovich ML, Morrow M.
Ann Surg Oncol 21(3):717–730, 2014

PAPER DESCRIPTION

- **Objective/Research Question**: This study was undertaken to systematically review the evidence on the association between surgical margins in breast conservation therapy and local recurrence (LR) for invasive breast cancer.

- **Design**: Meta-analysis.

- **Sample Size**: Thirty-three studies reporting on 28,162 patients who were eligible for inclusion and provided margin data. All studies were observational.

- **Inclusion Criteria**: Studies were eligible for inclusion if they reported data allowing calculation of the proportion of LR in relation to margin status and margin width, along with the following:
  1. Subjects had early-stage invasive breast cancer (clinical or pathologic stage I–II).
  2. Patients underwent breast-conserving therapy (BCT) and whole-breast radiotherapy.
  3. Studies reported quantitatively defined microscopic margins where negative margins, and relatively positive and/or close margins, were defined in terms of a distance from the cut edge of the specimen.
  4. Age data were provided.
  5. There was a minimum median or mean follow-up time of at least 4 years.

DOI: 10.1201/b23352-10

- **Exclusion Criteria**: Studies were excluded if they reported LR without quantifying margins, if subjects had all the same margin status or if they used nonstandard or unclear margin definitions.

- **Treatment Received**: Patients undergoing BCT and whole-breast radiotherapy.

- **Results**: LR was seen in 1,506 of 28,162 patients from 33 studies. The odds of ipsilateral breast tumour recurrence were found to be strongly associated with margin status but not margin distance.

EXPERT COMMENTARY BY LEAH KIM AND MEHRA GOLSHAN

Paper significance

It has been well established that breast conservation therapy (BCT) is an effective treatment strategy for invasive breast cancer and provides equivalence in survival compared to mastectomy with a slightly higher rate of LR. In addition, local control confers a survival benefit in the long term.[1-3] However, internationally there is a lack of consensus on what defines a negative margin in BCT, leading to significant variability between surgeons with respect to re-excision rates.[4] This study-level meta-analysis aimed to systematically review the existing evidence on the association between surgical margins in BCT and LR in invasive breast cancer to help develop consensus guidelines at the time of its publication in 2014.

For their analysis, Houssami and colleagues created two models to examine margin status and margin distance and its association with LR. The authors' standard classification for 'positive margins' was defined by the presence of invasive cancer at the transected or inked margin. 'Negative margins' were defined as the absence of tumour within a specified distance of the resection margin, and a 'close margin' had a tumour within that distance but not at the resection margin. In Model 1, margin status was analysed as a dichotomous variable (positive/close vs. negative), while margin distance was fitted as a categorical variable (as >0 mm, 1 mm, 2 mm or 5 mm), using 1 mm as a reference category. In Model 2, margin status was divided into three categories: positive versus close versus negative (reference category); distance was divided into 1 mm (reference category) versus 2 mm versus 5 mm.

After analysing 33 studies (with a LR in 1,506 of 28,162 patients), the odds of ipsilateral breast tumour recurrence were found to be strongly associated with margin status (model 1: OR = 1.96 for positive/close vs. negative; and model 2: OR = 1.74 for close vs. negative, 2.44 for positive vs. negative; $P <$ 0.001 for both models) but not margin distance (model 1: >0 mm vs. 1mm [referent] vs. 2 mm vs. 5 mm [$P = 0.12$]; and model 2: 1 mm vs. 2 mm vs.

5 mm [$P = 0.90$]). This association remained robust even after adjusting for additional radiation boosts, median follow-up time and endocrine therapy. Furthermore, they discovered that there was little to no evidence that the margin distance influenced the odds of local recurrence (model 1: 1 mm [OR = 1.0, referent], 2 mm [OR = 0.95], 5 mm [OR = 0.65], $P = 0.21$ for trend; and model 2: 1 mm [OR = 1.0, referent], 2 mm [OR = 0.91], 5 mm [OR = 0.77], $P = 0.58$ for trend).

Therefore, the authors concluded that a positive tumour margin is associated with more than a twofold increase in LR, while wider margins lack a positive impact on local recurrence. As a result, it laid the foundation by which the Society of Surgical Oncology (SSO) and the American Society for Radiation Oncology (ASTRO) published their consensus guidelines in 2014, stating that "no tumour on ink" is an adequate negative margin in an era of improving multidisciplinary cancer therapy.[5]

In context of the relevant current literature

One potential limitation in this study, however, is that there were only a small number of studies that provided data on 1 mm margins compared to data on wider margin widths. As a result, there is not an adequate statement on this margin definition, and there continues to be ongoing controversy on the topic of close margins.

For instance, a recent systematic review and meta-analysis by Bundred et al. suggested that at or close pathologic margins after BCS for early invasive breast cancer are associated with local and distant recurrence when compared to wider margins.[6] After analysing 68 studies (112,140 patients) from 1980 to 2021, they found that a close margin (<2 mm) is associated with increased distant recurrence (1.38, 95% CI = 1.13–1.69, $P < 0.001$) and local recurrence (2.09, 95% CI = 1.39–3.13, $P < 0.001$) when compared with negative margins, after adjusting for receipt of adjuvant chemotherapy and radiotherapy. Similarly, a recent single-institutional retrospective review has demonstrated that a close margin is a prognostic factor for local regional recurrence.[7] These studies suggest that the international guidelines be revisited and consider making 1 mm a minimum clear margin in early-stage invasive breast cancer.

Furthermore, there are clinical nuances, even in the setting of a negative margin, that may warrant a re-excision. For instance, the presence of an extensive intraductal component and coexistence of ductal carcinoma *in situ* (DCIS) in close margins can pose a challenge for surgeons, as the likelihood of residual disease is increased.[8] Additionally, it is well known that adjuvant chemotherapy, endocrine therapy and appropriate radiation reduce local recurrence and improve overall survival, but re-excision may be necessary in patients who are unable or unwilling to receive systemic therapy or radiation.[1,9]

Conclusions

In conclusion, the multidisciplinary approach to breast cancer is ever-changing as imaging modalities advance, surgical techniques improve and systemic therapies evolve. Therefore, it is recommended that surgeons should consider not only the margin width but also the tumour biology, patient characteristics and systemic therapy when discussing potential re-excision with their patients.

REFERENCES

1. Clarke M, et al. Effects of radiotherapy and of differences in the extent of surgery for early breast cancer on local recurrence and 15-year survival: An overview of the randomised trials. *Lancet*. 2005;366(9503):2087–106.

2. Veronesi U, et al. Twenty-year follow-up of a randomized study comparing breast-conserving surgery with radical mastectomy for early breast cancer. *N Engl J Med*. 2002;347(16):1227–32.

3. Fisher B, et al. Twenty-year follow-up of a randomized trial comparing total mastectomy, lumpectomy, and lumpectomy plus irradiation for the treatment of invasive breast cancer. *N Engl J Med*. 2002;347(16):1233–41.

4. McCahill LE, et al. Variability in reexcision following breast conservation surgery. *JAMA*. 2012;307(5):467–75.

5. Moran MS, et al. Society of Surgical Oncology–American Society for Radiation Oncology consensus guideline on margins for breast-conserving surgery with whole-breast irradiation in stages I and II invasive breast cancer. *Ann Surg Oncol*. 2014;21(3):704–16.

6. Bundred JR, et al. Margin status and survival outcomes after breast cancer conservation surgery: Prospectively registered systematic review and meta-analysis. *BMJ*. 2022;378:e070346.

7. Chae S, Min SY. Association of surgical margin status with oncologic outcome in patients treated with breast-conserving surgery. *Curr Oncol*. 2022;29(12):9271–83.

8. Boyages J, et al. Early breast cancer: Predictors of breast recurrence for patients treated with conservative surgery and radiation therapy. *Radiother Oncol*. 1990;19(1):29–41.

9. Early Breast Cancer Trialists' Collaborative Group (EBCTCG). Effects of chemotherapy and hormonal therapy for early breast cancer on recurrence and 15-year survival: An overview of the randomised trials. *Lancet*. 2005;365(9472):1687–717.

Ten Year Survival after Breast-Conserving Surgery plus Radiotherapy Compared with Mastectomy in Early Breast Cancer in the Netherlands: A Population-Based Study

van Maaren MC, de Munck L, de Back GH, Jobsen J, van Dalen T, Poortmans P, Strobbe LC, Siesling S.
Lancet Oncol 17:1258–1270, 2016

Historically, breast cancer was treated with mastectomy and axillary clearance, but in recent decades surgical de-escalation has reduced the morbidity of breast cancer surgery. The process started with trials such as the National Surgical Adjuvant Breast and Bowel Project (NSABP) B-06 trial showing that survival with breast-conserving surgery (BCS) (plus radiotherapy) gives equivalent survival rates to mastectomy, albeit with a higher rate of local recurrence. Since then, rates of local recurrence have progressively reduced due to improved surgery, radiotherapy and systemic therapy. This paper, and several similar articles, have re-evaluated survival rates according to type of breast surgery and suggest that survival may be better with BCS, although the observational nature of the data, despite adjusting for confounders, means it is not possible to make any definitive conclusions.

PAPER DESCRIPTION

- **Objective/Research Question**: To determine whether there is improved overall survival for BCS plus radiotherapy (i.e., breast-conserving therapy [BCT]) compared with mastectomy based on long-term observational data and adjustment for measurable confounding factors.

- **Design**: Population-based observational study.

- **Sample Size**: Trial included 37,207 patients for analysis of overall survival with a subcohort of 7,552 patients evaluated for cancer-specific survival.

- **Inclusion Criteria**: The study included all female patients diagnosed between 1 January 2000 and 31 December 2004 with primary invasive breast cancer (T1-2, N0-1, M0).

- **Exclusion Criteria**: Patients with Paget's disease or pure ductal carcinoma *in situ* were excluded, together with those receiving primary systemic therapy or postmastectomy radiotherapy.

- **Intervention or Treatment Received**: In the primary cohort, 21,734 (58%) patients received BCT and 15,473 (42%) underwent mastectomy, whilst in the subcohort the corresponding figures were 4,647 (62%) and 2,905 (38%), respectively. Adjustment for confounding variables was performed for a range of key variables including: age, socioeconomic status, hospital volume, region, sublocalisation of tumour, histological tumour type, differentiation grade, tumour size, number of positive lymph nodes, hormone receptor status and adjuvant systemic therapy.

- **Results**: A statistically significant overall survival advantage was associated with BCT compared with mastectomy for both unadjusted (hazard ratio [HR] = 0.51, 95% confidence interval [CI] = 0.49–0.53, $p < 0.0001$) and adjusted data (HR = 0.81, 95% CI = 0.78–0.85, $p < 0.001$), irrespective of tumour stage (T1N0 and T1N1; T2N0 and T2N1). No significant improvement in overall distant metastasis-free survival for BCT was observed in the subcohort after adjustment for confounding variables (HR = 0.88, 95% CI = 0.77–1.01, $p = 0.07$), but it was for the T1N0 subgroup (HR = 0.74, 95% CI = 0.58–0.94, $p = 0.14$). There was also improved overall relative survival for BCT in this subgroup, and this was likewise confined to T1N0 patients (HR = 0.60, 95% CI = 0.42–0.85, $p = 0.004$).

EXPERT COMMENTARY BY ISMAIL JATOI AND JOHN BENSON

Paper significance

For more than three decades, patients with primary breast cancer have been routinely informed that BCT consisting of lumpectomy and radiotherapy provides equivalent survival outcomes to mastectomy.[1] Six seminal randomised trials have assessed these two treatment options and found no difference in disease-free or overall survival.[2] This had prompted many surgeons to offer patients with likely equipoise the opportunity to choose between these two local therapy options without fear of detrimental survival outcomes for one over another. In the face of these entrenched beliefs, van Maaren and colleagues reported results of this observational study, showing an association of better 10-year overall survival for BCT when compared to mastectomy.[3] Based on this and related studies of nonrandomised design, should clinicians now inform patients that BCT may be associated with superior survival outcomes when compared with mastectomy? This is an important question that needs to be addressed from a historical perspective, with consideration of the potential limitations of observational data when compared to evidence derived from randomised controlled trials.

In the mid-20th century, two notable developments had a profound impact on approaches to the management of primary breast cancer. Firstly, there was burgeoning interest in radiotherapy as a modality for breast cancer treatment.[4] Specifically, it was believed that radiotherapy could enhance the local effects of lumpectomy, thereby avoiding the need for mastectomy. Secondly, randomised controlled clinical trials were widely acknowledged as the most robust method for determining optimal treatment strategies.[5] Randomisation ensures that the two study groups are balanced in terms of both known and unknown confounders.

Randomised trials were therefore undertaken to compare BCS (excision of the tumour and a variable amount of normal surrounding breast tissue) and radiotherapy versus mastectomy. These included the Milan trial, the NSABP B-06 trial, the US National Cancer Institute (NCI) trial, the Institute Gustaf Roussy (IGR) trial, the European Organisation for the Research and Treatment of Cancer (EORTC) 10801 trial and the Danish trial.[2] In total, there were approximately 4,061 patients enrolled in these six trials, with a pooled analysis revealing that BCT and mastectomy have comparable effects on mortality with long-term follow-up.[2] However, there was a significantly increased risk of local recurrence in patients treated with BCT that did not translate into any survival decrement. This latter point might be attributed to close follow-up of patients and timely mastectomy after detection of in-breast recurrence. Ultimately, these six trials served as the basis for the National Institutes of Health (NIH) Consensus Development Panel declaration in 1991.[6] This NIH consensus statement emphasised that BCT is preferred over mastectomy as a treatment option, and most surgeons would concur with this opinion, especially when there is likely better quality of life for breast preservation. Furthermore, this statement affirmed that survival was equivalent between the two treatment options based on evidence from these randomised trials of BCT. Yet, this study of van Maaren and colleagues along with other, more recent observational studies purport that BCT is associated with improved overall survival when compared to mastectomy.

Although the van Maaren paper adjusts for certain confounding variables such as age and smaller mean tumour size in the BCT group, it is impossible to take account of all potential confounders.[7] Investigators can only adjust for factors included in the dataset (i.e., measured confounders); it is unmeasured confounders that threaten the validity of observational studies. By contrast, confounding bias is less of a concern in large trials, where the process of randomisation ensures a better balance of variables between the study and control groups. In theory, any potential confounders (both measured and unmeasured) should be equally distributed between the study and control groups in randomised controlled trials of large sample size, but this does not apply to observational studies. Van Maaren and colleagues allude to this concern when pointing out that 10-year distant metastasis-free survival was improved for BCT compared with mastectomy in the T1N0 subgroup only, indicating a possible confounding by severity.[3] Hence, results of this study might partially be explained if surgeons performed more extensive resections (namely, mastectomy) for those patients with tumour characteristics associated with a worse prognosis. It might be surmised that many of these characteristics (some of which represent unmeasured confounders) were perhaps not available in the dataset.

In context of the relevant current literature

The threat of unmeasured confounders is illustrated in a study examining the association between contralateral prophylactic mastectomy (CPM) and breast cancer outcomes.[8] In numerous observational studies, CPM has been associated with reductions in breast cancer–specific mortality and all-cause mortality when compared to unilateral mastectomy alone. One of the authors utilised the Surveillance, Epidemiology, and End Results (SEER) dataset to examine the associations between CPM and breast cancer–specific mortality, all-cause mortality, and noncancer mortality. After adjusting for potential confounders reported in the SEER dataset, CPM was found to be associated with a lower breast cancer–specific mortality (HR = 0.84, 95% CI = 0.79–0.89) and lower all-cause mortality (HR = 0.83, 95% CI = 0.80–0.88), but was most strongly associated with reduction in noncancer mortality (HR = 0.71, 95% CI = 0.64–0.80). This latter finding suggests the existence of unmeasured confounders that limit interpretation and the conclusions that can be drawn from this observational study.

Several observational studies utilising large datasets from around the world have consistently shown that BCT is associated with improved survival outcomes when compared to mastectomy. Moreover, a meta-analysis of more than 1,500,000 patients revealed improved overall survival with BCT when compared to mastectomy.[9] However, in this large meta-analysis, the six aforementioned randomised trials represented only a fraction of patients (n = 4,061) included in this meta-analysis, with data for the remaining 1,496,000 patients pertaining to observational studies with much heterogeneity. Hence, results of this meta-analysis largely reflected those of observational studies. Furthermore, a high proportion of studies failed to balance the stage of disease with the type of surgery (BCS or mastectomy), and more recent studies incorporate screen-detected cancers that are detected earlier but potentially subject to lead-time bias. The latter can result in better survival estimates without any reduction in mortality. Finally, it should be mentioned that there has to be a biologically plausible explanation for any claims of a survival advantage for BCT. Interestingly, an abscopal (remote systemic effect of radiotherapy) effect could be invoked as a possible mechanism; hence, local breast radiotherapy could induce a systemic immune response involving the programmed cell death ligand (PDL) pathway that exerts effects on micro-metastases at distant sites that favour improved survival outcomes.[10]

Conclusions

Despite observational studies adjusting for numerous confounders in the dataset, they cannot supplant sacrosanct results from large, well-conducted, randomised controlled trials. Unmeasured confounders threaten the validity of all observational studies. At the present time, we should inform patients that BCT will likely improve quality of life compared to mastectomy, but level I evidence from randomised trials reveals no meaningful differences in survival.

REFERENCES

1. Jacobson JA, Danforth DN, Cowan KH, et al. Ten-year results of a comparison of conservation with mastectomy in the treatment of stage I and II breast cancer. *N Engl J Med.* 1995;332(14):907–11. doi:10.1056/NEJM199504063321402

2. Jatoi I, Proschan MA. Randomized trials of breast-conserving therapy versus mastectomy for primary breast cancer: A pooled analysis of updated results. *Am J Clin Oncol.* 2005;28(3):289–94. doi:10.1097/01.coc.0000156922.58631.d7

3. van Maaren MC, de Munck L, de Bock GH, et al. 10 year survival after breast-conserving surgery plus radiotherapy compared with mastectomy in early breast cancer in the Netherlands: A population-based study. *Lancet Oncol.* 2016;17(8):1158–70. doi:10.1016/S1470-2045(16)30067-5

4. Boyages J, Baker L. Evolution of radiotherapy techniques in breast conservation treatment. *Gland Surg.* 2018;7(6):576–95. doi:10.21037/gs.2018.11.10

5. Bhatt A. Evolution of clinical research: A history before and beyond James Lind. *Perspect Clin Res.* 2010;1(1):6–10.

6. NIH Consensus Conference. Treatment of early-stage breast cancer. *JAMA.* 1991;265(3):391–5.

7. Grimes DA, Schulz KF. Bias and causal associations in observational research. *Lancet.* 2002;359(9302):248–52. doi:10.1016/S0140-6736(02)07451-2

8. Jatoi I, Parsons HM. Contralateral prophylactic mastectomy and its association with reduced mortality: Evidence for selection bias. *Breast Cancer Res Treat.* 2014;148(2): 389–96. doi:10.1007/s10549-014-3160-y

9. De la Cruz Ku G, Karamchandani M, Chambergo-Michilot D, et al. Does breast-conserving surgery with radiotherapy have a better survival than mastectomy? A meta-analysis of more than 1,500,000 patients. *Ann Surg Oncol.* 2022;29(10):6163–88. doi:10.1245/s10434-022-12133-8

10. Jatoi I, Benson JR, Kunkler I. Hypothesis: Can the abscopal effect explain the impact of adjuvant radiotherapy on breast cancer mortality? *NPJ Breast Cancer.* 2018;4:8. doi:10.1038/s41523-018-0061-y

Twenty-Five-Year Follow-Up of a Randomized Trial Comparing Radical Mastectomy, Total Mastectomy, and Total Mastectomy followed by Irradiation

Fisher B, Jeong JH, Anderson S, Bryant J, Fisher ER, Wolmark N.
N Engl J Med 347(8):567–575, 2002

Breast surgery for cancer was always in the form of mastectomy and axillary node clearance until the 1990s, when pioneering surgeon Bernard Fisher[1] led a seminal, and at the time highly controversial, trial into axillary surgery. At the time, Fisher and his colleagues were pilloried by the surgical fraternity, but their data demonstrated that axillary surgery did not influence survival outcomes regardless of whether the nodes were involved or not and that axillary clearance was more likely to cause lymphoedema compared to axillary radiotherapy. The trial supports the use of sentinel node biopsy and further de-escalation strategies. This publication is the report of the long-term (25-year) follow-up data of the National Surgical Adjuvant Breast and Bowel Project (NSABP) B-04 trial.

PAPER DESCRIPTION

- **Objective/Research Question**: To determine whether less extensive axillary surgery with or without radiation therapy is as effective as the Halsted radical mastectomy for patients with either clinically negative or clinically positive axillary nodes.

- **Design**: Randomised trial.

- **Sample Size**: One thousand seven hundred and sixty-five women with primary operable breast cancer were randomly assigned to treatment from July 1971 to September 1974.

- **Inclusion Criteria**: Women with primary operable breast cancer able to provide written informed consent.

DOI: 10.1201/b23352-12

- **Exclusion Criteria**:
  - Pregnant or lactating
  - Previously treated for current neoplasm, or for prior or concomitant cancer other than basal or squamous cell skin tumour
  - Bilateral breast cancer
  - Pathology other than carcinoma
  - Inflammatory tumour
  - Skin ulceration > 2 cm
  - Peau d'orange involving more than one-third of breast skin
  - Presence of satellite or parasternal nodules
  - Fixation of axillary lymph nodes
  - Distant suspicious lymph nodes
  - Poor fitness precluding their suitability to any of the treatment options
  - Presence of non-malignant systemic disease making prolonged follow-up unlikely

- **Intervention or Treatment Received**: The original NSABP B-04 trial was set up as two parallel trials: one for patients with clinically node-negative disease and one for those with clinically node-positive disease (**Figure 12.1**). One thousand and seventy-nine patients with clinically node-negative disease were randomised to radical mastectomy (where axillary clearance is performed as part of the surgery) (*n* = 362), total mastectomy (where no axillary clearance is performed) with locoregional/axillary radiation (*n* = 352) or total mastectomy (no axillary clearance) alone with no axillary treatment (*n* = 365). Five hundred and eighty-six patients with clinically node-positive disease were randomised to radical mastectomy (*n* = 292) or total mastectomy plus radiation (*n* = 294). End points for comparison amongst treatment groups were: disease-free survival, relapse-free survival, distant-disease-free survival and overall survival.

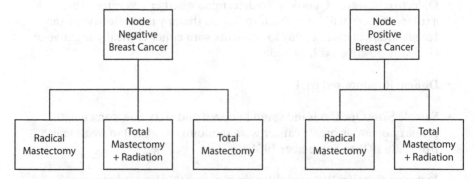

Figure 12.1   Schema for the National Surgical Adjuvant Breast and Bowel Project (NSABP) B-04 trial. (Reprinted with permission from Elsevier.)

- **Results**: This randomised study compared radical mastectomy to less extensive surgery. No significant difference in disease-free survival, relapse-free survival, distant-disease-free survival or overall survival was seen between the three groups of women with node-negative disease, or the two groups of women with node-positive disease. In women with initially negative nodes who had no axillary surgery and no radiotherapy, 19% subsequently had nodal disease identified clinically at a median of 15 months from their primary surgery, and rates of locoregional control differed between groups (5% versus 9% versus 15% for axillary clearance, axillary radiotherapy or no axillary treatment groups, respectively). There was no difference in locoregional recurrence rates in the clinically node-positive groups, where all patients had either axillary clearance or axillary radiotherapy.

EXPERT COMMENTARY BY EILIDH BRUCE AND BEATRIX ELSBERGER

Paper significance

This landmark trial was one of the first high-impact studies that supported the paradigm shift from radical to conservative axillary surgery. Led by investigators from the National Surgical Adjuvant Breast and Bowel Project, the original NSABP B-04 trial compared radical mastectomy to less extensive surgery. Follow-up at 3, 5, 10 and 25 years has shown no significant difference with respect to disease-free survival, distant-disease-free survival and overall survival amongst the three groups of patients with clinically node-negative disease or the two groups with clinically node-positive disease.

Study limitations

There was no assessment in this study of the impact of systemic therapy on survival outcomes. The study was also designed to detect a difference in survival of more than 10% between the treatment groups; therefore, smaller differences in survival may not have been detected, such as those which have since been reported for radiation therapy. The authors note that the estimate of overall mortality may also be less indicative of mortality related to breast cancer after 5 years, as the incidence of death unrelated to breast cancer increased at a faster rate than the incidence of death related to breast cancer.

In context of the relevant current literature

This landmark paper was originally published in 1977 and is now supported by robust 25-year follow-up data. At that time, standard treatment for invasive breast cancer was a Halsted radical mastectomy: en bloc resection of the breast, pectoral muscles and axillary contents. The futility of this radical approach was first confirmed by Fisher and colleagues in this paper which compared the Halsted mastectomy to total mastectomy. 'Total mastectomy' was defined as removal of breast tissue in the area bounded medially by the midline of the sternum, superiorly by the supraclavicular space, laterally along the lateral edge of the latissimus dorsi and inferiorly to the costal margin. The nipple–areola complex was excised, as was the pectoral fascia but not the muscles themselves. No operative intervention was permitted in the axilla beyond the border of the pectoral muscle.

In the node-negative group, patients who underwent total mastectomy plus radiation had a lower rate of locoregional recurrence (5%) than those who underwent radical mastectomy (9%) or total mastectomy (13%) alone ($p = 0.002$) without radiation. However, no similar difference was seen in the node-positive group.

With regard to the axilla, the findings of the NSABP-04 paper do not show any significant survival advantage from removing occult positive nodes at the time of initial surgery or from radiation therapy. Of the clinically node-negative patients, 40% of the group randomised to radical mastectomy had lymph node involvement in their surgical specimens. It can therefore be assumed that 40% of those with clinically node-negative disease who were randomised to total mastectomy also had nodal involvement. However, only 19% of patients with node-negative disease who underwent total mastectomy without radiation subsequently developed nodal disease and underwent axillary lymph node dissection. Given that there was no difference in overall survival between the treatment arms, this suggests that routine axillary lymph node dissection for patients with a clinically node-negative axilla will not have a significant impact on survival outcomes. A meta-analysis of trials comparing axillary clearance versus observation only has confirmed these findings.[5]

The final algorithm is shown in **Table 12.1**.

Table 12.1 VNPI scoring system

Parameter	Score 1	Score 2	Score 3
Size	15 mm or less	16–40 mm	Over 41 mm
Minimum surgical margin	10 mm or more	1–9 mm	Less than 1mm
Pathological grade	Non-high grade No necrosis	Non-high grade Necrosis	High grade With or without necrosis
Age	61 years of over	40–60 years	39 years or less

Source: Modified from Silverstein et al. [3].

Note: Scores of 1–3 for each parameter are then totalled to give the final Van Nuy's Prognostic Index (VNPI) and management allocated as follows:

- VNPI 4–6 = No benefit from RT so they could be considered for excision alone.
- VNPI 7–9 = RT provided a 15% lower local recurrence rate ($P = 0.03$), so consider RT or re-excision if the margin is less than 10 mm.
- VNPI 10–12 = RT provided benefit, but mastectomy was recommended since they had a 50% local recurrence rates.

Conclusions

This historic landmark trial with lengthy follow-up data underpins the practice of axillary conservation and started the trend towards sentinel lymph node biopsy and further axillary de-escalation. Sadly, clinical practice was slow to embrace the implications from these studies, with de-escalation being only recently adopted after many further similar trials (such as the AMAROS [After Mapping of the Axilla: Radiotherapy or Surgery][6] and the Z0011 trials[7]).

REFERENCES

1. Fisher B, Jeong JH, Anderson S, Bryant J, Fisher ER, Wolmark N. Twenty-five-year follow-up of a randomized trial comparing radical mastectomy, total mastectomy, and total mastectomy followed by irradiation. *N Engl J Med*. 2002;347(8):567–75.
2. Fisher B, Anderson S, Bryant J, Margolese RG, Deutsch M, Fisher ER, et al. Twenty-year follow-up of a randomized trial comparing total mastectomy, lumpectomy, and lumpectomy plus irradiation for the treatment of invasive breast cancer. *N Engl J Med*. 2002;347(16):1233–41.
3. Veronesi U, Banfi A, Salvadori B, Luini A, Saccozzi R, Zucali R, et al. Breast conservation is the treatment of choice in small breast cancer: long-term results of a randomized trial. *Eur J Cancer*. 1990;26(6):668–70.
4. Black DM, Mittendorf EA. Landmark trials affecting the surgical management of invasive breast cancer. *Surg Clin North Am*. 2013;93(2):501–18.
5. Sangha MS, Baker R, Ahmed M. Axillary dissection versus axillary observation for low risk, clinically node-negative invasive breast cancer: a systematic review and meta-analysis. *Breast Cancer*. 2021;28(6):1212–24.
6. Donker M, van Tienhoven G, Straver ME, Meijnen P, van de Velde CJ, Mansel RE, et al. Radiotherapy or surgery of the axilla after a positive sentinel node in breast cancer (EORTC 10981-22023 AMAROS): a randomised, multicentre, open-label, phase 3 non-inferiority trial. *Lancet Oncol*. 2014;15(12):1303–10.
7. Giuliano AE, Hunt KK, Ballman KV, Beitsch PD, Whitworth PW, Blumencranz PW, et al. Axillary dissection vs no axillary dissection in women with invasive breast cancer and sentinel node metastasis: a randomized clinical trial. *J Am Med Assoc*. 2011;305(6):569–75.

Effect of Axillary Dissection vs No Axillary Dissection on 10-Year Overall Survival among Women with Invasive Breast Cancer and Sentinel Node Metastasis: The ACOSOG Z0011 (Alliance) Randomized Clinical Trial

Giuliano AE, Ballman KV, McCall L, et al.
JAMA 318(10):918–926, 2017

Prior to the ACOSOG Z0011 trial (also known as the Z11 trial), the standard of care after identification of positive axillary lymph nodes following sentinel lymph node biopsy (SLNB) was a completion axillary clearance. This was despite the fact that the majority of such women have no further nodal disease, suggesting they have been overtreated. In addition, evidence from earlier trials such as the National Surgical Adjuvant Breast and Bowel Project (NSABP) B-04[1] had demonstrated no survival advantage when comparing axillary clearance, axillary radiotherapy or no further axillary treatment. The Z11 trial set out to demonstrate that completion axillary clearance may be safely omitted in women with low-risk cancers, thus reducing morbidity. Despite its flaws, it was perhaps the most highly impactful and practice-changing trial of recent years.

PAPER DESCRIPTION

- **Objective/Research Question**: To determine whether the 10-year overall survival of patients with sentinel lymph node (SLN) metastases treated with breast-conserving therapy and sentinel lymph node dissection (SLND) alone without axillary lymph node dissection (ALND) is non-inferior to that of women treated with axillary dissection.

- **Design**: Prospective multicentre randomised Phase III clinical trial.

- **Sample Size**: Eight hundred and fifty-six women from 115 institutions completed the trial and were randomised to SLND (*n* = 436) or ALND (*n* = 420) between May 1999 and December 2004. Enrolment was closed due to a lower than expected event rate (see below for the reasons for this).

- **Inclusion Criteria**: Adult women with histologically confirmed invasive breast carcinoma clinically 5 cm or less in size, no palpable lymphade-nopathy, with one or two SLNs containing metastatic breast cancer documented by frozen section, touch preparation or haematoxylin and eosin (H&E) staining on permanent section.

   All women were treated with breast conservation for their breast cancer and had tangential whole-breast radiotherapy afterwards.

- **Exclusion Criteria**:
  - Patients with metastases identified initially or solely with immunohistochemical staining (i.e., very small foci)
  - Three or more positive SLNs
  - Matted nodes
  - Gross extranodal disease
  - Receiving neoadjuvant hormonal or chemotherapy

- **Intervention or Treatment Received**: Before randomisation, all patients underwent lumpectomy and SLND. Eligible women were randomly assigned to ALND or no further axillary-specific intervention. ALND was defined as anatomic level I and II dissection including at least 10 nodes. All patients were then to receive tangential whole-breast irradia-tion and adjuvant systemic therapy. Third-field radiation (i.e., formal axillary radiotherapy) was prohibited. There was no difference in type of chemotherapy or proportion receiving endocrine therapy, chemotherapy or both between the groups.

- **Results**: Eight hundred and fifty-six patients completed the trial, with 446 in the SLND-alone group and 445 in the ALND group. At 10 years (median follow-up of 9.3 years), overall survival was 86.3% in the SLND group and 83.6% in the ALND group, which was found to be statistically non-inferior. There was no significant difference in 10-year disease-free survival between the groups.

EXPERT COMMENTARY BY EILIDH BRUCE AND BEATRIX ELSBERGER

Paper significance

Axillary treatment, particularly ALND, is associated with an increased risk of lymphoedema, shoulder movement restriction and sensorimotor disturbance. Prior to publication of this landmark ACOSOG Z0011 paper, there was a general consensus that specific axillary treatment (e.g., ALND or axillary radiotherapy) was essential as part of the treatment strategy for patients with SLN metastases. The Z11 trial was the first to challenge this mindset and has been highly influential in driving de-escalation of axillary surgery.

Study limitations

Results from the initial ACOSOG Z0011 randomised clinical trial, published in 2011, were criticised due to their relatively short period of follow-up (median = 6.3 years) which may not have detected late deaths, which are often seen in women with low-risk, oestrogen receptor–positive breast cancer. This has since been addressed by the longer-term follow-up outcomes which confirm the early follow-up findings.[2] The study is limited by the heterogeneous nature of breast cancer as a disease, in that not all biological subtypes are represented in large numbers. More significantly, the study did not meet its recruitment goal: 40% of patients had micro-metastases (which would not be an indication of completion clearance using modern management strategies), and there was a significant attrition rate (19.4% loss to follow-up). There was also a lack of radiation therapy quality assurance, and a number of patients did receive radiotherapy against protocol. Results of the Z11 trial are also not applicable to patients undergoing mastectomy. In addition, there was criticism that the findings of the study are not applicable using the study's own recruitment criteria, as the characteristics of recruited patients tended towards the better end of the scale for prognoses, probably because of selective recruitment by local investigators. This also resulted in the study being underpowered because this selective recruitment led to fewer breast cancer events than predicted.

In context of the relevant current literature

This trial showed that ALND may be omitted in a specific group of patients with fewer than three positive nodes undergoing breast-conserving surgery with whole-breast radiotherapy. The POSNOC (Positive Sentinel Node: Adjuvant Therapy Alone versus Adjuvant Therapy plus Clearance or Axillary Radiotherapy) trial[3] is now ongoing and aims to evaluate whether for women with early breast cancer and one or two nodes with macro-metastases, adjuvant therapy alone is non-inferior to adjuvant therapy plus axillary treatment (ANLD, or axillary radiotherapy). It is a randomised, multicentre trial based in the UK, Australia and New Zealand, and their primary outcome is 5-year axillary recurrence. The study includes patients treated with breast-conserving surgery and mastectomy, making the results more applicable to overall clinical practice.

Conclusions

Data from 10 years of follow-up from the Z0011 Alliance trial suggest that eliminating ALND does not affect overall survival or disease-free survival in women with one or two positive sentinel nodes (not palpable) and clinical T1 or T2 tumours who are treated with lumpectomy, whole-breast irradiation and systemic therapy. Due to its limitations, the trial was controversial but did result in significant changes in practice, with significant reductions in rates of completion axillary clearance globally.[4-6] The ongoing POSNOC was set up to address the unanswered questions and provide more robust data in this setting, although practice and guidelines have already changed as a result of the Z11 trial. The POSNOC trial has met its recruitment targets and will hopefully address some of the previous challenges faced by the Z11 trial.

REFERENCES

1. Fisher B, Jeong JH, Anderson S, Bryant J, Fisher ER, Wolmark N. Twenty-five-year follow-up of a randomized trial comparing radical mastectomy, total mastectomy, and total mastectomy followed by irradiation. *N Engl J Med*. 2002;347(8):567–75.
2. Giuliano AE, Ballman KV, McCall L, Beitsch PD, Brennan MB, Kelemen PR, et al. Effect of axillary dissection vs no axillary dissection on 10-year overall survival among women with invasive breast cancer and sentinel node metastasis: the ACOSOG Z0011 (Alliance) randomized clinical trial. *JAMA*. 2017;318(10):918–26.
3. Goyal A, Mann GB, Fallowfield L, Duley L, Reed M, Dodwell D, et al. POSNOC-POsitive Sentinel NOde: adjuvant therapy alone versus adjuvant therapy plus Clearance or axillary radiotherapy: a randomised controlled trial of axillary treatment in women with early-stage breast cancer who have metastases in one or two sentinel nodes. *BMJ Open*. 2021;11(12):e054365.
4. Poodt IGM, Spronk PER, Vugts G, van Dalen T, Peeters M, Rots ML, et al. Trends on axillary surgery in nondistant metastatic breast cancer patients treated between 2011 and 2015: a Dutch population-based study in the ACOSOG-Z0011 and AMAROS era. *Annals of Surgery*. 2018;268(6):1084–90.
5. Cha C, Kim EY, Kim SY, Ryu JM, Park MH, Lee S, et al. Impact of the ACOSOG Z0011 trial on surgical practice in Asian patients: trends in axillary surgery for breast cancer from a Korean Breast Cancer Registry analysis. *World J Surg Oncol*. 2022;20(1):198.
6. Joyce DP, Lowery AJ, McGrath-Soo LB, Downey E, Kelly L, O'Donoghue GT, et al. Management of the axilla: has Z0011 had an impact? *Ir J Med Sci*. 2016;185(1):145–9.

CHAPTER 14

Radiotherapy or Surgery of the Axilla after a Positive Sentinel Node in Breast Cancer (EORTC 10981-22023 AMAROS): A Randomised, Multicentre, Open-Label, Phase 3 Non-Inferiority Trial

Donker M, van Tienhoven G, Straver ME, et al.
Lancet Oncol 15(12):1303–1310, 2014

It has long been known that axillary surgery does not confer a survival advantage, following the seminal National Surgical Adjuvant Breast and Bowel Project (NSABP) B-04[1] (and other) trials, albeit at the expense of reduced rates of regional control. Sentinel node biopsy became the standard of care for staging women with clinically uninvolved axillae, but this was usually followed by completion axillary clearance in women with axillary metastases. The NSABP B-04 had also shown that axillary radiotherapy gave equivalent rates of survival as surgical clearance; however, it had not investigated quality of life or rates of lymphoedema. The AMAROS (After Mapping of the Axilla: Radiotherapy or Surgery?) trial set out to assess locoregional control and adverse events related to completion axillary clearance versus axillary radiotherapy in women with positive sentinel nodes.

PAPER DESCRIPTION

- **Objective/Research Question**: To determine whether axillary radiotherapy provides comparable regional control with fewer side effects compared with axillary lymph node dissection (ALND) in patients with T1–T2 primary breast cancer with a positive sentinel node.

- **Design**: Randomised, multicentre, Phase III non-inferiority trial.

- **Sample Size**: Four thousand eight hundred and six patients from 34 centres were randomised from February 2001 to April 2010. One thousand four hundred and twenty-five had a positive sentinel node and constituted the intention-to-treat population. The trial was specifically designed to recruit women *before* the results of the sentinel lymph node biopsy (SLNB) were known to reduce recruitment bias towards women with lower risk cancers. This is why the number recruited was much higher than the number of women randomised.

- **Inclusion Criteria**: Women with breast tumours of up to 3 cm, fit to undergo either of the treatment options and able to comply with follow-up.

- **Exclusion Criteria**: Patients with a medical history of previous malignancy, those who received neoadjuvant systemic treatment for primary breast cancer and patients who had received axillary surgery or radiotherapy.

  The protocol was updated in 2008 to adjust for developments in clinical practice. This included tumours up to 5 cm and patients with multifocal disease. The study group also deemed that sentinel nodes with only isolated tumour cells were no longer regarded as positive, although both micro- and macro-metastases were included in those eligible.

- **Intervention or Treatment Received**: Before randomisation, each centre had to fulfil surgical quality control. The sentinel node procedure had to be performed with the assistance of a radioactive isotope tracer, and preferably (but not mandatorily) this would be combined with the use of blue dye. Local treatment of the breast was either breast-conserving surgery with radiotherapy, or mastectomy with or without chest wall radiotherapy. In terms of axillary treatment, those randomised to ALND underwent dissection of at least levels I and II, including at least 10 nodes. Adjuvant axillary radiotherapy after ALND was permitted when at least four positive nodes were identified. Those randomised to axillary radiotherapy underwent treatment with 25 fractions of 2 Gy to the contents of all three levels of the axilla and medial part of the supraclavicular fossa.

  There was no significant change to regional radiotherapy utilisation rates between arms (internal mammary and supraclavicular fossa). There has been recent debate about whether not clearing the axilla may impact adjuvant abemaciclib use, but general consensus is that this will affect very few women and may be discussed on a case-by-case basis.

- **Primary and Secondary End Points**: The primary end point was a 5-year axillary recurrence rate. This was defined as tumour recurrence in the ipsilateral axillary lymph nodes, infraclavicular fossa or interpectoral area. Secondary end points were axillary recurrence-free survival, disease-free survival, overall survival, shoulder mobility, lymphoedema and quality of life.

- **Results**: Of the 1,425 patients with a positive sentinel node, 744 were randomly assigned to ALND and 681 to axillary radiotherapy. Median follow-up of these patients was 6.1 years. Thirty-three percent of patients in the ALND group had additional positive nodes within the surgical specimen. The planned non-inferiority test was underpowered due to a lower number of events within the follow-up time period. The 5-year axillary recurrence rate was 0.43% after ALND versus 1.19% after axillary radiotherapy. Lymphoedema in the ipsilateral arm was noted significantly more often after ALND than after radiotherapy. At 5 years, 23% of patients had lymphoedema after ALND and 11% after axillary radiotherapy. Range of movement at the shoulder did not differ between groups. Quality of life did not differ significantly in any of the relevant domains (arm symptoms, pain or body image).

EXPERT COMMENTARY BY EILIDH BRUCE AND BEATRIX ELSBERGER

Paper significance

Before the introduction of sentinel node biopsy, axillary radiotherapy was being implemented as an alternative to ALND for patients with clinically node-negative disease based on the results of the NSABP B-04 study. This became less relevant after the introduction of SLNB, which had the advantage over upfront axillary radiotherapy that it gave staging information, and until this trial there were few data comparing outcomes between ALND and axillary radiotherapy in patients with a positive sentinel node. The AMAROS trial was therefore the first to assess whether axillary radiotherapy provides comparable regional control with a better side effect profile than ALND in patients with T1–T2 disease, no palpable lymph-adenopathy but a positive sentinel node. The study found that radiotherapy did provide comparable locoregional control; however, the results were underpowered. Despite this, the study was powered to conclude that axillary radiotherapy is a less morbid alternative to ALND in this cohort of women with low-volume nodal disease. Subsequent follow-up to 10 years has confirmed this finding.

Study limitations

The primary outcome (5-year axillary recurrence) was far less common than was anticipated, and therefore the primary test of the AMAROS trial was underpowered to detect a difference in recurrence rates between the two groups. However, it was powered to evaluate the secondary outcomes of adverse effects. At the time of trial design, the risk of axillary recurrence was thought to be determined largely by the presence of a positive sentinel node. Therefore, data on tumour biology (e.g., receptor status), the presence of lymphovascular invasion and the extranodal extension of nodal disease were not recorded or included in analysis, and this may confound results.

In context of the relevant current literature

Further to this landmark paper, the monocentric OTOASOR trial[2] (Optimal Treatment of the Axilla—Surgery or Radiotherapy) confirmed the findings of the AMAROS trial. Within the OTOASOR trial, a study of 2,073 patients with early breast cancer and a positive sentinel node, axillary radiotherapy was non-inferior to ALND when evaluating survival and regional recurrence. The European Organisation for Research and Treatment of Cancer (EORTC) has subsequently published 10-year follow-up data for the AMAROS trial,[3] which confirmed the low rates of axillary recurrence after both axillary treatments, with no difference in overall survival, disease-free survival and locoregional control.

Both UK- and Europe-based breast cancer guidelines have been updated to reflect these findings. Current National Institute for Health and Care Excellence (NICE) guidelines state that clinicians should 'offer axillary treatment (axillary node clearance or axillary radiotherapy) after SLNB to people who have 1 or more sentinel lymph node macrometastases'. The European Society for Medical Oncology (ESMO) clinical practice guidelines for early breast cancer state that 'axillary radiation is a valid alternative in patients with positive SLNB, irrespective of the type of breast surgery'. This paper and the ACOSOG Z0011[4] paper have both been highly influential in changing practice in the management of the axilla, with rates of completion clearance falling markedly in the decade since they were published.

Conclusions

Findings from AMAROS have shown axillary recurrence after 10 years in patients with a positive sentinel lymph node undergoing adjuvant treatment with axillary radiotherapy to be rare, and not significantly different to the recurrence rate after ALND.

REFERENCES

1. Fisher B, Jeong JH, Anderson S, Bryant J, Fisher ER, Wolmark N. Twenty-five-year follow-up of a randomized trial comparing radical mastectomy, total mastectomy, and total mastectomy followed by irradiation. *N Engl J Med*. 2002;347(8):567–75.
2. Savolt A, Peley G, Polgar C, Udvarhelyi N, Rubovszky G, Kovacs E, et al. Eight-year follow up result of the OTOASOR trial: The Optimal Treatment Of the Axilla–Surgery Or Radiotherapy after positive sentinel lymph node biopsy in early-stage breast cancer: a randomized, single centre, phase III, non-inferiority trial. *Eur J Surg Oncol*. 2017;43(4):672–9.
3. Bartels SAL, Donker M, Poncet C, Sauve N, Straver ME, van de Velde CJH, et al. Radiotherapy or surgery of the axilla after a positive sentinel node in breast cancer: 10-year results of the randomized controlled EORTC 10981-22023 AMAROS trial. *J Clin Oncol*. 2023;41(12):2159–65.
4. Giuliano AE, Ballman KV, McCall L, Beitsch PD, Brennan MB, Kelemen PR, et al. Effect of axillary dissection vs no axillary dissection on 10-year overall survival among women with invasive breast cancer and sentinel node metastasis: the ACOSOG Z0011 (Alliance) randomized clinical trial. *JAMA*. 2017;318(10):918–26.

Sentinel Lymph Node Surgery after Neoadjuvant Chemotherapy in Patients with Node-Positive Breast Cancer: The ACOSOG Z1071 (Alliance) Clinical Trial

Boughey JC, Suman VJ, Mittendorf EA, et al.

JAMA 310(14):1455–1461, 2013

The use of neoadjuvant chemotherapy (NACT) has been one of the major advances in breast surgery of the past two decades, rendering inoperable disease operable and reducing mastectomy rates. Biological therapies and polychemotherapy regimes have been able to deliver very high rates of pathological complete response in the breast and even higher rates in the axilla. This prompted interest in whether women with clinically node-positive disease could safely avoid axillary node clearance if their nodal disease responded to treatment. Critical to this question was whether a sentinel lymph node biopsy (SLNB) would be accurate in women with clinically involved nodes, with concerns that the lymphatic pathways would be damaged by their disease and reduce the biopsy's accuracy. The ACOSOG Z1071 trial set out to determine the false-negative rate (FNR) of post-NACT SLNB by performing both a SLNB and a clearance and comparing the accuracy of the two techniques. It concluded that accuracy was slightly lower than an acceptable level, but subsequent modifications have yielded improved results such that this technique is now acceptable. These modifications include removal of at least three nodes, use of dual tracers and more recently using targeted axillary dissection (TAD). The study was a key stepping-stone in axillary de-escalation.

PAPER DESCRIPTION

- **Objective/Research Question**: To determine the FNR for sentinel lymph node (SLN) surgery following neoadjuvant chemotherapy in women presenting with biopsy-proven node-positive (cN1) breast cancer.

- **Design**: Prospective, multicentre, Phase II clinical trial.

- **Sample Size**: Six hundred and sixty-three women with clinical stage T0–T4, N1–N2, M0 breast cancer were enrolled between July 2009 and June 2011 from 136 institutions.

- **Inclusion Criteria**: Women over 18 years with histologically proven clinical stage T0–T4 N1–N2, M0 breast cancer who received neoadjuvant chemotherapy. Patients had to have an Eastern Cooperative Oncology Group (ECOG) performance status of 0 or 1.

- **Exclusion Criteria**: History of prior ipsilateral axillary surgery, prior SLN surgery or excisional lymph node biopsy for pathological confirmation of axillary status.

- **Intervention or Treatment Received**: Following neoadjuvant chemotherapy, patients underwent both SLN surgery and axillary lymph node dissection (ALND). Use of both blue dye and radiolabelled mapping agent was encouraged to identify the SLN.

- **Results**: Of 663 evaluable patients with cN1 disease, 649 underwent chemotherapy followed by both SLN surgery and ALND. A SLN could not be identified in 46 patients (7.1%). Only one SLN was excised in 78 patients (12%). Of the remaining 525 patients with two or more SLNs removed, no cancer was identified in the axillary lymph nodes of 215 patients, equating to a pathological complete nodal response of 41%. Cancer was not identified in the SLNs in 39 patients, but was then found in the nodes obtained with ALND. This equates to a FNR of 12.6%. The acceptable FNR threshold was set by the authors as 10%, and therefore the paper could not support the use of SLN surgery as an alternative to ALND.

EXPERT COMMENTARY BY EILIDH BRUCE AND BEATRIX ELSBERGER

Paper significance

Axillary lymph node status is an integral prognostic factor in the treatment of breast cancer and is used to guide decisions on local, regional and systemic treatments. Options for axillary lymph node staging after chemotherapy include SLN surgery or ALND, but the latter is significantly more morbid in terms of its postoperative outcomes. However, the concern with regard to SLN surgery in this context is for the potential of false-negative results. False-negative results can occur when the SLNs do not contain cancer, but cancer is found in nodes obtained from ALND. In comparison to ALND, the application of SLN surgery for staging the axilla following chemotherapy in patients with node-positive breast cancer was largely unknown, and this paper was one of the first to address this question.

Paper limitations

Results from this paper are limited by heterogeneity in its methodology, as the dual-agent mapping technique for SLN surgery was encouraged but not mandatory. The cohort was therefore a mix of patients who underwent SLN surgery with either a single- or dual-agent mapping technique. The dual-agent mapping technique had a significantly more acceptable FNR (10.8%) than the single-agent mapping technique (20.3%, $p = -0.05$). The method of patient enrolment in the study was also a limiting factor. Patients could be enrolled before, during or after their chemotherapy regardless of their length of therapy or nodal response. Therefore, patients who had significant residual nodal disease with poor response to chemotherapy, who were likely to be unsuitable for SLN surgery from the outset, were included within the cohort.

In context of the relevant current literature

This ACOSOG Z1071 landmark paper aimed to identify the FNR of SLN surgery in comparison to ALND in the setting of node-positive disease after neoadjuvant chemotherapy. However, we cannot address this topic without mention of the National Surgical Adjuvant Breast and Bowel Project (NSABP) B-32[1] study, which first evidenced SLN surgery as the safe and appropriate axillary strategy for node-negative breast cancer patients, published in 2010 in *Lancet Oncology*. This was a large study, in which 5,611 women were randomly assigned to sentinel node resection plus axillary dissection, or to sentinel node resection alone with axillary dissection only if the sentinel nodes were positive. In the B-32 study, blue dye and radioactive tracer were used for the SLN surgery. Overall survival, disease-free survival and regional control were statistically equivalent between groups.

The situation becomes more complex when we begin to consider the role of SLN surgery in patients with node-positive disease for restaging the axilla after neoadjuvant chemotherapy. In this setting, the patient cohort is more heterogeneous, including patients who have good clinical/radiological response and those who have not. This may somewhat explain the higher FNR demonstrated in the Z1071 paper. The SENTINA (SENTinel NeoAdjuvant)[2] multicentre cohort study set out to define the optimal timing of SLN surgery for patients undergoing neoadjuvant chemotherapy. The study included 1,737 patients in four different arms (**Figure 15.1**), and SLN surgery was performed with a radioactive tracer, with blue dye optional as a second tracer. The primary endpoint was the accuracy (FNR) of SLN surgery after neoadjuvant chemotherapy, for patients who converted from cN1 to ycN0 disease. In this group, the FNR of SLN surgery was 14.2%. The FNRs within this group were higher if only one or two sentinel nodes were removed.

Both the ACOSOG Z1071 and SENTINA studies found that the FNR in SLN surgery in patients' post-neoadjuvant chemotherapy was improved when three or more SLNs are evaluated. This mirrors results from the NSABP B-32 study in node-negative patients. Similarly, Hunt and colleagues[3] have provided more evidence to support the harvest of more than two SLNs to reduce the FNR in patients after neoadjuvant chemotherapy.

More recently, the concept of TAD[4] has become popular and enhances accuracy compared to SLNB alone. In this technique, the clinically involved node is marked before chemotherapy and is then localised at the time of SLNB, to ensure that the previously positive node is pathologically assessed. A number of techniques for node localisation have been successfully reported including Magseed, radioactive iodine seeds and cardon dye tattoo. Evidence suggests that the technique is safe and accurate and is becoming widely used.

The ongoing ATNEC [1] trial aims to build upon this evidence. ATNEC is a Phase III, open, randomised multicentre trial comparing standard axillary treatment (either ALND or axillary radiotherapy) with no axillary treatment for patients with early-stage breast cancer (T1–T3, N1, M0) and nodal metastases on needle biopsy, who after neoadjuvant chemotherapy have no evidence of residual nodal disease within the axilla on SLN surgery. After SLNB plus TAD, those with no evidence of nodal disease are then randomised to axillary clearance or no further axillary treatment. The study is recruiting, so it will be many years before the outcome is known.

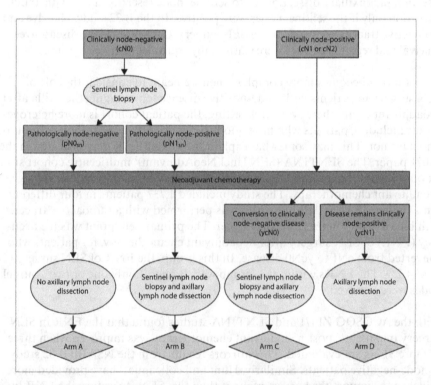

Figure 15.1   SENTINA (SENTinel NeoAdjuvant)[2] trial design. (Reprinted with permission from Elsevier.)

Conclusions

A body of evidence supports the use of SLN surgery in place of ALND in axillary staging of breast cancer patients with node-negative disease. The application of SLN surgery after neoadjuvant chemotherapy is far more complex. Across these studies, agreement exists that the safe and effective use of SLN surgery in patients having undergone neoadjuvant surgery will be very dependent upon patient selection (response to chemotherapy), dual-agent mapping and harvest of a number of sentinel nodes. The ATNEC trial will take this forward with the aim of de-escalating axillary treatment in a safe way without compromising recurrence or survival rates.

NOTE

1. (Axillary Management in T1-3N1M0 Breast Cancer Patients with Needle Biopsy—Proven Nodal Metastases at Presentation after Neoadjuvant Chemotherapy; see https://www.isrctn.com/ISRCTNISRCTN36585784.)

REFERENCES

1. Krag DN, Anderson SJ, Julian TB, Brown AM, Harlow SP, Ashikaga T, et al. Technical outcomes of sentinel-lymph-node resection and conventional axillary-lymph-node dissection in patients with clinically node-negative breast cancer: results from the NSABP B-32 randomised phase III trial. *Lancet Oncol.* 2007;8(10):881–8.
2. Kuehn T, Bauerfeind I, Fehm T, Fleige B, Hausschild M, Helms G, et al. Sentinel-lymph-node biopsy in patients with breast cancer before and after neoadjuvant chemotherapy (SENTINA): a prospective, multicentre cohort study. *Lancet Oncol.* 2013;14(7):609–18.
3. Hunt KK, Yi M, Mittendorf EA, Guerrero C, Babiera GV, Bedrosian I, et al. Sentinel lymph node surgery after neoadjuvant chemotherapy is accurate and reduces the need for axillary dissection in breast cancer patients. *Ann Surg.* 2009;250(4):558–66.
4. Boughey JC, Ballman KV, Le-Petross HT, McCall LM, Mittendorf EA, Ahrendt GM, et al. Identification and resection of clipped node decreases the false-negative rate of sentinel lymph node surgery in patients presenting with node-positive breast cancer (T0-T4, N1-N2) who receive neoadjuvant chemotherapy: results from ACOSOG Z1071 (Alliance). *Ann Surg.* 2016;263(4):802–7.

CHAPTER 16

Planning and Use of Therapeutic Mammaplasty: The Nottingham Approach

McCulley SJ, Macmillan RD.
Br J Plast Surg 58(7):889–901, 2005

Therapeutic mammaplasty (TM) describes the excision of breast cancer in combination with plastic surgical techniques to lift and reduce the breast. This technique may extend the boundaries of standard breast-conserving surgery (BCS) by reducing the risk of poor cosmetic outcomes or allowing some women to avoid mastectomy. This paper is one of the first to systematically describe methods for planning and performing TM procedures based on tumour location. Specifically, the authors describe type A and type B scenarios based on whether the tumour lies within the standard excision pattern of each technique, and they outline appropriate skin pattern and nipple pedicle selection based on tumour location.

PAPER DESCRIPTION

- **Objective/Research Question**: To provide guidance for the planning and use of TM based on tumour location.

- **Design**: Single-centre experience; technical description of surgical techniques and recommendations supported by case discussions.

- **Sample Size**: Based on the first 50 TMs performed in a single centre.

- **Results**:

EXPERT COMMENTARY BY DANIELLE BANFIELD AND SHELLEY POTTER

The authors offer an approach to planning and surgical techniques for TM. They describe both cosmetic and oncological advantages to TM and a variety of techniques which extend the use of this procedure to provide options for all possible tumour sites. Options for skin pattern and nipple pedicle selection are provided based on tumour location. Preoperative planning is aided by dividing the breast into nine zones oriented around mammaplasty markings. The authors propose a categorisation of procedures into Scenario A, where the tumour lies within a routine reduction mammaplasty excision and no adaptations of the technique are required, and Scenario B, where the tumour lies outside of the expected mammaplasty techniques and adaptations are needed. The paper uses six clinical cases to describe approaches to these tumour types.

Paper significance

This paper by McCulley and Macmillan underpins the modern practice of oncoplastic breast-conserving surgery (OPBCS) by providing clear guidelines on how standard TM techniques can be extended to allow tumour excision in any area of the breast, extending the scope of TM and allowing it to be offered to a wider range of patients.

Paper limitations

This paper is predominantly a technical report of the evolution of a surgical technique based on 50 consecutive cases performed at a single expert centre, supported by case discussions. The authors have not presented data on key outcomes such as complication rates or the need for re-excision. Furthermore, outcomes in a single specialist centre may not be widely applicable to everyday practice. The follow-up term of 3 years is limited, and the study does not include any patient-reported outcome measures. The paper cites the onco-cosmetic benefits of radiotherapy to a smaller breast following TM, but there is currently no robust evidence to support this. There is a need for further long-term evidence regarding both clinical and patient-reported outcomes for TM.[1]

In context of the relevant current literature

This paper builds on the previously published work by Clough and colleagues, which provided a bilevel classification and per-quadrant atlas,[2] by describing how mammaplasty techniques can be modified to facilitate tumour excision and reduce mastectomy rates. This is a growing trend, facilitated by TM, by neoadjuvant systemic therapy and more recently by use of perforator flaps.

The key benefits of TM include improving outcomes for women with breast cancer and reducing re-excision rates. It has been shown to be an oncologically safe option[3,4] and may allow women who are not suitable for standard BCS to avoid mastectomy. Evidence to support these proposed benefits, however, remains limited.

A recent Cochrane Review by Nanda and colleagues[5] included 78 non-randomised studies reporting outcomes in 178,813 women and compared the outcomes of OPBCS with (1) standard BCS, (2) mastectomy only and (3) mastectomy and breast reconstruction. They conclude that OPBCS is associated with a reduced risk of re-excision compared to standard BCS but a higher risk of complications, but there is limited evidence on patient-reported outcomes. There was insufficient evidence to compare OPBCS with mastectomy +/– implant breast reconstruction (IBR). The authors concluded that 'this review highlighted the deficiency of well-conducted studies to evaluate efficacy, safety and patient-reported outcomes following OPBCS' and the need for further research.

In the UK, a combined analysis of 2,916 women having OPBCS or mastectomy +/– IBR showed that TM was associated with a lower rate of complications than mastectomy and was successful at allowing women to avoid mastectomy in 87% of cases. Studies to support improvements in key patient-reported outcomes following TM remain limited,[6,7] and more research is needed.

Conclusions

Therapeutic mammaplasty offers a breast-conserving alternative to mastectomy and immediate breast reconstruction in suitable patients. The Therapeutic Mammaplasty (TeaM) and Implant Breast Reconstruction Evaluation Phase 2 (iBRA-2) groups showed it is a safe and effective alternative and may have lower complication rates than mastectomy and reconstruction. This paper allows application of TM to a wider range of breast types and tumour locations. However, as evidenced by the 2021 Cochrane Review, there is little robust evidence for oncological outcomes of TM, and further work is needed to assess the long-term clinical and patient-reported outcomes of this procedure.

REFERENCES

1. Potter S, Trickey A, Rattay T, O'Connell RL, Dave R, Baker E, et al., on behalf of the TeaM and iBRA-2 Steering Groups, the Breast Reconstruction Research Collaborative, and the Mammary Fold Academic and Research Collaborative. Therapeutic mammaplasty is a safe and effective alternative to mastectomy with or without immediate breast reconstruction. *Br J Surg.* 2020;107(7):832–44.
2. Clough KB, Kaufman GJ, Nos C, Buccimazza I, Sarfati IM. Improving breast cancer surgery: a classification and quadrant per quadrant atlas for oncoplastic surgery. *Ann Surg Oncol.* 2010;17(5):1375–91.
3. Campbell EJ, Romics L. Oncological safety and cosmetic outcomes in oncoplastic breast conservation surgery, a review of the best level of evidence literature. *Breast Cancer.* 2017;9:521–30.
4. Mansell J, Weiler-Mithoff E, Stallard S, Doughty JC, Mallon E, Romics L. Oncoplastic breast conservation surgery is oncologically safe when compared to wide local excision and mastectomy. *Breast.* 2017;32:179–85.
5. Nanda A, Hu J, Hodgkinson S, Ali S, Rainsbury R, Roy PG. Oncoplastic breast-conserving surgery for women with primary breast cancer. *Cochrane Database Syst Rev.* 2021;10(10).
6. Rose M, Svensson H, Handler J, Hoyer U, Ringberg A, Manjer J. Patient-reported outcome after oncoplastic breast surgery compared with conventional breast-conserving surgery in breast cancer. *Breast Cancer Res Treat.* 2020;180(1):247–56.
7. Ritter M, Oberhauser I, Montagna G, Zehnpfennig L, Schaefer K, Ling BM, et al. Comparison of patient-reported outcomes among different types of oncoplastic breast surgery procedures. *J Plast Reconstr Aesthet Surg.* 2022;75(9):3068–77.

Oncoplastic Breast-Conserving Surgery for Women with Primary Breast Cancer

Nanda A, Hu J, Hodgkinson S, Ali S, Rainsbury R, Roy PG.
Cochrane Database Syst Rev (10):CD013658, 2021

PAPER DESCRIPTION

- **Objective/Research Question**: To review evidence examining the effect of oncoplastic breast-conserving surgery (OPBCS) on cancer-related outcomes (local recurrence, disease-free survival and overall survival), quality of life (QoL) and cosmesis in women with breast cancer.

- **Design**: A Cochrane Review undertaken using robust Cochrane methodology. This included systematic searches of the Cochrane Breast Cancer Group's Specialist Register, the Cochrane Central Register of Controlled Trials (CENTRAL), MEDLINE (via OVID), Embase (via OVID), the World Health Organization's International Clinical Trials Registry Platform and ClinicalTrials.gov to identify relevant papers. At least two authors reviewed each study and undertook independent data extraction. Data were assessed for risk of bias (using the Risk of Bias in Non-Randomised Studies of Interventions [ROBINS-I] tool), confounding and heterogeneity (I^2). Meta-analysis of data was undertaken where appropriate, and the Grading of Recommendations Assessment, Development and Evaluation (GRADE) working group approach[1] was used to assess the certainty of evidence of the main outcomes.

- **Sample Size**: Seventy-eight non-randomised observational studies including 178,813 women were included in the qualitative synthesis, with 71 studies in the meta-analysis.

- **Intervention or Treatment Received**: Women undergoing OPBCS for primary breast cancer.

- **Results**: Seventy-eight non-randomised observational studies including 178,813 women were included in the qualitative synthesis, with 71 studies in the meta-analysis. Three major comparisons were made:
  1. *OPBCS versus standard breast-conserving surgery (BCS)*: There was little or no difference in oncological outcomes, including local

DOI: 10.1201/b23352-17

recurrence-free survival up to 5 years (hazard ratio [HR] = 0.90, 95% confidence interval [CI] = 0.61–1.43, four studies, 7,600 participants) or disease-free survival (HR = 1.06, 95% CI = 0.89–1.26, seven studies, 5,532 participants), when compared to standard BCS, though with very low or low certainty of evidence, respectively.

OPBCS may reduce the chance of re-excision (risk ratio [RR] = 0.76, 95% CI = 0.69–0.85, 38 studies, 13,341 participants), but the evidence is very uncertain. For the clinical outcomes, the data showed that OPBCS may increase the number of women who have at least one complication (RR = 1.19, 95% CI = 1.10–1.27, 20 studies, 118,005 participants) but with very low-certainty evidence. A meta-analysis was not possible for cosmesis or the patient-reported outcome measures (PROMs), but no significant differences were found in QoL scores using BREAST-Q. However, the data tended to favour OPBCS in terms of cosmetic satisfaction, though with very low certainty of evidence.

2. *OPBCS versus mastectomy*: Oncological outcomes favoured OPBCS in terms of local recurrence-free survival, compared with mastectomy, but the evidence was very uncertain (HR = 0.55, 95% CI = 0.34–0.91, two studies, 4,713 participants). The evidence of impact on disease-free survival was also very uncertain, as only one observational study (1,193 participants) was included in the analysis (RR = 0.58, 95% CI = 0.41–0.82). OPBCS may reduce complications compared to mastectomy, but the evidence was very uncertain (RR = 0.75, 95% CI = 0.67–0.83, four studies, 4,839 participants). In terms of PROMs, no conclusions were possible, as the evidence was from a single observational study.

3. *OPBCS versus mastectomy and immediate breast reconstruction*: OPBCS demonstrated little or no difference in oncological outcomes, including local recurrence-free survival (HR = 1.37, 95% CI = 0.72–2.62, one study, 3,785 participants) or disease-free survival (HR = 0.45, 95% CI = 0.09–2.22, one study, 317 participants), both with very low-certainty evidence when compared to mastectomy with reconstruction. OPBCS may reduce complications compared to mastectomy and reconstruction, but the evidence was very uncertain (RR = 0.49, 95% CI = 0.45–0.54, five studies, 4,973 participants). A comparison of cosmetic outcomes and PROMs was not possible due to data paucity, methodological diversity and a high risk of bias.

In conclusion, the oncological evidence for OPBCS compared to other types of surgery for breast cancer was very uncertain, but significantly, inferiority of OPBCS was not demonstrated. OPBCS may reduce the need for re-excision but increase the rate of complications compared to standard BCS, and it may reduce the rate of complications compared to mastectomy with and without reconstruction, but again the evidence was very uncertain. The authors deduced that no certain conclusions could be made to help inform policymakers, that joint decision making including appropriate personalised discussion was needed to determine the choice of surgical procedure and that there was a lack of well-conducted studies to evaluate efficacy, safety and PROMS following OPBCS.

EXPERT COMMENTARY BY KATHERINE FAIRHURST AND SHELLEY POTTER

Paper significance

OPBCS describes the practice of both removing the breast tumour and utilising plastic surgery techniques to reconstruct the breast. OPBCS can be broadly divided into two categories: (1) volume displacement techniques, including therapeutic mammaplasty using breast reduction and/or mastopexy techniques, which are most commonly used for women with large and/or ptotic breasts; and (2) volume replacement techniques, for example using local chest wall perforator flaps, which tend to be suitable for women with smaller non-ptotic breasts, and less commonly require symmetrisation to the contralateral breast.

In context of the relevant current literature

OPBCS techniques have grown exponentially in popularity as surgeons endeavour to push the boundaries of breast conservation to avoid deformity and/or mastectomy and improve cosmetic outcomes and QoL. However, there is a paucity of high-quality comparative evidence for OPBCS versus other surgical techniques, and the need for further research has been identified repeatedly in the literature over the past 5 years.

The need to evaluate the clinical and cost-effectiveness of OPBCS was identified in the updated 2018 breast surgery gap analysis led by the Association of Breast Surgery.[2] The 2019 Oncoplastic Breast Consortium meeting also identified key research gaps as evaluating the impact of OPBCS versus mastectomy on QoL, determining the best measurement tools and establishing what the most accurate quality indicators are for OPBCS versus standard BCS or mastectomy.[3] The James Lind Alliance Priority Setting Partnership in Breast Cancer Surgery published in 2023 identified 59 key research priorities in breast cancer surgery agreed by all key stakeholders including patients. Among these priorities were outcomes of OPBCS versus standard BCS and mastectomy with and without reconstruction and, importantly, how best to discuss this with patients, as well as the safety of avoiding mastectomy for multicentric breast cancer.[4]

In 2021, the GRETA (Group for REconstructive and Therapeutic Advancements) group, comprising 21 academics and clinicians from across the world, used the GRADEpro tool[1] to deliberate and prioritise benefits and harms for OPBCS and then evaluate the evidence to formulate recommendations.[5] The group defined a list of critical outcomes for decision making including health-related QoL, patient satisfaction with cosmetic outcomes and depression, along with oncological and clinical outcomes. Interestingly, GRETA concluded that OPBCS should be recommended for those who are suitable for standard BCS despite this being with a very low certainty of evidence.

Conclusions

This comprehensive review and meta-analysis have shown that the safety, efficacy and effect on QoL of OPBCS remain uncertain, although the data available do not suggest any adverse safety signal. Well-designed, prospective comparative studies that use standardised outcome-reporting measures are needed to address this uncertainty. Randomised controlled trials (RCTs) are the gold standard, but studies comparing OPBCS and mastectomy are unlikely to be feasible due to patient and surgeon preference.[6] Methodologically robust, large-scale registry and/or prospective cohort studies, including outcomes of importance to patients, are probably the preferred design to realise timely results. Such studies will generate reliable and standardised information to inform enhanced patient and clinician decision making regarding OPBCS and, most importantly, improve long-term outcomes for patients.

REFERENCES

1. Group GW. [cited 2023 28th June 2023]; Available from: https://www.gradeworkinggroup. org.
2. Cutress RI, et al. Opportunities and priorities for breast surgical research. *Lancet Oncol.* 2018;19(10):e521–33.
3. Weber WP, et al. Knowledge gaps in oncoplastic breast surgery. *Lancet Oncol.* 2020;21(8): e375–85.
4. Potter S, et al. Identifying research priorities in breast cancer surgery: a UK priority setting partnership with the James Lind Alliance. *Breast Cancer Res Treat.* 2023;197(1):39–49.
5. Rocco N, et al. Should oncoplastic breast conserving surgery be used for the treatment of early stage breast cancer? Using the GRADE approach for development of clinical recommendations. *Breast.* 2021;57:25–35.
6. Ingram J, et al. The challenge of equipoise: qualitative interviews exploring the views of health professionals and women with multiple ipsilateral breast cancer on recruitment to a surgical randomised controlled feasibility trial. *Pilot Feasibility Stud.* 2022;8(1):46.

CHAPTER 18

Short-Term Safety Outcomes of Mastectomy and Immediate Implant-Based Breast Reconstruction with and without Mesh (iBRA): A Multicentre, Prospective Cohort Study

Potter S, Conroy EJ, Cutress RI, et al.
Lancet Oncol 20:254–266, 2019

This prospective, multicentre cohort study aimed to assess the short-term safety of immediate implant-based breast reconstruction (IBBR) performed with and without mesh. It included 2,108 women who underwent 2,655 implant-based reconstructions at 81 UK centres between February 2014 and June 2016. Of these, 182 (9%, 95% confidence interval [CI] = 8–10) experienced implant loss, 372 (18%, 95% CI = 16–20) required readmission to hospital and 370 (18%, 95% CI = 16–20) required return to theatre for complications within 3 months of their initial surgery. Five hundred and twenty-two patients (25%, 95% CI = 23–27) required treatment for an infection. The authors concluded that these complications were higher than those recommended by national standards and that a clinical trial was required to determine the optimal approach to IBBR.

PAPER DESCRIPTION

- **Objective/Research Question**: To determine the short-term safety of immediate IBBR performed with and without mesh to inform the feasibility of a future randomised clinical trial.

- **Design**: A multicentre, prospective cohort study.

- **Sample Size**: Two thousand one hundred and eight women undergoing 2,655 IBBR procedures.

- **Inclusion Criteria**: Women aged 16 and older who had mastectomy with immediate implant-based reconstruction with any technique.

- **Exclusion Criteria**: Patients undergoing delayed reconstruction, flap-based implant reconstruction or revision surgery were excluded.

- **Treatment or Intervention Received**: Mastectomy and immediate implant-based reconstruction using any technique with or without mesh.

- **Results**: Two thousand one hundred and eight women underwent 2,655 IBBR procedures. Of these, 54% had biological mesh-assisted reconstruction, 12% underwent synthetic mesh-assisted reconstruction, 9% were treated with a traditional subpectoral implant without mesh and 21% received a subpectoral implant with a dermal sling. Pre-pectoral reconstruction with mesh was performed in the later stages of the study, accounting for 2% of patients. The remainder underwent a combination of techniques (3%) or had no technique specified (7%). A total of 14 different mesh products were used throughout the course of the study.

  Two thousand and eighty-one patients (99%) were followed up to 3 months postoperatively. Implant loss was experienced by 182 patients (9%). Five hundred and twenty-two patients (25%) had a postoperative infection requiring treatment, and 372 patients (18%) were readmitted for a complication of their reconstruction within 3 months, with 370 (18%) requiring further surgery.

  These four outcomes were compared with data from the National Mastectomy and Breast Reconstruction Audit (NMBRA) and UK National Quality Criteria for Breast Reconstruction. Implant loss rates were equivalent to the NMBRA published data but higher than National Quality Standards. Both postoperative infection and readmission rates were again consistent with NMBRA data and higher than National Quality Standards. The number of patients requiring reoperation was higher than that reported in the NMBRA data.

  Exploratory analysis identified an association between higher body mass index (BMI) and smoking and all four clinical outcomes; it also identified an apparent association between infection and previous radiotherapy, and between reoperation and operative time. Age, neoadjuvant chemotherapy, bilateral surgery, indication for surgery, nipple-sparing procedures, insertion of a definitive fixed-volume implant and type of reconstruction were not identified as significant risk factors for any of the four key outcomes.

EXPERT COMMENTARY BY DANIELLE BANFIELD AND SHELLEY POTTER

Paper significance

IBBR is the most commonly performed reconstruction in the UK. Mesh-assisted techniques were introduced with the aim of improving outcomes for patients, specifically avoiding the need for painful and time-consuming tissue expansion and the need for a second operation with standard two-stage techniques, and improving cosmetic outcomes by allowing better lower pole projection.

Mesh was introduced without robust evaluation, and the Implant Breast Reconstruction Evaluation (iBRA) was the largest prospective evaluation of mesh-assisted IBBR worldwide. It provided large-scale real-world data to suggest that complications following the procedure were high and improvements were required to improve outcomes for patients. Exploratory analysis emphasised the importance of careful patient selection for IBBR but did not suggest that the use of mesh impacted complications. Subsequent analysis of patient-reported outcomes assessed using the validated BREAST-Q at 18 months post reconstruction also demonstrated similar scores across all domains irrespective of whether IBBR was performed with or without mesh,[1] suggesting the proposed benefits of mesh-assisted IBBR were not being realised. The study highlighted the need for further research, ideally a well-designed randomised clinical trial to establish best practice for implant-based procedures. The results of the iBRA study influenced updated joint Association of Breast Surgery (ABS) and British Association of Plastic, Reconstructive and Aesthetic Surgeons (BAPRAS) guidelines for the practice of mesh-assisted IBBR in the UK.[2]

Paper limitations

This was a prospective observational study based on current standard practice and therefore subject to bias. The study was pragmatic and did not specify patient selection criteria or provide guidelines for how the procedure should be performed. There was therefore the potential for considerable variation in practice between sites. Despite pre-specifying outcomes prior to commencing the study, changes in practice during the study, such as the introduction of implant salvage, may have led to over- or underreporting of complications. Furthermore, the paper only reported a 3-month follow-up, so complications occurring during chemotherapy or adjuvant radiotherapy would not have been captured. Finally, IBBR is a rapidly evolving technique. Newer pre-pectoral techniques were introduced towards the end of the study, but insufficient cases were included for a meaningful comparison to be made, and the study mainly included subpectoral mesh-assisted techniques.

In context of the relevant current literature

Data from the real-world iBRA study are consistent with the findings of two small multicentre randomised controlled trials (RCTs) comparing traditional two-stage expander implant reconstruction and single-stage direct-to-implant mesh-assisted reconstruction. These trials suggest that mesh use fails to improve the patient-reported outcomes of IBBR[3-7] but may be associated with increased patient harm and higher complication rates.[3] Irrespective of the published evidence, however, mesh-assisted reconstruction has become the standard of care in the UK, and the technique has continued to evolve.

Pre-pectoral reconstruction, in which the implant, wrapped in mesh, is placed on top of rather than underneath the pectoral muscle, is now becoming standard practice in the UK. Pre-pectoral reconstruction aims to avoid the distressing implant animation that is seen when the implant is placed in a subpectoral pocket, reduce postoperative pain and improve cosmetic outcomes as the implant is placed in an anatomical position. Observational data[8] suggest that the complication rates of pre-pectoral reconstruction are similar to those of subpectoral techniques, but long-term outcome data including patient-reported outcomes are lacking.

Robust evaluation to establish the benefits of the technique is required, particularly in light of the Cumberledge Report, but Best-BRA (Is Subpectoral or Pre-Pectoral Implant Placement Best in Immediate Breast Reconstruction?, ISRCTN10081873),[9] a UK-based RCT trial comparing pre- and subpectoral IBBR, was not found to be feasible due to the rapid evolution of practice and loss of community equipoise. OPBC-02/PREPEC (Pre- versus Sub-Pectoral Implant-Based Breast Reconstruction after Skin-Sparing Mastectomy or Nipple-Sparing Mastectomy), a large-scale pragmatic international RCT[10] comparing the techniques, however, has been able to recruit successfully and will generate data to support practice. Accrual is almost complete, and the study is due to report in 2025.

Conclusions

The iBRA study aimed to generate high-quality evidence to support the practice of IBBR, the most commonly performed type of breast reconstruction in the UK. IBBR, however, is a rapidly evolving technique, and ongoing robust evaluation is required to provide evidence to support practice and avoid patient harms.

REFERENCES

1. Sewart E, et al. Patient-reported outcomes of immediate implant-based breast reconstruction with and without biological or synthetic mesh. *BJS Open*. 2021;5(1).
2. Whisker L, et al. Biological and synthetic mesh assisted breast reconstruction procedures: Joint guidelines from the Association of Breast Surgery and the British Association of Plastic, Reconstructive and Aesthetic Surgeons. *Eur J Surg Oncol*. 2021.
3. Dikmans REG, et al. Two-stage implant-based breast reconstruction compared with immediate one-stage implant-based breast reconstruction augmented with an acellular dermal matrix: an open-label, phase 4, multicentre, randomised, controlled trial. *Lancet Oncol*. 2017;18(2):251–8.
4. Negenborn VL, et al. Quality of life and patient satisfaction after one-stage implant-based breast reconstruction with an acellular dermal matrix versus two-stage breast reconstruction (BRIOS): primary outcome of a randomised, controlled trial. *Lancet Oncol*. 2018;19(9):1205–14.
5. Lohmander F, et al. Implant based breast reconstruction with acellular dermal matrix: safety data from an open-label, multicenter, randomized, controlled trial in the setting of breast cancer treatment. *Ann Surg*. 2019;269(5):836–41.

6. Lohmander F, et al. Quality of life and patient satisfaction after implant-based breast reconstruction with or without acellular dermal matrix: randomized clinical trial. *BJS Open*. 2020;4(5):811–20.

7. Lohmander F, et al. Effect of immediate implant-based breast reconstruction after mastectomy with and without acellular dermal matrix among women with breast cancer: a randomized clinical trial. *JAMA Netw Open*. 2021;4(10):e2127806.

8. Harvey KL, et al. Short-term safety outcomes of mastectomy and immediate prepectoral implant-based breast reconstruction: Pre-BRA prospective multicentre cohort study. *Br J Surg*. 2022;109(6):530–8.

9. Roberts K, et al. Best-BRA (Is subpectoral or pre-pectoral implant placement best in immediate breast reconstruction?) A protocol for a pilot randomised controlled trial of subpectoral versus pre-pectoral immediate implant-based breast reconstruction in women following mastectomy. *BMJ Open*. 2021:(in press).

10. Kappos EA, et al. Prepectoral versus subpectoral implant-based breast reconstruction after skin-sparing mastectomy or nipple-sparing mastectomy (OPBC-02/PREPEC): a pragmatic, multicentre, randomised, superiority trial. *BMJ Open*. 2021;11(9):e045239.

CHAPTER 19

Improving Breast Cancer Surgery: A Classification and Quadrant per Quadrant Atlas for Oncoplastic Surgery

Clough KB, Kaufman GJ, Nos C, Buccimazza I, Sarfati IM.
Ann Surg Oncol 17:1375–1391, 2010

PAPER DESCRIPTION

- **Objective/Research Question**: To develop novel guidelines to support appropriate patient selection with the implementation of a bilevel classification system and quadrant-per-quadrant atlas, advising the optimal choice of surgical technique for patients with breast cancer undergoing oncoplastic breast-conserving surgery (OPBCS).

- **Design**: This paper describes a classification system and atlas based on expert opinion.

- **Sample Size**:

- **Inclusion Criteria**: Clough and colleagues describe three factors to identify patients who would benefit from OPBCS. These are (1) excision volume, (2) tumour location and (3) glandular density.
  1. **Excision volume**: Excision volume is the most crucial determinant of the outcome of breast-conserving surgery (BCS), with poorer cosmetic outcomes reported as excision volumes increase. Excisions that exceed 20% of breast volume are at high risk of subsequent deformity. Clough and colleagues emphasised the importance of estimating the total excision volume relative to the overall size of the breast preoperatively during the decision-making process.
  2. **Tumour location**: Tumour location is the second most important factor in determining the need for OPBCS, as there are areas of the breast that are at high risk of deformity, even if relatively small volumes of tissue are removed. The upper inner quadrant and lower central breast are two areas at particularly high risk of subsequent deformity. If resection of a tumour from these areas is planned, an oncoplastic procedure should be considered based on the quadrant-per-quadrant atlas proposed by the authors.

3. **Glandular density**: This is the final factor that should be considered when assessing the suitability of a patient for OPBCS. The Breast Imaging Reporting and Data System (BI-RADS) scoring system is used to classify breast density on mammogram. It is a four-point scale that ranges from 1 (fatty) to 4 (extremely dense). Certain oncoplastic techniques (e.g., level-1 procedures) require significant undermining of the breast from both the skin and pectoralis muscle (dual-plane mobilisation). Use of these techniques is not recommended in patients with low-density breast tissue (BI-RADS category 1–2) due to the high risk of fat necrosis.

• **Oncoplastic Classification System**: The authors propose a bilevel classification of OPBCS based on excision volume and reshaping complexity.

Level-1 OPBCS procedures involve resection of less than 20% breast tissue with dual-plane undermining including nipple–areolar complex (NAC) recentralisation if nipple deviation is anticipated. These procedures are not recommended in patients with fatty breasts due to the high risk of fat necrosis. All breast surgeons should be able to perform these techniques. The six steps for level-1 OPBCS are described as: (1) the skin incision, (2) skin undermining, (3) NAC undermining, (4) full-thickness excision, (5) glandular re-approximation and (6) de-epithelialisation, with NAC repositioning (if required).

Level-2 OPBCS procedures involve excision of 20%–50% of the breast volume and can be used in all patients, irrespective of breast density. They require excision of excess skin to reshape the breast, and as they are based on mammaplasty techniques, they are often called 'therapeutic mammaplasty'. Clough and colleagues propose an atlas to guide technique selection based on the position of the tumour in the breast **(Table 19.1)**.

• **Results**:

Table 19.1 Level-2 oncoplastic breast-conserving surgery (OPBCS): Quadrant-per-quadrant atlas (Orientation for left breast)

Clock position	Procedures
5–7 o'clock Lower pole	Superior pedicle mammoplasty/Inverted T or vertical scar
7–8 o'clock Lower inner quadrant	Superior pedicle mammoplasty/V scar
9–11 o'clock Upper inner quadrant	Batwing
12 o'clock Upper pole	Inferior pedicle mammoplasty or round block mammoplasty
1–2 o'clock Upper outer quadrant	Racquet mammoplasty/Radial scar
4–5 o'clock Lower outer quadrant	Superior pedicle mammoplasty/J scar
Central subareolar	Inverted T or vertical-scar mammoplasty with NAC resection

Source: Reprinted with permission from Springer Nature.

EXPERT COMMENTARY BY DAVID STARK AND SHELLEY POTTER

Paper significance

OPBCS combines plastic surgical techniques with oncological resection to preserve breast shape and appearance while effectively treating breast cancer, often extending the boundaries of standard breast-conserving surgery (BCS) or allowing patients to avoid mastectomy. This landmark paper describes a bilevel OPBCS classification system and quadrant-per-quadrant atlas to guide appropriate patient and procedure selection for women undergoing OPBCS for breast cancer.

The article was the first description of standardised guidelines to support optimal patient selection and surgical decision making in OPBCS. The bilevel OPBCS classification (levels 1 and 2) and atlas have been widely adopted into clinical practice and contributed to improved surgical outcomes with breast tissue preservation, reduced re-excision rates and enhanced cosmetic results. This landmark paper supported surgeons to integrate plastic surgical techniques into breast cancer surgery and led to the wider adoption of OPBCS into routine clinical practice. This, ultimately, has led to better patient satisfaction and quality of life.

Paper limitations

The description of OPBCS techniques and guidelines for patient selection reflect the outcomes of surgery performed by world-leading experts in the field and may not be representative of outcomes in less expert hands without further training. Importantly, the paper does not address potential complications or long-term outcomes associated with OPBCS techniques. Further research and long-term follow-up studies are needed to assess the outcomes of these surgical approaches.

In context of the relevant current literature

This paper was the first to describe a step-by-step guide to patient and procedure selection in OPBCS. To further understand the evolving landscape of OPBCS, it is beneficial to consult additional papers and current literature in the field. Rainsbury's article offers a historical perspective on the evolution of OPBCS, tracking the transition into the reconstruction of defects by either volume replacement or displacement.[1] This contribution provides additional context to the techniques presented in Clough et al.'s work.[3] Munhoz et al.'s paper investigates the outcomes of immediate and delayed BCS reconstruction with mastectomy.[2] The findings add valuable insights into the timing and potential benefits of various approaches, which are relevant to the application of Clough et al.'s classification and atlas. Clough et al.'s paper originally emphasised the utilisation of oncoplastic techniques with concomitant symmetrisation of the contralateral breast to enable extensive resections for BCS.[7] This study complements the classification and atlas by highlighting the advantages and outcomes associated with the integration of OPBCS into breast-conserving treatment strategies.

Although OPBCS aims to improve outcomes for patients having BCS by reducing the rate of re-excision by allowing larger volumes of tissue to be removed and improving cosmetic outcomes, several systematic reviews have highlighted that high-quality evidence to support these proposed positives are lacking. A recent Cochrane Review compared the outcomes of OPBCS with standard BCS and with mastectomy +/– reconstruction.[4] This review including 178,813 women suggested that OPBCS may result in a reduced rate of re-excision surgery but may lead to more complications and a greater recall rate than conventional BCS. Hasan et al.'s meta-analysis also demonstrated that re-excision significantly favoured conventional BCS, but local recurrence, close surgical margins and need for mastectomy showed no significant difference between both techniques.[5]

There are increasing data to support the oncological safety of OPBCS, particularly in patients having larger tumours excised using level-2 procedures. Clough et al. investigated the outcomes of level-2 oncoplastic techniques and demonstrated a 2.2% 5-year local recurrence rate, which is at the lower end of the literature reporting on local recurrence after OPBCS.[7] De Lorenzi et al. completed a 10-year follow-up series showing a 6.7% recurrence rate in OPBCS in comparison to 4.2% in the conventional group.[8] Mohamedahmed et al.'s systematic review aimed to evaluate comparative outcomes between these methods, concluding that the available literature clearly demonstrates superior or at least equivalent outcomes when comparing OPBCS to conventional BCS, although there is a lack of level-1 evidence.[9] OPBCS may provide better patient satisfaction with the appearance of the breast, as it aims to avoid deformity following surgery. However, the evidence to support these benefits is of poor quality.[4]

Conclusions

This paper proposed an OPBCS classification and atlas to enhance patient selection, promote a standardised approach for surgeons and offer specific solutions for diverse scenarios, ultimately refining outcomes in breast conservation. Further evidence to support the potential clinical, oncological and patient-reported outcomes of these techniques remains elusive.

REFERENCES

1. Rainsbury RM. Surgery insight: oncoplastic breast-conserving reconstruction—indications, benefits, choices, and outcomes. *Nat Clin Pract Oncol.* 2007;4(11):657–64.

2. Munhoz AM, Aldrighi CM, Montag E, Arruda E, Brasil JA, Filassi JR, et al. Outcome analysis of immediate and delayed conservative breast surgery reconstruction with mastopexy and reduction mammaplasty techniques. *Ann Plast Surg.* 2011;67(3):220–5.

3. Clough KB, Lewis JS, Couturaud B, Fitoussi A, Nos C, Falcou MC. Oncoplastic techniques allow extensive resections for breast-conserving therapy of breast carcinomas. *Ann Surg.* 2003;237(1):26–34.

4. Nanda A, Hu J, Hodgkinson S, Ali S, Rainsbury R, Roy PG. Oncoplastic breast-conserving surgery for women with primary breast cancer. *Cochrane Database Syst Rev.* 2021;10(10).

5. Hasan MT, Hamouda M, Khashab MKE, Elsnhory AB, Elghamry AM, Hassan OA, et al. Oncoplastic versus conventional breast-conserving surgery in breast cancer: a pooled analysis of 6941 female patients. *Breast Cancer.* 2023;30(2):200–14.

6. Nizet JL, Maweja S, Lakosi F, et al. Oncological and surgical outcome after oncoplastic breast surgery. *Acta Chir Belg.* 2015;115:33–41.

7. Clough KB, van la Parra RFD, Thygesen HH, Levy E, Russ E, Halabi NM, et al. Long-term results after oncoplastic surgery for breast cancer: a 10-year follow-up. *Ann Surg.* 2018;268(1):165–71.

8. De Lorenzi F, Hubner G, Rotmensz N, Bagnardi V, Loschi P, Maisonneuve P, et al. Oncological results of oncoplastic breast-conserving surgery: Long term follow-up of a large series at a single institution: a matched-cohort analysis. *Eur J Surg Oncol.* 2016;42(1):71–7.

9. Mohamedahmed AYY, Zaman S, Zafar S, Laroiya I, Iqbal J, Tan MLH, et al. Comparison of surgical and oncological outcomes between oncoplastic breast-conserving surgery versus conventional breast-conserving surgery for treatment of breast cancer: a systematic review and meta-analysis of 31 studies. *Surg Oncol.* 2022;42.

CHAPTER 20

Gene Expression Patterns of Breast Carcinomas Distinguish Tumor Subclasses with Clinical Implications

Sørlie T, Perou CM, Tibshirani R, Aas T, Geisler S, Johnsen H, et al.
Proc Natl Acad Sci 98(19):10869–10874, 2001

The purpose of this study was to classify breast carcinomas based on variations in gene expression patterns derived from DNA microarrays, and to correlate tumour characteristics to clinical outcomes. A total of 85 DNA microarray experiments representing 78 cancers, three fibroadenomas and four samples of normal breast tissue were analysed by grouping tumours together based on their genetic similarity when looking at a large number (thousands) of genes (hierarchical clustering) and their clinical outcomes. Genes were analysed according to whether they were overexpressed or underexpressed, which was then correlated with survival. The cancers could be classified into a basal epithelial-like group, an *ERBB2*-overexpressing group and a normal breast–like group based on variations in gene expression, and two separate luminal types could be distinguished. Survival analyses on a subgroup of patients with locally advanced breast cancer uniformly treated in a prospective study showed significantly different outcomes for the patients belonging to the various groups, including a poor prognosis for the basal-like subtype and a significant difference in outcomes for the two oestrogen receptor–positive groups.

PAPER DESCRIPTION

- **Objective/Research Question**: The study aimed to classify breast tumours based on gene expression profiles using genomic microarrays and to correlate this with tumour characteristics and clinical outcomes including prognosis.

- **Design**: Tissue analysis of 78 breast carcinomas (71 ductal, five lobular and two ductal carcinomas *in situ* obtained from 77 different individuals; two independent tumours from one individual diagnosed at different times), three fibroadenomas and four normal breast tissue samples, three of which were pooled normal breast samples from multiple individuals.

DOI: 10.1201/b23352-20

- **Sample Size**: Eighty-five tissue samples representing 84 individuals.

- **Follow-Up**: Median clinical follow-up time of 66 months.

- **Intervention or Treatment Received**: Tissue samples from breast cancers, benign breast lesions and normal tissue were analysed for the expression of thousands of genes simultaneously using complementary DNA (cDNA) microarray technology. This involves isolating messenger RNA from tissues using reverse transcription polymerase chain reaction (RT-PCR) to create cDNA and labelling it with fluorescent tags before introducing it to the array. The microarray contains thousands of gene probes which hybridise with the complementary tissue cDNA. Fluorescent images were then obtained. This was scanned to create computer-generated images which represent gene expression. Information about gene expression obtained from cDNA microassay testing was interpreted mathematically using significance analysis of microarrays (SAM). For negative scores, higher expression of a gene correlated with longer survival. Conversely, higher expression of a gene with a positive score correlated with shorter survival.

- **Results**: The group's previous work had identified three distinct subtypes of breast cancer: basal-like, *HER2*+ and normal breast–like. Based on differences in microarray studies performed in this study, luminal tumours were further divided into at least two distinct subgroups (luminal A and B); a third subgroup, luminal C, was also proposed. The expression of several distinct genes was found to be associated with different tumour subtypes. For example, high levels of gene expression for keratins 5 and 17 and *ERBB2* were associated with basal-like and *HER2*+ subtypes, respectively. *TP53* gene mutations have previously been identified as correlating with poor prognosis. Over 40% of tumours tested were found to have a *TP53* mutation ($n = 30$), but the distribution between the subtypes was uneven. Luminal A tumours were significantly less likely to possess a *TP53* mutation compared to *HER2*+ or basal-like subtypes. Different tumour subgroups were found to have prognostic value regarding both overall and relapse-free survival. More than 75% of tumour samples analysed remained in the same subgroup after analysis against a different sample set of genes, adding to the validity and reproducibility of the results.

EXPERT COMMENTARY BY CLIONA KIRWAN AND RACHEL FOSTER

Paper significance

Improving our understanding of the genomics of breast cancer heterogenicity has led to the classification of five distinct breast cancer subtypes which represent biologically distinct disease entities with separate prognostic and therapeutic implications. This paper was key to our modern classification of breast cancer, although further work has now identified several further distinct subgroups, such as within the triple-negative group, all with different prognostic significance.

Paper limitations

Clinical outcomes were based on only 49 patients with locally advanced disease, so this may not reflect the more common early breast cancer population with later presentation of metastatic disease. This limited patient cohort, treated in the early 1990s, had not been exposed to modern drug regimens which could markedly alter prognosis in modern practice.

In context of the relevant current literature

Breast cancer is a complex and heterogeneous disease resulting from somatic gene mutations as well as changes in gene and protein expression. As our understanding of breast cancer molecular genetics has increased, so too has the complexity of the classification systems used. A traditional histopathological classification based on tumour type, such as invasive ductal or lobular carcinoma, has been widely adopted into multidisciplinary team practice. With most tumours falling into a small number of types, this offers little potential for personalisation of treatment. Biological classification was then introduced with factors such as hormone receptor status, *HER2* overexpression or amplification and Ki67 percentage score.

In 2000, Perou and colleagues were the first to classify breast cancers into distinct subtypes based on their gene expression profiles,[1] and they initially identified three subtypes: basal-like, *HER2*+ and normal breast–like. Basal-like tumours represent an aggressive molecular subtype, lacking in the expression of oestrogen, progesterone and *HER2* receptors.[2] Oestrogen receptor–positive tumours have been further divided into luminal A and luminal B subtypes. Luminal A tumours are hormone receptor–positive and *HER2* receptor–negative, and they have a low proliferative index. Normal breast–like tumours closely resemble luminal A tumours. Luminal B tumours are hormone receptor–positive and *HER2*-positive or -negative, with a higher proliferative index than luminal A tumours. Clinical outcomes such as tumour response to cytotoxic chemotherapy as well as overall prognosis have been shown to correlate with breast cancer subtype.[3]

Extensive research using microarray assays and hierarchical clustering has resulted in the identification of multiple gene sets that are able to classify tumours into discrete subtypes. Testing a predetermined subset of genes identified by hierarchical clustering provides results which are comparable with those achieved by whole gene set testing. Using different gene sets to test the same tumour have been shown to produce equivalent subtype and survival predictions.[4] The Prediction Analysis of Microarray 50 (PAM50) quantitative RT-PCR (qRT-PCR) assay test was developed which uses the expression profile of 50 genes to identify a tumour's subtype.[5] This test has been shown to add benefit in terms of prognostic information compared to standard tests using tumour stage, grade and molecular markers.[6]

The commercially available Prosigna® gene expression assay incorporates the PAM50 subtype analysis into its 10-year recurrence prediction test. The test is validated for use in patients with early hormone receptor–positive, *HER2*-negative, invasive breast cancer. It incorporates the size and grade of cancer, nodal status, and hormone and *HER2* receptor status along with the PAM50 gene expression assay. The results of the test include risk group classification (low, intermediate or high), risk of recurrence score (0–100) and intrinsic subtype (luminal A, luminal B, *HER2*-enriched or basal-like). The National Institute for Health and Care Excellence (NICE) recommends the Prosigna® test as an option for guiding adjuvant chemotherapy decisions in patients who have a hormone receptor–positive, *HER2*-negative, node-negative breast cancer and have an intermediate risk of recurrence based on validated tools such as PREDICT or the Nottingham Prognostic Index (NPI).[7]

Conclusions

Breast cancers can be classified into five different subtypes (basal-like, *HER2+* and luminal A, B and C) based on their complex gene expression signatures which are then associated with different clinical outcomes and prognoses. This important study paved the way for future researchers to determine the link between gene expression profiles and variation in clinical phenotype including response to treatments, likelihood of disease recurrence and metastasis.

REFERENCES

1. Perou CM, Sørlie T, Eisen MB, van de Rijn M, Jeffrey SS, Rees CA, et al. Molecular portraits of human breast tumours. *Nature*. 2000;406(6797):747–52.
2. Schneider BP, Winer EP, Foulkes WD, Garber J, Perou CM, Richardson A, et al. Triple-negative breast cancer: risk factors to potential targets. *Clin Cancer Res*. 2008;14(24):8010–8.
3. Troester MA, Hoadley KA, Sørlie T, Herbert B-S, Børresen-Dale A-L, Lønning PE, et al. Cell-type-specific responses to chemotherapeutics in breast cancer. *Cancer Res*. 2004;64(12):4218–26.
4. Fan C, Oh DS, Wessels L, Weigelt B, Nuyten DSA, Nobel AB, et al. Concordance among gene-expression–based predictors for breast cancer. *N Engl J Med*. 2006;355(6):560–9.
5. Dowsett M, Sestak I, Lopez-Knowles E, Sidhu K, Dunbier AK, Cowens JW, et al. Comparison of PAM50 risk of recurrence score with oncotype DX and IHC4 for predicting risk of distant recurrence after endocrine therapy. *J Clin Oncol*. 2013;31(22):2783–90.
6. Parker JS, Mullins M, Cheang MC, Leung S, Voduc D, Vickery T, et al. Supervised risk predictor of breast cancer based on intrinsic subtypes. *J Clin Oncol*. 2009;27(8):1160–7.
7. NICE. Tumour profiling tests to guide adjuvant chemotherapy decisions in early breast cancer. 2018.

CHAPTER 21

Comprehensive Molecular Portraits of Human Breast Tumours

The Cancer Genome Atlas Network.
Nature 490:61–70, 2012

This study undertook complex analysis of over 800 breast cancers using a range of different molecular techniques. These looked at DNA, RNA, microRNA, protein expression and epigenetic changes (DNA methylation). The aim was to understand the underlying molecular changes that differentiate the four major breast cancer subtypes. These are the oestrogen receptor (ER)-positive high- and low-proliferation subgroups (luminal A and B), *HER2*-amplified and triple-negative type. Data from the different types of analysis were correlated and analysed together to increase the depth of analysis. The paper confirmed the existence of four main breast cancer classes when combining data from the five platforms, each of which showed significant molecular heterogeneity. They were able to identify somatic (acquired or non-inherited) mutations in three genes (*TP53*, *PIK3CA* and *GATA3*) that occurred at > 10% incidence across all breast cancers; however, there were numerous subtype-associated and novel gene mutations, including the enrichment of specific mutations in *GATA3*, *PIK3CA* and *MAP3K1* with the luminal A subtype. They also identified two novel protein-expression-defined subgroups, possibly produced by stromal/microenvironmental elements, and integrated analyses identified specific signalling pathways dominant in each molecular subtype, including a *HER2*/phosphorylated *HER2*/*EGFR*/phosphorylated *EGFR* signature within the *HER2*-enriched expression subtype. Comparison of basal-like breast tumours with high-grade serous ovarian tumours showed many molecular commonalities, indicating a related aetiology and similar therapeutic opportunities. The biological finding of the four main breast cancer subtypes caused by different subsets of genetic and epigenetic abnormalities raises the hypothesis that much of the clinically observable plasticity (ability to change phenotype and adapt, for example to become endocrine- or chemo-resistant) and heterogeneity occur within, and not across, these major biological subtypes of breast cancer. This is important in understanding how cancers develop and evolve, which has implications for understanding and treating recurrence and for the identification of new treatment targets.

PAPER DESCRIPTION

- **Objective/Research Question**: To advance the understanding of the genomics underpinning the development of breast cancer by performing detailed molecular analyses of breast tumours and normal tissue using a range of different technologies.

- **Design**: Multifaceted molecular analysis of patients with invasive breast cancer.

- **Sample Size**: Eight hundred and twenty-five patients.

- **Follow-Up**: Median follow-up of 17 months.

- **Inclusion Criteria**: Newly diagnosed invasive breast cancers between 1988 and 2011 undergoing surgical resection.

- **Exclusion Criteria**: Patients who had received prior treatment (chemotherapy or radiotherapy).

- **Intervention or Treatment Received**: Patients diagnosed with invasive breast cancer had specimens taken from tumour and normal tissue, from which RNA and DNA were obtained. These were subject to analysis using one or more genomic assays. These high-throughput assays examine the expression of a range of individual genes associated with breast cancer as well as detect single-nucleotide polymorphisms (SNPs) and epigenetic alterations such as methylation (changes not to the sequence of bases or genetic code, but to molecules bound to the DNA which influence gene expression).

- **Results**: Five hundred and ten tumours were subject to whole-genome sequencing identifying 30,626 somatic mutations. The Mutational Significance in Cancer (MuSiC) package was applied, which identifies mutations responsible for disease processes as distinct to background mutations, with little significance.[1] This identified 35 significantly mutated genes, including most of the previously recognised breast cancer genes as well as several novel mutated genes. Differences were noticed in the types of mutation of a particular gene across different breast cancer subtypes; for example, in basal-like tumours, *TP53* mutations were mostly nonsense or frame shift compared to missense mutations in luminal A and B tumours.

  Analysis of DNA from the normal tissue of 507 patients identified 47 with germline genetic variant mutations representing nine different genes: *ATM, BRCA1, BRCA2, BRIP1, CHEK2, NBN, PTEN, RAD51C* and *TP53*. This supports the theory that approximately 10% of sporadic breast cancers have a strong germline contribution.

  Identifying genomic changes offers the potential for new therapeutic targets. Luminal ER-positive tumours showed a high frequency of mutation in the *PIK3CA* gene; therefore, targeting this activated kinase or downstream signalling may be of potential benefit. Similar findings were reported for the *ATK1* gene. For the *BRCA1* and *BRCA2* gene mutations, poly (ADP-ribose) polymerase (PARP) inhibitors were identified as potential therapeutic targets.

Approximately 20% of breast cancers are *HER2+* which results in a more aggressive phenotype and a worse prognosis. In genomic assessment of patients with *HER2+* tumours, additional somatic mutations were identified including a high frequency of *PIK3CA* (39%), *EGFR* and *HER3* as well as losses of *PTEN* and *INPP4B*. Clinically, *HER2+* tumours are targeted with a combination treatment of pertuzumab and trastuzumab.[2] This study also suggests targeting *HER2–EGFR* as a potential new combined therapeutic target.

EXPERT COMMENTARY BY RACHEL FOSTER AND CLIONA KIRWAN

Paper significance

The use of high-information genetic assays allows a more in-depth understanding of the molecular architecture of breast cancer, including the genetic and epigenetic abnormalities responsible for the clinical differences seen within the four main breast cancer subtypes.

Paper limitations

Due to the time scale when the data were collected (1988–2011), there were changes to guidelines and thresholds during the study period. For example, prior to 2010, there was no universal standard for defining ER positivity, which is now defined as nuclear staining > 1%; therefore, local hospitals used their own thresholds. Similarly, updates to the American Joint Committee on Cancer staging guidelines were made during the study period. Researchers mapped all staging to the seventh edition for standardisation.

In context of the relevant current literature

Hanahan and Weinberg summarised the hallmarks of cancer development into the acquisition of six capabilities: self-sustained growth, insensitivity to anti-growth signals, ability to invade and metastasise, limitless replicative potential, sustained angiogenesis and the ability to evade programmed cell death.[3] Understanding the complex genomic alterations, including changes in DNA methylation and microRNA expression, which underpin tumorigenesis offers potential diagnostic, classification and treatment opportunities.

In 2013, at the St Gallen International Breast Cancer Conference, the classification of breast cancers into four distinct subtypes was agreed: luminal A, luminal B, basal-like and *HER2* overexpression.[4] Differences in clinical outcomes, including survival, between breast cancer subtypes have been well documented.[5] Research has become increasingly focussed on the heterogenicity of tumours within each of the breast cancer subtypes. Up to 80% of basal-like tumours are triple-negative, lacking in overexpression of oestrogen, progesterone and human epidermal growth factor 2 (*HER2*) receptors. These receptors are the target for treatments in luminal breast cancers. Triple-negative breast cancers have traditionally been treated empirically with cytotoxic chemotherapy. An improved understanding of the heterogenicity of triple-negative disease has led to the identification of specific biomarkers including the programmed death ligand-1 (PDL1) which can be targeted with pembrolizumab to improve disease-free survival in advanced triple-negative disease.[6,7]

HER2 overexpression is associated with *HER2* and luminal subtypes of breast cancer.[8] The *HER2* oncogene codes for a transmembrane tyrosine kinase receptor, and complex downstream signalling results in cell proliferation. Tumours with overexpression of *HER2* are associated with a more aggressive phenotype and poorer prognosis.[9] There are several techniques for assessing tumour DNA, RNA or protein to determine *HER2* status, with immunohistochemistry being the most commonly used in the UK. Equivocal results are then further analysed using fluorescent *in situ* hybridisation (FISH). Accurate *HER2* testing is needed for targeted treatments such as trastuzumab and lapatinib. Prospective trials have identified biomarkers of trastuzumab resistance which may be useful for predicting clinical outcomes.[10]

Triple-negative, *BRCA*-positive breast cancers traditionally had limited adjuvant treatment options beyond standard chemotherapy. The PARP inhibitor olaparib has been shown to reduce breast cancer recurrence and prevent progression to metastatic disease when given in the adjuvant setting for early *BRCA1* and *BRCA2* mutant breast cancers.[11] *BRCA1* and *BRCA2* tumour suppressor genes play a key role in homologous recombination which is required for the repair of DNA double-strand breaks. Olaparib can target *BRCA* mutant cells, causing cell death.

Conclusions

Whole-genome sequencing of breast cancers has increased our understanding of the heterogenicity of breast tumours between different subgroups and within each subgroup, offering the potential for research into new therapeutic targets.

REFERENCES

1. Dees ND, Zhang Q, Kandoth C, Wendl MC, Schierding W, Koboldt DC, et al. MuSiC: identifying mutational significance in cancer genomes. *Genome Res.* 2012;22(8):1589–98.

2. Baselga J, Cortés J, Kim S-B, Im S-A, Hegg R, Im Y-H, et al. Pertuzumab plus Trastuzumab plus Docetaxel for Metastatic Breast Cancer. *New Engl J Med*. 2011;366(2):109–19.
3. Hanahan D, Weinberg RA. The Hallmarks of Cancer. *Cell*. 2000;100(1):57–70.
4. Goldhirsch A, Winer EP, Coates AS, Gelber RD, Piccart-Gebhart M, Thürlimann B, et al. Personalizing the treatment of women with early breast cancer: highlights of the St Gallen International Expert Consensus on the Primary Therapy of Early Breast Cancer 2013. *Ann Oncol*. 2013;24(9):2206–23.
5. Sørlie T, Perou CM, Tibshirani R, Aas T, Geisler S, Johnsen H, et al. Gene expression patterns of breast carcinomas distinguish tumor subclasses with clinical implications. *Proc Natl Acad Sci USA*. 2001;98(19):10869–74.
6. Lehmann BD, Bauer JA, Chen X, Sanders ME, Chakravarthy AB, Shyr Y, et al. Identification of human triple-negative breast cancer subtypes and preclinical models for selection of targeted therapies. *J Clin Invest*. 2011;121(7):2750–67.
7. Schmid P, Cortes J, Pusztai L, McArthur H, Kümmel S, Bergh J, et al. Pembrolizumab for early triple-negative breast cancer. *New Engl J Med*. 2020;382(9):810–21.
8. Perou CM, Sørlie T, Eisen MB, van de Rijn M, Jeffrey SS, Rees CA, et al. Molecular portraits of human breast tumours. *Nature*. 2000;406(6797):747–52.
9. Ross JS, Slodkowska EA, Symmans WF, Pusztai L, Ravdin PM, Hortobagyi GN. The HER-2 receptor and breast cancer: ten years of targeted anti-HER-2 therapy and personalized medicine. *Oncologist*. 2009;14(4):320–68.
10. Musolino A, Naldi N, Bortesi B, Pezzuolo D, Capelletti M, Missale G, et al. Immunoglobulin G fragment C receptor polymorphisms and clinical efficacy of trastuzumab-based therapy in patients with HER-2/neu-positive metastatic breast cancer. *J Clin Oncol*. 2008;26(11):1789–96.
11. Tutt ANJ, Garber JE, Kaufman B, Viale G, Fumagalli D, Rastogi P, et al. Adjuvant olaparib for patients with BRCA1- or BRCA2-mutated breast cancer. *New Engl J Med*. 2021;384(25):2394–405.

70-Gene Signature as an Aid to Treatment Decisions in Early-Stage Breast Cancer

Cardoso F, van't Veer LJ, Bogaerts J, et al. for the MINDACT Investigators.
N Engl J Med 375(8):717–729, 2016

The MammaPrint test is a gene array containing 70 different genes which can improve prediction of breast cancer outcomes in early-stage disease.

PAPER DESCRIPTION

- **Objective/Research Question**: To assess the degree of concordance between clinical risk (calculated using Adjuvant! Online) and genomic risk (calculated using MammaPrint). When a discordance between risk scores is identified, the study aimed to assess which method was best in predicting benefit from adjuvant chemotherapy. The study was powered to determine if adjuvant chemotherapy can be safely omitted in a subgroup of clinically high-risk, genomically low-risk patients, as determined by distal metastasis-free survival (DMFS) at 5 years.

- **Design**: International, prospective, randomised, Phase III non-inferiority study. The primary test group were patients who had discordance between the clinical and genomic risk assessment scores.

- **Sample Size**: A total of 6,693 patients were enrolled in the study between 2007 and 2011. Two thousand one hundred and forty-two patients were identified as having discordance between their clinical and genomic risk assessment and were randomised to receive adjuvant chemotherapy or not. One thousand four hundred and ninety-seven (22.4%) of the patients enrolled in the study were clinically high risk and genomically low risk.

- **Follow-Up**: Five-year follow-up period.

- **Inclusion Criteria**:
  1. Age between 18 and 70 years at the time of randomisation
  2. Primary unilateral invasive breast cancer: T1, T2, or T3 and operable
  3. Surgery to include breast-conserving surgery (with adjuvant radiotherapy) or mastectomy, with sentinel lymph node biopsy (SLNB) or axillary node clearance (ANC)
  4. World Health Organization (WHO) performance status of 0 or 1

- **Exclusion Criteria**:
  1. Previous or concurrent cancer
  2. Previous chemotherapy, radiotherapy or hormonal therapy

- **Intervention or Treatment Received**: Women with early-stage breast cancer had a clinical recurrence score calculated using Adjuvant! Online (which is no longer available, making study comparisons difficult) and a genomic risk assessment using MammaPrint, a 70-gene assay. Patients with concordant low-risk results had chemotherapy omitted, and patients with concordant high-risk results were given chemotherapy. The primary test group were patients with discordant clinical and genomic risk outcomes; they were centrally randomised to receive chemotherapy or not. Randomisation was stratified for institution, risk group, hormone receptor status, age (< 50 vs. ≥ 50 years), *HER2* status, type of axillary surgery (SLNB vs. ANC) and type of surgery (mastectomy vs. breast conservation surgery). The primary aim was to determine the non-inferiority of no chemotherapy in the high-clinical-risk/low-genomic-risk subgroup.

- **Results**: Adjuvant! Online stratified patients into clinically high- and low-risk groups with an approximately equal divide. Genomic risk assessment using MammaPrint identified 64% of patients as being low risk and the remaining 36% as high risk. Concordance between clinical and genomic results was seen in 68% of all patients, but it was more likely for low-risk than high-risk patients. Twenty-three percent of all patients had a high clinical risk and low genomic risk ($n = 1,550$). Randomisation of this subgroup to either receive chemotherapy or not resulted in a DMFS rate of 95.9% versus 94.4%, respectively ($p = 0.27$). The lack of a statistically significant difference between patients in the clinically high-risk, genomically low-risk subgroup who did and did not receive chemotherapy supports the hypothesis that MammaPrint low-risk patients can safely be spared adjuvant chemotherapy even in the presence of high-clinical-risk factors.

  Almost half (48%) of patients in the primary test group were node-positive (1–3 nodes), but there was no statistically significant difference in DMFS at 5 years between patients who did and did not receive adjuvant chemotherapy (96.3% vs. 95.6%, $p = 0.72$). This suggests that genomically low-risk patients with 1–3 positive nodes can safely avoid chemotherapy, even in the presence of high-clinical-risk factors.

  Overall, using the MammaPrint genomic risk score to guide adjuvant chemotherapy decisions allowed 46% of clinically high-risk patients to safely avoid chemotherapy. This allows a large number of patients to avoid the morbidity associated with chemotherapy, as well as the potential health economic implications.

EXPERT COMMENTARY BY CLIONA KIRWAN AND RACHEL FOSTER

Paper significance

This study provides strong evidence to support the clinical use of the 70-gene assay MammaPrint in early hormone receptor–positive, *HER2*-negative, N0/N1 breast cancer to guide adjuvant chemotherapy decisions. This has the potential to reduce overtreatment of genomically low-risk patients and, in doing so, reduce significant short- and long-term health sequelae of chemotherapy and associated healthcare costs.

Paper limitations

Whilst the study effectively demonstrated that a low-risk MammaPrint score predicted no significant benefit from adjuvant chemotherapy, a high-risk MammaPrint score is not able to predict a benefit from adjuvant chemotherapy. For this to occur, all patients enrolled in the study with a high-risk genomic score would require randomisation to chemotherapy or no chemotherapy, which would be ethically unacceptable.

The study population included a small subset of 645 patients who were *HER2*-positive, of which 176 (27.3%) had no chemotherapy and 469 (72.7%) had chemotherapy. These numbers are relatively small but contribute to the overall data pool.

The benefits of chemotherapy are seen early; however, the risk of local or distal disease recurrence persists beyond the 5-year follow-up period, and longer-term data are required for full assessment.

The node-positive group represented only 20.9% of the overall patients in the study; of these, 801 patients had one positive node, and 405 patients had two or three positive nodes. In the study, micro-metastases were counted in the node-positive group whilst isolated tumour cells were considered node-negative; this differs with UK clinical practice, where micro-metastases are considered to be node-negative from a surgical perspective but impact on chemotherapy decision making. The numbers of positive nodes (macro-metastasis) therefore represent only a small number of patients in the study, making interpretation of the results of this subgroup more difficult.

Only 20 patients (1.3%) in the study were aged 35 or younger with a high clinical and low genomic risk; therefore, extrapolating the results of the study to younger patients is more difficult. Further work needs to be undertaken to assess this population in more detail and with larger numbers.

In context of the relevant current literature

Investigators at the Netherlands Cancer Institute published evidence to support the use of MammaPrint DNA microarray analysis to predict the risk of distal metastasis in a well-defined subset of breast cancer patients.[1] This was independently validated in two further large cohort studies published in 2006 and 2009, respectively.[2,3] Analysis of the 70 genes incorporated into the MammaPrint assay has led to an improved understanding of the evolution of breast cancer, including the metastatic process.[4]

The use of adjuvant chemotherapy in early breast cancer is based on estimates of the likelihood of disease recurrence or distal metastasis. Factors such as patient age, menopause status, tumour size and grade, hormone receptor status and human epidermal growth factor receptor 2 (*HER2*) have been used to estimate the risk of recurrence. Several prognostic calculation tools including the Nottingham Prognostic Index (NPI), PREDICT and Adjuvant! Online have become incorporated into clinical practice and are used to guide decisions around adjuvant therapy. As chemotherapy is associated with significant short- and long-term morbidity, identifying patients who can safely avoid chemotherapy prevents overtreatment and reduces chemotherapy-associated healthcare costs.

Studies have linked specific gene alterations with clinical outcomes and response to treatment. One example of this is the *HER2* oncogene, which codes for a transmembrane growth factor receptor associated with a poor clinical outcome but strong response to chemotherapy.[5,6] Sørlie and Perou's work led to the identification of five intrinsic molecular subtypes of invasive breast cancer: luminal A, luminal B, luminal B–like, *HER2*-enriched and basal-like.[7] This work led to the development of commercially available multigene prognostic assessment tools including Oncotype Dx, MammaPrint, Prosigna and Endopredict. A range of genes, including those involved in regulation of the cell cycle, invasion and angiogenesis, are assessed.[1] Use of these tests is more powerful at predicting recurrence than standard clinical and pathological factors.[8]

MammaPrint assesses the expression of 70 genes, the highest number of any test currently available. It is calculated independently of clinical or pathological factors. A simple binary classification system of low or high risk for recurrence is generated. Several prospective studies measured the impact of the 70-gene assay on decision making regarding adjuvant treatment in early breast cancer patients.[9-11] The MINDACT study provides high-level evidence to support the use of the 70-gene assay in early hormone receptor–positive breast cancer to guide adjuvant chemotherapy decisions. Similarly, the TAILORx (Trial Assigning Individualized Options for Treatment [Rx]) trial supported the use of the 21-gene assay Oncotype Dx to predict disease recurrence and benefit from chemotherapy in a similar study population.[12]

Clinicians' confidence in decision making regarding adjuvant chemotherapy is significantly improved with the use of multigene assays in clinical practice.[10,11] The IMPACt study showed a 60% reduction in the number of genomically low-risk patients subsequently being recommended adjuvant therapy.[11] Furthermore, adjuvant treatment recommendations for intermediate-risk patients based on Oncotype Dx testing were changed in approximately a third of cases (33.6%) following the addition of the 70-gene assay MammaPrint.[13] Newer generation prognostic tests which incorporate genomic, clinical and pathological factors have since been developed including Endopredict and Prosigna.

Conclusions

The 70-gene signature MammaPrint was the first genomic assay to be validated in a randomised trial, assigning a low- or high-risk score for the development of distant metastasis in early node-negative or node-positive (1–3 nodes) breast cancer. Clinically it has been proven to be of benefit in identifying patients who traditionally would have been offered chemotherapy based on clinical risk but who can safely avoid chemotherapy.

REFERENCES

1. van't Veer LJ, Dai H, van de Vijver MJ, He YD, Hart AA, Mao M, et al. Gene expression profiling predicts clinical outcome of breast cancer. *Nature*. 2002;415(6871):530–6.
2. Buyse M, Loi S, van't Veer L, Viale G, Delorenzi M, Glas AM, et al. Validation and clinical utility of a 70-gene prognostic signature for women with node-negative breast cancer. *J Natl Cancer Inst*. 2006;98(17):1183–92.
3. Bueno-de-Mesquita JM, Linn SC, Keijzer R, Wesseling J, Nuyten DS, van Krimpen C, et al. Validation of 70-gene prognosis signature in node-negative breast cancer. *Breast Cancer Res Treat*. 2009;117(3):483–95.
4. Tian S, Roepman P, Van't Veer LJ, Bernards R, de Snoo F, Glas AM. Biological functions of the genes in the mammaprint breast cancer profile reflect the hallmarks of cancer. *Biomark Insights*. 2010;5:129–38.
5. Ciocca DR, Fujimura FK, Tandon AK, Clark GM, Mark C, Lee-Chen G-J, et al. Correlation of HER-2/neu amplification with expression and with other prognostic factors in 1103 breast cancers. *J Natl Cancer Inst*. 1992;84(16):1279–82.
6. Tandon AK, Clark GM, Chamness GC, Ullrich A, McGuire WL. HER-2/neu oncogene protein and prognosis in breast cancer. *J Clin Oncol*. 1989;7(8):1120–8.
7. Sørlie T, Perou CM, Tibshirani R, Aas T, Geisler S, Johnsen H, et al. Gene expression patterns of breast carcinomas distinguish tumor subclasses with clinical implications. *Proc Natl Acad Sci USA*. 2001;98(19):10869–74.
8. van de Vijver MJ, He YD, van't Veer LJ, Dai H, Hart AA, Voskuil DW, et al. A gene-expression signature as a predictor of survival in breast cancer. *N Engl J Med*. 2002;347(25):1999–2009.
9. Wuerstlein R, Kates R, Gluz O, Grischke EM, Schem C, Thill M, et al. Strong impact of MammaPrint and BluePrint on treatment decisions in luminal early breast cancer: results of the WSG-PRIMe study. *Breast Cancer Res Treat*. 2019;175(2):389–99.

10. Drukker CA, Bueno-de-Mesquita JM, Retèl VP, van Harten WH, van Tinteren H, Wesseling J, et al. A prospective evaluation of a breast cancer prognosis signature in the observational RASTER study. *Int J Cancer*. 2013;133(4):929–36.
11. Soliman H, Shah V, Srkalovic G, Mahtani R, Levine E, Mavromatis B, et al. MammaPrint guides treatment decisions in breast cancer: results of the IMPACt trial. *BMC Cancer*. 2020;20(1):81.
12. Sparano JA, Gray RJ, Ravdin PM, Makower DF, Pritchard KI, Albain KS, et al. Clinical and genomic risk to guide the use of adjuvant therapy for breast cancer. *New Engl J Med*. 2019;380(25):2395–405.
13. Tsai M, Lo S, Audeh W, Qamar R, Budway R, Levine E, et al. Association of 70-gene signature assay findings with physicians' treatment guidance for patients with early breast cancer classified as intermediate risk by the 21-gene assay. *JAMA Oncol*. 2018;4(1):e173470.

CHAPTER 23

21-Gene Assay to Inform Chemotherapy Benefit in Node-Positive Breast Cancer (RxPonder)

Kalinsky K, Barlow WE, Gralow JR, et al.
New Engl J Med 385:2336–2347, 2021

PAPER DESCRIPTION

- **Objective/Research Question**: To assess the effect of chemotherapy on invasive disease–free survival (IDFS) in women with 1–3 node-positive, hormone receptor–positive, *HER2*-negative, invasive breast cancer. It also looked to establish if a relationship exists between a higher recurrence score (RS) and increased benefit from chemotherapy.

- **Design**: Phase III randomised controlled trial.

- **Sample Size**: Five thousand and eighty-three women underwent randomisation, and 5,018 participated in the trial.

- **Follow-Up**: Fifteen years.

- **Inclusion Criteria**:
  1. Female and over 18 years of age
  2. Positive oestrogen +/– progesterone receptors
  3. *HER2*-negative
  4. 1–3 nodes positive following sentinel lymph node biopsy (SLNB) or axillary node clearance (ANC)
  5. Had breast-conserving surgery (with clear margins) and planned for radiotherapy or mastectomy
  6. Able to receive taxane- and/or anthracycline-based chemotherapy
  7. Has not had an aromatase inhibitor or tamoxifen within 5 years

- **Exclusion Criteria**:
  1. Inflammatory or metastatic breast cancer
  2. Underwent chemotherapy prior to study registration
  3. Requires chronic treatment with systemic steroids or immune suppressants
  4. Male breast cancer patients

DOI: 10.1201/b23352-23

- **Intervention or Treatment Received**: Patients were randomised to either chemotherapy and endocrine therapy or endocrine therapy alone. Approved endocrine therapies for pre- and postmenopausal women were specified (tamoxifen, ovarian suppression or ablation, aromatase inhibitor). Endocrine treatment was given for a minimum of 5 years but could be extended, and switching from one therapy to another was allowed. Patients were stratified for RS (0–13 vs. 14–25), menopause status (premenopausal versus postmenopausal) and type of nodal surgery (ANC vs. SLNB).

- **Results**: Two thousand three hundred and fifty-three women were randomised to the endocrine therapy–only arm, and 2,085 women to chemo-endocrine therapy. It had been hypothesised that the RS would be predictive of response to adjuvant chemotherapy. However, for women with a RS of 0–25, the RS value did not significantly predict a benefit from chemotherapy in terms of IDFS. The RS was found to be independently prognostic, with a lower RS being associated with a longer invasive disease–free survival independently of menopause status.

  Chemotherapy benefit to IDFS differed between pre- and postmenopausal women. In postmenopausal women (67%), there was no statistically significant difference in IDFS at 5 years regardless of whether they received chemotherapy or not (91.3% vs. 91.9%). In contrast, premenopausal women who received chemotherapy had a relative increase in IDFS of 40% and a relative increase in distant relapse-free survival (DRFS) of 42%. This benefit was independent of RS.

  Subgroup analysis did not demonstrate a significant benefit of chemotherapy for postmenopausal women who had axillary node dissection compared to sentinel node biopsy. Furthermore, there was no benefit seen for chemotherapy based on the number of involved nodes (1 vs. 2 vs. 3). In contrast, in premenopausal women, chemotherapy was beneficial to patients undergoing axillary node dissection but not women having sentinel node biopsy. A slight benefit was seen in premenopausal women receiving chemotherapy in the node-positive subgroup for one node but not for two or three nodes.

  The number of recorded adverse events in the chemo-endocrine group totalled 1,336 and 717 for post- and premenopausal women, respectively. In the endocrine-only treatment group, the number of adverse events totalled 1,577 and 751 in the post- and premenopausal subgroups.

EXPERT COMMENTARY BY CLIONA KIRWAN AND RACHEL FOSTER

Paper significance

Postmenopausal, but not premenopausal, women with hormone receptor–positive, *HER2*-negative, 1–3 node-positive breast cancer with a RS between 0 and

25 can safely avoid the use of adjuvant chemotherapy, as it does not offer additional benefit beyond taking endocrine therapy in this group of patients.

Paper limitations

It remains unclear in this study if the benefit of chemotherapy in premenopausal women is due to its direct cytotoxic effects on cancer cells or its effect on inducing menopause, which could also be achieved by using ovarian suppression. The addition of ovarian suppression to standard endocrine treatment in premenopausal women was shown to improve disease-free survival in the Suppression of Ovarian Function Trial (SOFT) and the Tamoxifen and Exemestane Trial (TEXT).[1] A randomised controlled trial would be required to compare endocrine therapy and ovarian function suppression against endocrine therapy and chemotherapy.

The follow-up period in the study was limited to 5 years; this relatively short follow-up period was addressed in the study, referencing previous meta-analysis data which demonstrated the maximum benefit of chemotherapy occurring mainly within the first 5 years.[2] However, reviewing longer-term follow-up data would be useful.

In context of the relevant current literature

Women with early breast cancer are offered a range of adjuvant treatments following surgery including endocrine therapy, chemotherapy and targeted therapies with the aim of reducing local and distal disease recurrence. Several tools have been developed based on clinical and histological factors, such as tumour size and grade as well as hormone receptor and nodal status, to predict prognosis and guide adjuvant treatments. These include the Nottingham Prognostic Index (NPI),[3] PREDICT Plus[4] and Adjuvant! Online.[5] Women who are identified as being at intermediate risk have a less clear benefit from adjuvant chemotherapy.

Several multigene expression tumour-profiling tests are commercially available to facilitate treatment decisions based on individual tumour biology. These tests include Oncotype Dx,[6] Prosigna[7] and MammaPrint,[8] which assess a combination of different genes to assign an individual tumour RS. The Translational Arm of the Arimidex, Tamoxifen, Alone or in Combination (TransATAC) study demonstrated that RSs can be used to predict distant disease recurrence for hormone receptor–positive, node-positive or -negative breast cancer.[9] Retrospective studies demonstrated that patients with a high RS (> 31) had a benefit from adjuvant chemotherapy.[10,11] The number of patients with early breast cancer requiring adjuvant chemotherapy can be reduced by up to 85% by using multigene assays, avoiding overtreatment and sparing patients the side effects of cytotoxic chemotherapy.

The Trial Assigning Individualized Options for Treatment (TAILORx) validated the use of the 21-gene RS generated by Oncotype Dx for node-negative, hormone receptor–positive, early breast cancer. It classifies patients as being at low, intermediate, or high risk of disease recurrence.

Women with a low RS (< 11) could be safely treated with hormone therapy alone; women with a high RS (> 25) benefited from both chemotherapy and endocrine therapy. For women with a RS of 11–25, having endocrine therapy alone was not inferior to having chemo-endocrine therapy.[12] Some chemotherapy benefit was seen for women aged 50 years or younger.

RxPONDER went on to assess Oncotype Dx–calculated RSs in a similar population of women with node-positive (1–3 nodes) early breast cancer. The findings are concordant with TAILORx regarding the benefits of chemotherapy for premenopausal women and not postmenopausal women with mid-range RSs. Similarly, the MINDACT multicentre, randomised, Phase III trial concluded that patients with a high clinical risk such as node positivity, but low genomic risk assessed using the MammaPrint 70-gene assay, had an excellent distal disease-free survival rate when given endocrine therapy alone.[8]

Both the TAILORx and MINDACT studies reported a correlation between higher RS and increased benefit of adjuvant chemotherapy; however, this was not found in the RxPONDER trial.

Conclusions

The RxPONDER trial validated the use of the 21-gene Oncotype Dx RS to inform adjuvant systemic therapy recommendations for patients with hormone receptor–positive, *HER2*-negative breast cancer. Postmenopausal women with a RS < 25 may safely avoid chemotherapy. Conversely, premenopausal women with the same tumour characteristics gain significant benefit from adjuvant chemotherapy. A RS of 0–25 was identified as being of prognostic value for both pre- and postmenopausal women. It was anticipated that a higher RS would predict increased benefit from chemotherapy; however, this was not demonstrated in the study. Furthermore, the study did not address the mechanism by which chemotherapy benefits premenopausal women; this could be due directly to its cytotoxic effects or due to ovarian suppression.

REFERENCES

1. Francis PA, Pagani O, Fleming GF, Walley BA, Colleoni M, Láng I, et al. Tailoring adjuvant endocrine therapy for premenopausal breast cancer. *New Engl J Med.* 2018;379(2):122–37.
2. Peto R, Davies C, Godwin J, Gray R, Pan HC, Clarke M, et al. Comparisons between different polychemotherapy regimens for early breast cancer: meta-analyses of long-term outcome among 100,000 women in 123 randomised trials. *Lancet.* 2012;379(9814):432–44.

3. Haybittle JL, Blamey RW, Elston CW, Johnson J, Doyle PJ, Campbell FC, et al. A prognostic index in primary breast cancer. *Br J Cancer*. 1982;45(3):361–6.
4. Wishart GC, Bajdik CD, Dicks E, Provenzano E, Schmidt MK, Sherman M, et al. PREDICT Plus: development and validation of a prognostic model for early breast cancer that includes HER2. *Br J Cancer*. 2012;107(5):800–7.
5. Ravdin PM, Siminoff LA, Davis GJ, Mercer MB, Hewlett J, Gerson N, et al. Computer program to assist in making decisions about adjuvant therapy for women with early breast cancer. *J Clin Oncol*. 2001;19(4):980–91.
6. Kalinsky K, Barlow WE, Gralow JR, Meric-Bernstam F, Albain KS, Hayes DF, et al. 21-gene assay to inform chemotherapy benefit in node-positive breast cancer. *New Engl J Med*. 2021;385(25):2336–47.
7. Wallden B, Storhoff J, Nielsen T, Dowidar N, Schaper C, Ferree S, et al. Development and verification of the PAM50-based Prosigna breast cancer gene signature assay. *BMC Med Genomics*. 2015;8(1):54.
8. Cardoso F, van't Veer LJ, Bogaerts J, Slaets L, Viale G, Delaloge S, et al. 70-gene signature as an aid to treatment decisions in early-stage breast cancer. *N Engl J Med*. 2016;375(8):717–29.
9. Dowsett M, Cuzick J, Wale C, Forbes J, Mallon EA, Salter J, et al. Prediction of risk of distant recurrence using the 21-gene recurrence score in node-negative and node-positive postmenopausal patients with breast cancer treated with anastrozole or tamoxifen: a TransATAC study. *J Clin Oncol*. 2010;28(11):1829–34.
10. Paik S, Tang G, Shak S, Kim C, Baker J, Kim W, et al. Gene expression and benefit of chemotherapy in women with node-negative, estrogen receptor-positive breast cancer. *J Clin Oncol*. 2006;24(23):3726–34.
11. Albain KS, Barlow WE, Shak S, Hortobagyi GN, Livingston RB, Yeh IT, et al. Prognostic and predictive value of the 21-gene recurrence score assay in postmenopausal women with node-positive, oestrogen-receptor-positive breast cancer on chemotherapy: a retrospective analysis of a randomised trial. *Lancet Oncol*. 2010;11(1):55–65.
12. Sparano JA, Gray RJ, Makower DF, Pritchard KI, Albain KS, Hayes DF, et al. Adjuvant chemotherapy guided by a 21-gene expression assay in breast cancer. *New Engl J Med*. 2018;379(2):111–21.

PREDICT: A New UK Prognostic Model That Predicts Survival Following Surgery for Invasive Breast Cancer

Wishart GC, Azzato EM, Greenberg DC, et al.
Breast Cancer Res 12:R1–R10, 2010

PAPER DESCRIPTION

- **Objective/Research Question**: To validate the use of PREDICT, a breast cancer prognostication tool for use in early breast cancer to predict overall and breast cancer–specific survival for women treated for breast cancer in the UK.

- **Design**: Data were collected from women treated for invasive breast cancer in East Anglia between 1999 and 2003, and they were followed up for a period of up to 8 years. These data were used to develop the PREDICT model, which was then validated on patient data from a second UK cancer registry.

- **Sample Size**: Cancer registration data from 5,694 women with breast cancer (Eastern Cancer Registration and Information Centre [ECRIC]) were used to develop PREDICT. Data from a further cohort of 5,468 women in a different UK region (West Midlands Cancer Intelligence Unit [WMCIU]) were used to validate the PREDICT tool.

- **Follow-Up**: Median length of follow-up was 5.6 years, with a maximum of 8 years follow-up.

- **Inclusion Criteria**: The test dataset included all female breast cancer cases that were treated surgically for invasive breast cancer as identified on the ECRIC database between 1999 and 2003. The validation dataset comprised women with invasive breast cancer diagnosed between 1999 and 2003 within the boundaries of the WMCIU.

- **Exclusion Criteria:**
  1. No surgery or incomplete local therapy (e.g., breast-conserving surgery without radiotherapy)

DOI: 10.1201/b23352-24

2. Patients with fewer than four nodes excised with a diagnosis of node-negative disease
3. Ductal carcinoma *in situ* (DCIS) or lobular carcinoma *in situ* (LCIS) only

- **Intervention or Treatment Received**: Data obtained from the ECRIC database were used to develop prognostic models for oestrogen receptor–positive and oestrogen receptor–negative cancers. Prognostic factors included in the models were the number of positive nodes (0, 1, 2–4, 5–9 or 10+), tumour size (mm), tumour grade (low, intermediate or high), detection by screening, chemotherapy and hormone therapy use. Breast cancer–specific mortality was modelled independently to all other causes of mortality. A second UK dataset (WMCIU) was used to validate the PREDICT models.

- **Results**: The PREDICT model was developed using data from over 5,000 patients (ECRIC); this was then validated against another large dataset of UK breast cancer patients (WMCIU). Overall, this validated model worked well, with a high degree of discrimination.

  Data from both ECRIC and WMCIU showed a tendency for the model to overpredict mortality. The ECRIC data showed a difference between actual and predicted survival of less than 1% at 5 and 8 years, compared to the WMCIU data which showed a 2% difference.

  ECRIC data showed that at 5 years, actual deaths were 841 and predicted deaths were 890 (14.8% vs. 15.6%, $p = 0.10$). Similarly, at 8 years, actual deaths were 1,075 and predicted deaths were 1,082 (18.9% vs. 19.0%, $p = 0.83$). The validated WMCIU dataset showed that at 5 years, actual deaths were 862 and predicted deaths were 950 (15.8 vs. 17.4%, $p = 0.004$). At 8 years, actual deaths were 955 and predicted were 1,006 (17.5% vs. 18.4%, $p = 0.11$).

  The model fit was noted to be less accurate for some subgroups of women, including those younger than 35 years with oestrogen receptor–positive disease. Similarly, a less good fit was achieved for women with oestrogen receptor–negative disease with negative nodes, a tumour of 30–49 mm in size and of high grade.

EXPERT COMMENTARY BY RACHEL FOSTER AND CLIONA KIRWAN

Paper significance

This study validated the use of the PREDICT model (https://breast.predict.nhs.uk) based on a UK population for clinical use in early breast cancer to guide decisions regarding adjuvant treatments.

Paper limitations

The ECRIC data were collected from 5,694 women from over 10 UK hospitals including two teaching hospitals with high engagement in research. These real-world data are likely to be representative of UK practice as a whole. It was independently validated on another large dataset of over 5,468 patients showing reproducibility in its accuracy.

For certain subgroups of patients in the study, the PREDICT model was found to be less accurate. In data from both the ECRIC and WMCIU, predicted mortality was found to be lower than observed mortality for women older than 75. A study was performed in the Netherlands looking at PREDICT in a cohort of 2,012 older women (median age = 75 years), which identified that 5-year predicted survival was accurate but that 10-year survival tended to be overestimated.[1]

The ECRIC dataset included 111 women younger than 35 years, and for those with oestrogen receptor–positive disease, predicted survival was found to be less accurate. The UK POSH (Prospective Outcomes in Sporadic versus Hereditary Breast Cancer) study investigated this further and found that whilst PREDICT is a useful tool for providing 10-year overall survival estimates for younger patients, it is less accurate regarding short-term recurrence risk.[2]

Another subgroup of patients who need further consideration and research are patients receiving neoadjuvant chemotherapy. Evidence has shown that PREDICT overestimates survival in this group of patients.[3]

Therefore, a degree of caution needs to be used when interpreting the results of PREDICT in patients at the extremes of age, and those having neoadjuvant chemotherapy; in these subgroups of patients, further research with larger numbers of patients is required.

In context of the relevant current literature

A range of prognostic tools have been developed to guide clinician decision making about adjuvant treatments, including chemotherapy, to ensure it is offered to those who are likely to gain a significant benefit and avoid systemic toxicity for those who are unlikely to benefit.

In 1982, the Nottingham Prognostic Index (NPI) was developed by Galea and colleagues using a retrospective multivariate study which incorporated simple clinical data including lymph node stage, tumour size and pathological grade to predict prognosis.[4] Initially, patients were divided into three prognostic subgroups based on predicted 10-year survival rates. This has since been redefined into four groups (excellent, good, moderate and poor). The use of the NPI has been validated in multiple different patient populations including a recent long-term follow-up study of over 9,000 patients.[5]

Since the introduction of the NPI, a range of more complex web-based prognostic models have been developed internationally. A recent systematic review identified 58 different prognostic models for breast cancer.[6] Online prognostic tools can enhance shared decision making between patients and clinicians about adjuvant treatment options. Adjuvant! Online, an internet-based prediction model, was introduced in 2001 and was based on data collected from the US Surveillance, Epidemiology and End Results (SEER) registry.[7] It calculates prognosis using patient age, menopause status, comorbidity, tumour stage, number of nodes and oestrogen receptor status. In contrast, PREDICT is based on UK cancer registry data. In addition to the standard tumour characteristics, PREDICT incorporates *HER2*[8] and Ki67[9] status, as well as the method of cancer detection (screen-detected vs. symptomatic), which improves its performance. More recently it began to incorporate extended endocrine treatment into its prognostic model, following the publication of the ATLAS (Adjuvant Tamoxifen: Longer against Shorter) and aTTom (Adjuvant Tamoxifen—To Offer More?) trials. The PREDICT model has now been validated in multiple studies in both UK and international populations.[1,3,9–11]

For patients found to be at intermediate risk of disease recurrence using NPI or PREDICT, a range of commercially available genomic assay tests have been developed to further guide adjuvant treatment decision making. Three genomic assay tests (Endopredict, Oncotype Dx and Prosigna) are currently approved by the National Institute for Health and Care Excellence (NICE) to guide adjuvant chemotherapy decision making for patients with hormone receptor–positive, *HER2*-negative early breast cancer when found to have an intermediate risk of distant recurrence using a validated tool (PREDICT or NPI).

Conclusions

PREDICT is an online prognostication tool which was developed using data from women in the UK and has been validated on a second UK patient cohort. The tool is largely accurate but with limitations in some subgroups, particularly for older and younger women. The tool is now widely used in clinical practice globally and is regularly updated, most recently with the addition of bisphosphonates to clinical treatment options.

REFERENCES

1. de Glas NA, Bastiaannet E, Engels CC, de Craen AJ, Putter H, van de Velde CJ, et al. Validity of the online PREDICT tool in older patients with breast cancer: a population-based study. *Br J Cancer*. 2016;114(4):395–400.

2. Maishman T, Copson E, Stanton L, Gerty S, Dicks E, Durcan L, et al. An evaluation of the prognostic model PREDICT using the POSH cohort of women aged ≤40 years at breast cancer diagnosis. *Br J Cancer*. 2015;112(6):983–91.

3. Wong HS, Subramaniam S, Alias Z, Taib NA, Ho GF, Ng CH, et al. The predictive accuracy of PREDICT: a personalized decision-making tool for Southeast Asian women with breast cancer. *Medicine*. 2015;94(8):e593.

4. Haybittle JL, Blamey RW, Elston CW, Johnson J, Doyle PJ, Campbell FC, et al. A prognostic index in primary breast cancer. *Br J Cancer*. 1982;45(3):361–6.

5. Balslev I, Axelsson CK, Zedeler K, Rasmussen BB, Carstensen B, Mouridsen HT. The Nottingham Prognostic Index applied to 9,149 patients from the studies of the Danish Breast Cancer Cooperative Group (DBCG). *Breast Cancer Res Treat*. 1994;32(3):281–90.

6. Phung MT, Tin Tin S, Elwood JM. Prognostic models for breast cancer: a systematic review. *BMC Cancer*. 2019;19(1):230.

7. Ravdin PM, Siminoff LA, Davis GJ, Mercer MB, Hewlett J, Gerson N, et al. Computer program to assist in making decisions about adjuvant therapy for women with early breast cancer. *J Clin Oncol*. 2001;19(4):980–91.

8. Wishart GC, Bajdik CD, Dicks E, Provenzano E, Schmidt MK, Sherman M, et al. PREDICT Plus: development and validation of a prognostic model for early breast cancer that includes HER2. *Br J Cancer*. 2012;107(5):800–7.

9. Wishart GC, Rakha E, Green A, Ellis I, Ali HR, Provenzano E, et al. Inclusion of KI67 significantly improves performance of the PREDICT prognostication and prediction model for early breast cancer. *BMC Cancer*. 2014;14:908.

10. Wishart GC, Bajdik CD, Azzato EM, Dicks E, Greenberg DC, Rashbass J, et al. A population-based validation of the prognostic model PREDICT for early breast cancer. *Eur J Surg Oncol*. 2011;37(5):411–7.

11. Engelhardt EG, van den Broek AJ, Linn SC, Wishart GC, Rutgers EJT, van de Velde AO, et al. Accuracy of the online prognostication tools PREDICT and Adjuvant! for early-stage breast cancer patients younger than 50 years. *Eur J Cancer*. 2017;78:37–44.

CHAPTER 25

Genomic Analysis Defines Clonal Relationships of Ductal Carcinoma In Situ *and Recurrent Invasive Breast Cancer*

Lips EH, Kumar T, Megalios A, Visser LL, Sheinman M, Fortunato A, et al.
Grand Challenge PRECISION Consortium. Nature Genet 54:850–860, 2022

Ductal carcinoma *in situ* (DCIS) is often detected during routine mammography and represents 20% of all screen-detected breast cancers. Despite treatment, approximately 5% develop an invasive recurrence and 4% develop a DCIS recurrence over a period of 10 years. Since most DCIS lesions will never progress to invasive disease, there is a need to develop management strategies that avoid overtreatment.

We have limited knowledge on whether invasive recurrences are genetically related to the initial DCIS disease, making accurate evaluation of the risk of progression and the assessment of the prognostic value challenging. To date, this question has been difficult to address, due to the challenges in collecting matched ipsilateral longitudinal samples that are years to decades apart, and the technical challenges in performing genomic assays on archival formalin-fixed paraffin-embedded (FFPE) materials of this age.

PAPER DESCRIPTION

- **Objective/Research Question**: The study explored whether the initial DCIS and subsequent 'recurrence' share a common genetic lineage (i.e., are 'clonally related') or, alternatively, represent genetically independent diseases that emerge from different initiating cells in the same breast.

- **Design**: Multicentre case–control study.

- **Sample Size**: The study used 129 DCIS recurrence pairs.

DOI: 10.1201/b23352-25

- **Inclusion Criteria**: The authors used samples from patients with DCIS who subsequently developed an ipsilateral invasive breast cancer, enrolled in:
  1. *The Sloane project*: A national audit of women with non-invasive neoplasia within the UK National Health Service Breast Screening Programme (NHS BSP);
  2. *The Dutch DCIS cohort study*: A nationwide, population-based patient cohort derived from the Netherlands Cancer Registry; or
  3. *The Duke Hospital cohort.*

- **Exclusion Criteria**: Samples were excluded if:
  1. Only one sample of a pair was available,
  2. DNA quantity was insufficient, or
  3. Quality control analyses for either of the genetic profiling methods failed.

- **Intervention or Treatment Received**: The authors performed extensive genomic characterization of the primary tumour and matched recurrence. They used three profiling methods—whole-exome sequencing (WES), copy number (CN) profiling and targeted sequencing—to determine genomic clonality between the primary DCIS and the recurrent cancer.

  WES is a high-throughput technology that sequences all protein-coding regions of the genome (the exome). The exome represents only 1%–2% of a cell's genome but contains most genetic variants that are known to cause or contribute to disease, including cancers. CN profiling looks for deletions or duplications in DNA segments in the genome which may have a role in tumorigenesis or cancer progression, using either single-nucleotide polymorphism (SNP) arrays or low-pass whole-genome sequencing (lpWGS), a low-depth and therefore more cost-effective form of WGS. Targeted sequencing focuses on specific regions of interest in the genome, increasing coverage and accuracy for those specific regions, thereby compensating for lpWGS.

  The authors developed and used a statistical tool called Breakclone to assess genetic relatedness. The tool factors in the population frequency of different genetic abnormalities, meaning it considers how often specific genetic changes or mutations occur in the general population, not just within the cancer being analysed. This ensures that relevant clonal genetic changes are identified which are key drivers for uncontrolled cell proliferation (cancer), and it reduces background noise and overemphasis of recurrent aberrations that would recur independently in many tumours of a similar type across individuals. Breakclone computes a 'clonal relatedness score' and a p-value based on a permutation test, designating a pair as being either related ($p < 0.05$), ambiguous ($0.05 < p < 0.1$) or unrelated.

Single-cell DNA sequencing (scDNA-seq) was used in a small subset of cases for validation (2,294 cells obtained from four primary and recurrent DCIS tumour pairs). scDNA-seq enables researchers to unravel cellular heterogeneity and sequence rare cell populations.

- **Results**: Of the 129 DCIS recurrence pairs in the study, 95 had developed an ipsilateral invasive (INV) recurrence and 34 had an ipsilateral DCIS recurrence. The median patient age at diagnosis of the primary DCIS was 57 years, and median time to the recurrence was 4 years. Radiotherapy had been received by only 13% (12/95) of cases of primary DCIS that developed an INV recurrence, in contrast to 53% (18/34) of those that recurred as pure DCIS.

  In terms of clonality, 24 DCIS–INV pairs were assessed using WES, 71 DCIS–INV pairs were assessed using CN profiling, and 45 of these 71 underwent targeted sequencing. Combined results for the 95 DCIS–INV pairs showed that 71/95 (75%) were clonally related, 17/95 (18%) unrelated and 7/95 (7%) ambiguous. For the 34 DCIS pairs, which recurred as pure DCIS, 85% were clonally related, 9% unrelated and 6% ambiguous. This suggests that a subset of invasive cancer recurrences in patients who previously had DCIS are in fact independent tumours emerging in the same breast, whereas pure DCIS recurrences are more frequently clonal, likely to represent residual DCIS that was not detected preoperatively or remained *in situ* following surgery. DCIS–DCIS cases in this study also tended to recur earlier than DCIS–INV recurrences (mean 36 vs. 65 months, respectively, $p = 0.0003$). scDNA-seq validated the clonality classification based on tumour bulk DNA sequencing.

  The clonal relatedness in 10 INV recurrences with sufficient adjacent DCIS to the invasive component for separate genetic analysis was also investigated. In all cases, recurrent DCIS was clonally related to the adjacent recurrent INV tumour. However, in 2 out of 10 cases, recurrent INV and DCIS were unrelated to the primary DCIS, which indicates *de novo* tumours arising from new independent DCIS rather than a progression from primary DCIS.

  To estimate population risks of ipsilateral and contralateral INV breast cancer in patients with primary DCIS undergoing wide local excision (WLE) with and without adjuvant radiotherapy, the authors calculated age-standardized incidence ratios (SIRs) using the Dutch Cancer Registry data. Based on their results of clonal relatedness, assuming that 18% of ipsilateral versus 100% of contralateral recurrences were new primaries, the SIR for patients who underwent WLE only was 2.10, and it was 1.85 for patients who underwent WLE and radiotherapy. Both incidence ratios indicate that the rate of *de novo* breast cancer following primary DCIS is significantly increased compared to that of the general population.

In terms of specific genetic changes in the clonally related pairs, most of the genetic changes detected in INV recurrences were already present in the primary DCIS. Similarly, frequency analysis of CN aberrations across all DCIS and INV recurrences showed highly similar chromosomal gains and losses across the patient cohort. This suggests that most CN events and driver mutations had already occurred at the early stages of DCIS progression, many years before the emergence of the invasive disease, and were not associated with invasive recurrence. Nevertheless, there was some evidence that INV recurrences had acquired additional genetic alterations, representing clonal evolution.

In terms of clinical and pathological characteristics, whilst unrelated clonal pairs were more likely to have discordant oestrogen receptor (ER) status and occurred distant to the site of primary DCIS, there was no significant association of clonal relatedness with time to recurrence, age at diagnosis of primary DCIS, radiotherapy, ER and *HER2* receptor status, or grade of primary DCIS.

EXPERT COMMENTARY BY THOMAS SEDDON, PAVNEET S. KOHLI AND TIM RATTAY

Paper significance

Cancers arising in the same breast are often termed 'recurrences', and previous genetic studies of synchronous invasive and *in situ* disease have indicated a similar mutation profile, albeit with a lower number of genetic aberrations, in pure DCIS compared to INV tumours.[1] At the same time, the genetic mechanisms of progression from DCIS to INV tumour are diverse and probably vary from case to case.[2] In contrast, a study of metachronous tumour pairs from the same breast suggested that CN aberrations of primary DCIS and subsequent INV recurrences were in fact not concordant in a significant minority of patients.[3] This larger study confirms that invasive 'recurrences' can arise from both clonally related and unrelated primary DCIS, and a significant minority are likely to be *de novo* cancers.

So, what is the biological explanation for patients to have a clonally different cancer in the same breast over time? One possibility is that the cancer 'field effect' in the breast increases the probability of developing new cancers compared with the general population. Other factors such as lifestyle factors including obesity and alcohol, taking hormone replacement therapy (HRT) and previous radiotherapy may also play a role. Further research is needed into the mechanisms and contributing risk factors for invasive progression.

The finding that nearly one in five ipsilateral INV cancers following DCIS are not clonally related has several clinical implications. Primary DCIS is not just a precursor lesion to invasive cancer, but may also be considered a risk factor for *de novo* breast cancer (akin to lobular carcinoma *in situ* [LCIS]). We may have also overestimated the risk of 'recurrence' from the same population of *in situ* tumour cells, thereby confounding the potential benefit from radiotherapy, as radiation inhibits the growth of already existing cancer cells but might not prevent the emergence of new invasive cells. Along the same lines, the effect of surgery for DCIS in reducing the overall breast cancer risk may be questioned in this subset of patients, and systemic approaches to breast cancer risk reduction such as hormone therapy (see the National Surgical Adjuvant Breast and Bowel Project [NSABP] B-35[4] and IBIS-II DCIS trials[5]) or even immunotherapy[6] may be more important than we thought. Finally, molecular markers or genetic signatures, currently used in the clinic to discriminate high- and low-risk patients with DCIS in order to inform decisions about adjuvant radiotherapy,[7] may be irrelevant for clonally unrelated DCIS or INV recurrences.

Conclusions

DCIS is pre-invasive breast cancer which may harbour invasive disease at presentation and, if left untreated, may develop into invasive cancer. Despite treatment, local recurrence occurs in 5%–10% of DCIS cases and is invasive in 50% of these cases. This paper studies the molecular changes in the parent DCIS and the recurrence to determine if the disease was clonally related or represented new primary disease using genomic analysis. Paired samples of the original DCIS and recurrent tumours from 95 patients were analysed. This demonstrated that in 75% of cases, the recurrence was clonally related to the initial DCIS, suggesting that tumour cells were not eliminated during the initial treatment. A further 18% were clonally unrelated to the DCIS, suggesting new independent lineages, and 7% of cases were ambiguous. These data further our understanding of the biology of DCIS recurrence, risk prediction and the identification of new biomarkers for DCIS.

REFERENCES

1. Bergholtz H, et al. Comparable cancer-relevant mutation profiles in synchronous ductal carcinoma *in situ* and invasive breast cancer. *Cancer Rep*, 2020;3:e1248.
2. Pareja F, et al. Whole-exome sequencing analysis of the progression from non-low-grade ductal carcinoma *in situ* to invasive ductal carcinoma. *Clin Cancer Res.* 2020;26(14):3682–93.
3. Gorringe KL, et al. Copy number analysis of ductal carcinoma *in situ* with and without recurrence. *Mod Pathol.* 2015;28(9):1174–84.
4. Wolmark. Primary results, NSABP B-35/NRG Oncology: a clinical trial of anastrozole vs tamoxifen in postmenopausal patients with DCIS undergoing lumpectomy plus radiotherapy A randomized clinical trial. *Lancet.* 2016;387:849–56.

5. Cuzick J; et al. Use of anastrozole for breast cancer prevention (IBIS-II): long-term results of a randomised controlled trial. *Lancet*. 2020;395(10218):117–22.
6. Glencer AC, et al. Modulation of the immune microenvironment of high-risk ductal carcinoma *in situ* by intralesional pembrolizumab injection. *NPJ Breast Cancer*. 2021;7:59.
7. Ouattara D, et al. Molecular signatures in ductal carcinoma *in situ* (DCIS): a systematic review and meta-analysis. *J Clin Med*. 2023;12(5).

CHAPTER 26

Pathological Features of 11,337 Patients with Primary Ductal Carcinoma In Situ (DCIS) and Subsequent Events: Results from the UK Sloane Project

Shaaban AM, Hilton B, Clements K, Provenzano E, Cheung S, Wallis MG, et al.

Br J Cancer 2021 Mar;124(5):1009–1017

PAPER DESCRIPTION

- **Objective/Research Question**: This study analysed in detail the pathological features of a large prospective cohort of well-characterised screen-detected ductal carcinoma in situ (DCIS), and it mapped the changes in diagnosis and management over time and the development of subsequent ipsilateral, contralateral and distant metastases.

- **Design**: Prospective cohort study of screen-detected DCIS diagnosed during 2003–2012 with detailed follow-up.

- **Sample Size**: A total of 11,337 women, who were a representative one-third of all screen-detected DCIS diagnosed between 2003 and 2012 through the UK National Health Service Breast Screening Programme (NHS BSP).

- **Inclusion Criteria**: All women diagnosed with DCIS through the UK NHS BSP were eligible for prospective voluntary data collection by individual breast-screening units.

- **Exclusion Criteria**: Women who subsequently had the diagnosis upgraded to invasive breast cancer within 6 months, or for whom DCIS was diagnosed symptomatically, were excluded.

- **Results**: The cohort data included demographic, pathology, surgery and adjuvant therapy meticulously annotated and compared over time and with outcomes on national electronic data records. Highlighted changes included an increase in histological size, particularly DCIS over 40 mm; the grade of DCIS also increased over time, with overall 64% high grade.

Women with high-grade DCIS and indeed flat or micropapillary DCIS were more likely to undergo mastectomy. For breast conservation patients, margin involvement (tumour cells at the margin) was only 3%, with a further 3% having disease < 1 mm from the margin and 8% having disease 1–1.9 mm from it. While invasive cancer concomitant with DCIS was excluded, 7% of women had microinvasive disease which was less common over time.

For women diagnosed with a second event after 6 months, in a subset of 9,191 women from England, 12% re-presented with DCIS or developed invasive cancer (two-thirds of recurrences) in the ipsilateral (7%) or contralateral (5%) breast; 46 women (0.5%) developed distant recurrence at a median of 9.2 years. DCIS grade was not associated with the likelihood of recurrence. There was a significantly lower rate of recurrence after breast conservation surgery where a margin of ≥ 2 mm was achieved; for high-grade DCIS, the margin status was particularly significant.

The risk of recurrence of DCIS was about 0.5% per year up to 5 years and then tailed off, while the risk of invasive disease in the same breast was a consistent 0.5% per year to beyond 10 years. The protective effect of radiotherapy halved the rate of recurrence and was seen for both DCIS and invasive breast cancer, and it persisted after excluding the 14% of women who received adjuvant endocrine therapy.

EXPERT COMMENTARY BY STACEY CARTER, ELIZABETH BONEFAS, KAREN CLEMENTS AND ALASTAIR THOMPSON

Paper significance

DCIS is a heterogeneous, non-obligatory precursor of invasive breast cancer. This large, prospective cohort of 11,337 patients with screen-detected DCIS describes the features and clinical management over two decades. DCIS pathology informed surgical management and use of radiation therapy. Ipsilateral recurrence of DCIS lessened after 5 years, while the most common ipsilateral event, invasive cancer, was consistent to beyond 10 years at 0.5% per year with a median time to development of 62 months. Understanding the biology of DCIS and tailoring individual patient treatment remain key challenges in surgical oncology.

Paper limitations

This paper reports on one-third of all screen-detected DCIS in the UK, representative of the breast-screened population in general.[1] However, since women were age 46 and older for breast screening, younger women, DCIS detected as symptomatic disease and DCIS coincidental with invasive breast cancer were not considered in the cohort evaluated. Furthermore, the breast screening programme from which the women were identified screens every 3 years, and digital mammography was implemented later in the study, so the generalisability of the findings to other healthcare settings may be limited.

In context of the relevant current literature

The unique Sloane Project, reported in this paper and conducted over two decades, is the largest prospective cohort study in the setting of DCIS. It raises questions about the underlying biology of DCIS, the possible connections between DCIS and subsequent invasive breast cancer in the same breast and the power of and how to select for adjuvant interventions—radiation therapy and endocrine therapy—to modify the clinical course.

The underlying biology of DCIS likely involves epithelial abnormalities and stromal changes underpinning histopathological features, including grade and DCIS subtype, that have been associated with risk of invasive breast cancer.[2] Detailed analyses comparing DCIS with subsequent invasive breast cancer in the same breast have demonstrated that similar DNA mutations are apparent in both settings, and single-cell analyses can demonstrate clonal evolution from DCIS to invasive disease.[3] Interestingly, some 80% of invasive breast cancer has the same genomic changes as the original DCIS. Better targeting of the common molecular changes (such as *PIK3CA*, *P53* and nuclear factor I [NFI]) could have a clinical impact on the original DCIS to prevent subsequent invasion. However, in 20% of cases, the DCIS and invasive cancer are genomically distinct (suggesting that DCIS is a 'risk lesion' rather than a predisposing focus).

Whether all DCIS needs to be treated in a similar manner to invasive breast cancer remains contentious. If DCIS is not resected, then for high-grade DCIS, invasive cancer may well occur within a decade, while for low-grade DCIS, invasion rarely occurs over time.[4] This has led to multiple trials of active monitoring of DCIS that on clinical grounds is at low risk of developing into invasive cancer (reviewed in Ref. 2), with one successful randomised trial of active monitoring versus conventional surgery, the COMET (Comparison of Operative versus Monitoring and Endocrine Therapy) trial,[5] now complete, with outcomes awaited.

A key surgical metric remains clear margins of resection following breast conservation for DCIS, with the definition of clear margins varying over time but currently 2 mm circumferentially for pure DCIS in internationally recognised guidelines (Society of Surgical Oncology [SSO] and American Society of Clinical Oncology [ASCO] guidelines). While the extent of clear margins continues to be debated, following complete surgical removal, adjuvant radiotherapy is beneficial to reduce local recurrence for all groups of DCIS in a meta-analysis of the randomised trials (Oxford overview), reflected in the UK Sloane Project reviewed here. Refining who will, or will not, benefit from adjuvant radiation treatment after complete resection of DCIS has been the target of the Oncotype

Dx and PreludeDx assays performed on the DCIS but has not yet been widely adopted.[8] Adjuvant endocrine therapy also reduces the potential for further DCIS or invasive breast cancer after a diagnosis of DCIS,[9] although the finer points of which endocrine therapy to use, adherence to prescription of the drug and even whether oestrogen receptor testing is performed on the DCIS all impact the relatively low use of endocrine adjuvant therapy, at least in a UK setting.

Conclusions

DCIS is increasingly recognised as a heterogeneous condition with a variable clinical behaviour for which we do not fully understand the biology, and it requires thoughtful management. Understanding the biology of clinically indolent DCIS versus DCIS which then develops into invasive breast cancer, focussing on targeting which patients benefit most from adjuvant therapy and evolving to manage DCIS differently from invasive breast cancer remain contemporary challenges.

REFERENCES

1. Clements K, Dodwell D, Hilton B, Stevens-Harris I, Pinder S, Wallis MG, et al. Cohort profile of the Sloane Project: methodology for a prospective UK cohort study of >15 000 women with screen-detected non-invasive breast neoplasia. *BMJ Open.* 2022;12(12):e061585. doi: 10.1136/bmjopen-2022-061585. Erratum in: *BMJ Open.* 2023;13(1):e061585corr1. PMID: 36535720; PMCID: PMC9764674.
2. Casasent A, Almekinders M, Mulder C, Bhattacharjee P, Collyar D, Thompson AM, et al., Grand Challenge Precision Consortium. Biology of DCIS and its relationship to breast cancer. DCIS: When cancer is not really cancer? *Nat Rev Cancer.* 2022;22(12):663–78. doi:10.1038/s41568-022-00512-y. Epub 2022 Oct 19. PMID: 3626170.
3. Lips E, Kumar T, Megalios A, Visser L, Sheinman M, Fortunato A, et al., Grand Challenge Precision Consortium. Genomic analysis defines clonal relationships of ductal carcinoma *in situ* and recurrent invasive breast cancer. *Nat Genet.* 2022;54:850–60. doi:10.1038/s41588-022-01082-3
4. Maxwell A, Hilton B, Clements K, Dodwell D, Dulson-Cox J, Kearins O, et al. Unresected screen detected ductal carcinoma *in situ*: outcomes of 311 women in the Forget-me–not 2 study. *Breast.* 2022;61:145–55. doi:10.1016/j.breast.2022.01.001. Epub 2022 Jan 4. PMID: 34999428.
5. Hwang ES, Hyslop T, Lynch T, Frank E, Pinto D, Basila D, et al. The COMET (Comparison of Operative versus Monitoring and Endocrine Therapy) trial: a phase III randomised controlled clinical trial for low-risk ductal carcinoma *in situ* (DCIS). *BMJ Open.* 2019;9(3):e026797. doi:10.1136/bmjopen-2018-026797. PMID: 30862637.
6. Morrow M, Van Zee KJ, Solin LJ, Houssami N, Chavez-MacGregor M, Harris JR, et al. Society of Surgical Oncology-American Society for Radiation Oncology-American Society of Clinical Oncology Consensus Guideline on Margins for breast-conserving surgery with whole-breast irradiation in ductal carcinoma *in situ*. *Ann Surg Oncol.* 2016;23(12):3801–10. doi:10.1245/s10434-016-5449-z. Epub 2016 Aug 15. PMID: 27527714.

7. Early Breast Cancer Trialists' Collaborative Group (EBCTCG); Correa C, McGale P, Taylor C, Wang Y, Clarke M, Davies C, et al. Overview of the randomized trials of radiotherapy in ductal carcinoma *in situ* of the breast. *J Natl Cancer Inst Monogr.* 2010;2010(41):162–77. doi:10.1093/jncimonographs/lgq039. PMID: 20956824.
8. Rakovitch E, Bonefas E, Nofech-Mozes S, Thompson, AM. Ductal carcinoma *in situ* (DCIS)—precision medicine for de-escalation. *Curr Breast Cancer Rep.* 2021;13:1–7. doi:10.1007/s12609-021-00407-1
9. Cuzick J, Sestak I, Forbes JF, Dowsett M, Cawthorn S, Mansel RE, et al., Howell A on behalf of the IBIS II investigators. Use of anastrozole for breast cancer prevention (IBIS II) long term results of a randomised controlled trial. *Lancet.* 395:117–22.

CHAPTER 27

Effect of Tamoxifen and Radiotherapy in Women with Locally Excised Ductal Carcinoma In Situ: Long-Term Results from the UK/ANZ DCIS Trial

Cuzick J, Sestak I, Pinder SE, Ellis IO, Forsyth S, Bundred NJ, et al.
Lancet Oncol 12(1):21–29, 2011

The introduction of breast screening has resulted in a substantial increase in the diagnosis of ductal carcinoma *in situ* (DCIS). The characteristics of DCIS detected via screening are less aggressive than in women who present with symptomatic disease. Approximately 20% of cases will be upgraded to invasive disease after surgical excision, and although the rate of progression of DCIS if left untreated is uncertain, it is thought to be relatively low even after several decades. Treatment therefore needs to be tailored to avoid overtreatment for a disease which rarely causes death but upstages to invasive disease in half of all recurrences. Breast cancer–related mortality after a diagnosis of screen-detected DCIS is ~2% higher than in women in the general population on long-term follow-up. Local treatment with mastectomy or breast-conserving surgery with or without adjuvant radiotherapy helps provide local control. Similarly, adjuvant anti-oestrogens help reduce rates of local recurrence and contralateral disease. The UK, Australia, and New Zealand Ductal Carcinoma *In Situ* (UK/ANZ DCIS) trial (and the similar National Surgical Adjuvant Breast and Bowel Project [NSABP] B-24 trial) explored the impact of radiotherapy and anti-oestrogen therapy, and also the combination of both, in women with screen-detected DCIS treated with breast conservation surgery.

PAPER DESCRIPTION

- **Objective/Research Question**: The UK/ANZ DCIS trial aimed to assess the effectiveness of adjuvant radiotherapy and tamoxifen in women with DCIS treated with breast conservation surgery.

- **Design**: The study was a randomised 2 × 2 factorial trial of radiotherapy, tamoxifen, neither or both, with participants recruited between May 1990 and August 1998. However, clinicians and patients had a choice to omit or proceed with either of these treatments, and the analysis was

DOI: 10.1201/b23352-27

restricted to patients who were randomly assigned to that treatment based on intention to treat (what they were randomised to, rather than what they actually received). Patients were also offered the option to take part in only one of the two randomisations and pre-specify whether they had the other treatment. The primary outcome was ipsilateral invasive breast cancer (IBC) for the radiotherapy randomisation and any new breast event, including contralateral invasive or *in situ* disease, for tamoxifen.

- **Sample Size**: In total, 1,701 women were randomised into the trial, with 1,694 eligible for analysis. Of these, 912 were fully randomised to both treatments (2 × 2 randomisation). There were 782 women who elected to have one of the treatments and were only randomised to the other treatment. Numbers were roughly equal in the 2 × 2 randomisation groups. In the selective subgroups, 664 wanted to control their decision about having radiotherapy and only accepted tamoxifen randomisation. Of these, the majority (603) elected to have no radiotherapy.

- **Inclusion Criteria**: Patients with unilateral or bilateral DCIS who underwent breast conservation surgery with clear margins on both radiology of the surgical specimen and histological examination were eligible for the trial.

  Hormone receptor status was not incorporated into the study's inclusion criteria.

- **Exclusion Criteria**: Patients with uncertain pathological disease margins or other pathologies such as Paget's disease of the nipple, lobular carcinoma *in situ* and atypical ductal hyperplasia without DCIS were excluded, as were those with a reduced life expectancy.

- **Intervention Received**: Patients who received radiotherapy had the recommended dose of 50 Gy in 25 fractions over 5 weeks, whilst those who received tamoxifen were prescribed 20 mg daily for 5 years. After treatment, all patients were followed up with annual mammography for the first 7 years, and biennially thereafter.

- **Results**: Patients were followed up for a median of 12.7 years. Radiotherapy resulted in an absolute reduction in new breast events by 12.6% and reduced the incidence of both ipsilateral invasive disease (0.32, 95% confidence interval [CI] = 0.19–0.56, $p < 0.0001$) and ipsilateral DCIS (0.38, 95% CI = 0.22–0.63, $p < 0.0001$), but not contralateral breast cancer (0.84, 95% CI = 0.45–1.58, $p = 0.6$). Tamoxifen resulted in an absolute 10-year reduction in new breast events by 6.5%, and although it did not affect ipsilateral invasive disease (0.95, 95% CI = 0.66–1.38, $p = 0.8$), it did reduce the incidence of both recurrent ipsilateral DCIS

(0.70, 95% CI = 0.51–0.86, p = 0.03) and contralateral tumours (0.44, 95% CI = 0.25–0.77, p = 0.005). Use of tamoxifen alongside radiotherapy did not provide additional benefit in terms of either ipsilateral or contralateral recurrences. No impact on death rates was reported in any group; however, specifically looking at women who died of cardiovascular disease, radiotherapy indicated a small but significant negative impact (cardiovascular deaths 0–1% without radiotherapy vs. 1–2% with it, p < 0.008), although the numbers were small.

EXPERT COMMENTARY BY NICOLE JAMES AND GURDEEP MANNU

Paper significance

For both endocrine therapy and radiotherapy in DCIS, the UK/ANZ trial has had an important clinical impact and helped to not only change international practice but also shape subsequent research questions. It was one of two trials examining the effect of adjuvant tamoxifen after breast-conserving surgery in women with DCIS, with subsequent trials examining the role of aromatase inhibitors versus tamoxifen and the benefits of aromatase inhibitors versus not. The UK/ANZ trial was also the third trial examining adjuvant radiotherapy versus no radiotherapy after breast-conserving surgery in women with DCIS to complete accrual, and it found no significant differences in new breast events between patients randomly assigned to radiotherapy and tamoxifen and those randomised to radiotherapy alone. The 2018 National Institute for Health and Care Excellence (NICE) guidelines were updated to recommend consideration of endocrine therapy after breast-conserving surgery for women with oestrogen receptor (ER)-positive DCIS if radiotherapy is recommended but not received, or if radiotherapy is not recommended.[1] Radiotherapy trials building on the UK/ANZ trial have subsequently examined whole-breast versus partial-breast radiotherapy, whole-breast radiotherapy +/– boost, radiotherapy fractionations and radiotherapy techniques in women with DCIS.

Paper limitations

There was no information on margin distance collected by the trial, only whether it was clear or involved. Margin distance is associated with IBC recurrence rates in women with DCIS after treatment.[2] Nor was patient selection based on ER receptor status, which may mean the effect size of tamoxifen therapy may be slightly higher solely in ER-positive disease than that shown in this trial. As the trial started soon after the introduction of the National Health Service Breast Screening Programme (NHS BSP) in the UK, its findings may be less applicable to patients who are diagnosed with DCIS through symptoms, where disease tends to be higher grade, larger and more often associated with invasive foci.

In context of the relevant current literature

The only other trial investigating the use of tamoxifen in DCIS amongst patients receiving radiotherapy was the NSABP B-24 trial.[3] While the UK/ANZ trial solely included women with surgical resection margins clear of disease, one in four women recruited into the NSABP B-24 trial had positive tumour margins. In NSABP B-24, the 15-year invasive ipsilateral breast tumour recurrence rate in the radiotherapy-alone arm was 17.4% in women with positive surgical margins compared to 7.4% in those with negative margins. On the other hand, in the radiotherapy and tamoxifen group, the incidence of ipsilateral IBC was lower at 11.5%, but the risk in those with positive margins remained around 7.5%, providing evidence of the role of clear surgical resection margins prior to consideration of adjuvant endocrine therapy.

The benefit of radiotherapy and endocrine therapy shown in this trial has since been shown to translate into women in the general population by a population-based cohort study of all women diagnosed with DCIS through the NHS BSP between 2000 and 2014.[4] It confirmed the higher risks of IBC (relative risk [RR] = 1.43, 95% CI = 1.05–1.96) in women receiving breast-conserving surgery without radiotherapy seen in the UK/ANZ trial compared with women who received radiotherapy, as well as indicating a potentially beneficial role of endocrine therapy. The UK/ANZ trial helped to shift the paradigm in DCIS treatment. At the time of its publication, the natural history of DCIS was more unclear. Several ongoing trials of non-operative treatment in low-risk DCIS (e.g., LORIS[5] and LORD[6]), or with the addition of endocrine therapy in the Comparison of Operative versus Monitoring and Endocrine Therapy (COMET[7]) and may result in a further paradigm shift in DCIS treatment over the coming years.

Conclusions

Studies such as the UK/ANZ DCIS trial have shaped our management of women with DCIS. However, there is emering evidence that DCIS may be more of a heterogeneous entity than previously considered. Prospective studies which utilise novel techniques, including genomic profiling,[8] have the potential to further individualise therapies for DCIS. The goal of ongoing and future research should be to focus on separating lower risk lesions, where non-operative treatment may be feasible, from higher risk disease where adjuvant therapies may be tailored to the individual patient.[9]

REFERENCES

1. National Institute of Clinical Excellence. Early and locally advanced breast cancer: diagnosis and management NICE guideline [NG101] 2018.

2. Van Zee K, Subhedar P, Olcese C, Patil S, Morrow M. Relationship between margin width and recurrence of ductal carcinoma *in situ*: analysis of 2996 women treated with breast-conserving surgery for 30 years. *Ann Surg*. 2015;262:623–31.

3. Wapnir IL, Dignam JJ, Fisher B, Mamounas EP, Anderson SJ, Julian TB, Land SR, Margolese RG, Swain SM, Costantino JP, Wolmark N. Long-term outcomes of invasive ipsilateral breast tumor recurrences after lumpectomy in NSABP B-17 and B-24 randomized clinical trials for DCIS. *J Natl Cancer Inst*. 2011 Mar 16;103(6):478–88. doi: 10.1093/jnci/djr027. Epub 2011 Mar 11. PMID: 21398619; PMCID: PMC3107729.

4. Mannu G, Wang Z, Broggio J, Charman J, Cheung S. Invasive breast cancer and breast cancer mortality after ductal carcinoma *in situ* in women attending for breast screening in England, 1988-2014: population based observational cohort study. *Br Med J*. 2020;369:m1570.

5. Francis A, Fallowfield L, Rea D. The LORIS trial: addressing overtreatment of ductal carcinoma *in situ*. *Clin Oncol*. 2015;27(1):6–8.

6. Elshof L, Tryfonidis K, Slaets L, van Leeuwen-Stok A, Skinner V, Dif N. Feasibility of a prospective, randomised, open-label, international multicentre, phase III, non-inferiority trial to assess the safety of active surveillance for low risk ductal carcinoma *in situ* —The LORD study. *Eur J Cancer*. 2015;51(12):1497–510.

7. Hwang E, Hyslop T, Lynch T, Frank E, Pinto D, Basila D. The COMET (Comparison of Operative versus Monitoring and Endocrine Therapy) trial: a phase III randomised controlled clinical trial for low-risk ductal carcinoma *in situ* (DCIS). *BMJ Open*. 2019;9(3):e026797.

8. Rakovitch E, Sutradhar R, Nofech-Mozes S, et al. 21-gene assay and breast cancer mortality in ductal carcinoma *in situ*. *J Natl Cancer Inst*. 2021;113(5):572–9.

9. Mannu G, Groen E, Wang Z, Schaapveld M, Lips E, Chung M. Reliability of preoperative breast biopsies showing ductal carcinoma *in situ* and implications for non-operative treatment: a cohort study. *Breast Cancer Res Treat*. 2019;178(2):409–18.

A Prognostic Index for Ductal Carcinoma In Situ of the Breast

Silverstein MJ, Lagios MD, Craig PH, et al.

Cancer 77(11):2267–2274, 1996

Ductal carcinoma *in situ* (DCIS) represents about 20% of all breast malignancies but with a very low breast cancer–specific mortality rate due to either occult invasive disease or invasive recurrence. Treatment is with local surgery in the form of mastectomy alone or breast-conserving surgery (BCS) with, or without, radiotherapy (RT). However, risk-stratified treatment is important to prevent overtreatment of low-risk disease and undertreatment of high-risk disease. Local recurrence rates were high before RT in BCS. Therefore, the National Surgical Adjuvant Breast and Bowel Project (NSABP) group recommended RT after BCS following the NSABP B-17 trial which had shown high rates of recurrence after BCS which were reduced by RT, but disease characteristics were not stratified.[1] Following this, the Silverstein group in Van Nuys, California, used real-world data relating to DCIS to develop a predictive index for local recurrence, helping to shape surgical and radiotherapeutic management with stratification according to DCIS size, grade and margin width (and, in a later publication, patient age). The proposed Van Nuys Prognostic Index (VNPI) was widely used for decades in clinical practice but has now fallen out of favour as newer margin thresholds and algorithms have been adopted. Emerging technology on DCIS molecular profiling, combined with clinical parameters, may well see further changes in practice. Similarly, ongoing trials (LORIS, Low-Risk DCIS [LORD] and Comparison of Operative versus Monitoring and Endocrine Therapy [COMET]) may see the future emergence of nonsurgical management for very low-risk cases.

PAPER DESCRIPTION

- **Objective/Research Question**: Development of a predictive index for local recurrence of DCIS, with stratification according to DCIS size, grade and margin width (and, in a later publication, patient age), to help to determine surgical and radiotherapeutic management.

- **Design**: This was a retrospective, observational cohort study to determine treatment stratification factors for women with DCIS who were treated with BCS at two hospitals in California, USA. Multivariate analysis of three risk factors (DCIS size, grade and margin width, all grades from 1 to 3) was used to determine cutoffs for recurrence risk strata.

DOI: 10.1201/b23352-28

• **Sample Size**: Two cohorts of patients were initially studied: an initial cohort (recruited between 1979 and 1995) and a validation cohort of 79 patients (1972–1987). The two cohorts had similar characteristics and outcomes and were combined into a single cohort of 333 patients with 79 months of follow-up.

• **Results**: Using Cox's regression analysis, tumour size, grade and margin status were all shown to significantly predict recurrence risk. They used this to allocate scores to different ranges of each and developed a formula to predict outcomes. This formula was converted to a simple scoring system where a minimum score of 3 or a maximum score of 9 could be allocated and which was predictive of recurrence risk.

Using these scores, they created Kaplan–Meier survival scores of low risk (scores of 3 or 4), intermediate risk (5, 6 or 7) and high risk (8 or 9) when given RT or not. There was little benefit to low-risk women regardless of whether RT was used, and hence this group were not felt to benefit from RT. There was benefit for the intermediate-risk group, and hence RT was advised for this group. For the high-risk group, the risk of recurrence was very high, and mastectomy was advised.

The final algorithm is as follows:

• *VNPI 3–4*: RT provided no significant benefit (100% vs. 97%, p = nonsignificant), so they could be considered for excision alone.
• *VNPI 5–7*: RT provided a significant 17% reduction in the local recurrence rate (85% vs. 68%, p = 0.017).
• *VNPI 8–9*: RT provided benefit, but since more than 60% developed local recurrence, they were recommended mastectomy.

Further work was done after publication of the initial paper. A modified index was published 7 years later (2003),[2] in which age was added as a further stratification factor. The revised algorithm was developed on 706 patients with 12 years of follow-up. Age categories were ≤39, 40–60 and ≥61 years (scoring 1, 2 or 3, respectively).

The final algorithm is shown in **Table 28.1**.

Table 28.1   Van Nuys Prognostic Index (VNPI) scoring system

Parameter	Score 1	Score 2	Score 3
Size	15 mm or less	16–40 mm	Over 41 mm
Minimum surgical margin	10 mm or more	1–9 mm	Less than 1 mm
Pathological grade	Non-high-grade No necrosis	Non-high-grade Necrosis	High-grade With or without necrosis
Age	61 years or older	40–60 years	39 years or younger

Source: Modified from Silverstein et al.[3]

Scores of 1–3 for each parameter are then totalled to give the final VNPI and management allocated as follows:

- *VNPI 4–6*: No benefit from RT, so they could be considered for excision alone.
- *VNPI 7–9*: RT provided a 15% lower local recurrence rate ($p = 0.03$), so consider RT or re-excision if the margin is less than 10 mm.
- *VNPI 10–12*: RT provided benefit, but mastectomy was recommended since they had a 50% local recurrence rate.

Further fine-tuning was also published in 2010, with a more nuanced approach to margin widths,[4] with <3, 3–5 and >5 mm margins being considered.

EXPERT COMMENTARY BY AMIT AGRAWAL AND MAHMOUD SOLIMAN

Paper significance

The paper had an impact in that it initiated prognostication in DCIS. Direct application of the paper published two decades ago may be limited now in resource-rich healthcare systems, as discussed later in this chapter. Nonetheless, it continues to have a role as an inexpensive simple guide for a safe, modern (surgical) practice in DCIS. Certainly, the increasingly modified University of Southern California (USC)/VNPI score reminds the treating team about the importance of margins. In an era when digital mammograms and magnetic resonance imaging (MRI) in DCIS were not available, a wider margin was prudent to ensure the success of safe oncological conservation, more so in DCIS due to its discontinuous pattern in the ductal architecture. If there were doubts, mastectomy was deemed oncologically safe over disfiguring BCS since extreme oncoplastic surgery, now embraced by Professor Silverstein himself, was not in vogue at the time.[5]

Paper limitations

The dataset on which the VNPI was based was retrospective and collected in an era predating digital mammography, and indeed screening and hence recurrence rates are likely to be lower in modern practice. The recommendation of mastectomy for high-risk scores would now be moderated by the availability of oncoplastic BCS and even extreme oncoplasty.[5,6] In addition, modern de-escalation trends have sparked research trials of observation only (plus or minus anti-oestrogens), and so the very low-risk group may in future require less surgery, depending on the results of the LORIS,[7] LORD[8] and COMET[9] trials. The impact of increasing use of MRI in the management of DCIS may also affect the validity of the index, although it may lead to more mastectomies.[10]

In context of the relevant current literature

Modern surgical practice has now moved on, and MRI has become more widely used in the assessment of DCIS extent,[10] showing more accurate estimation than mammography alone but not improving rates of reoperation and increasing mastectomy rates (63% vs. 23%, $p < 0.0001$).[11] In addition, the optimal margin width with DCIS has been the subject of debate, and the optimal 10 mm margin of the VNPI is no longer regarded as necessary. UK, US and European guidelines have now largely agreed that 2 mm is acceptable for DCIS, which undermines the value of the VNPI which is now used infrequently.[12]

More information is also now available about the role of RT in DCIS, including stratification by risk group. A meta-analysis of four large multicentre randomised trials[13] showed that whole-breast RT following BCS for DCIS provided a 15.2% absolute benefit by reducing the 10-year non-invasive local recurrence rate from 28.1% to 12.9%. In contrast to the landmark and associated papers, RT was effective regardless of the age at diagnosis, the extent of BCS, use of tamoxifen, the method of DCIS detection, margin status, focality, grade, comedo necrosis, architecture or tumour size. During 1999–2006, the omission of RT in 'good-risk' DCIS was investigated in NRG Oncology's RTOG-9804 randomised trial. At a median of 13.9 years of follow-up, in low- to intermediate-grade DCIS with <2.5 cm and >3 mm margins, the local recurrence rate was significantly higher (15% without RT vs. 7% with RT, 95% confidence interval [CI] = 0.20–0.66, $p = 0.0007$). The real-world UK Sloane prospective data of screen-detected DCIS ($n = 9,938$) showed a 3.1% absolute difference (7.2% with RT vs. 4.1% without, $p < 0.001$) in local recurrence independent of the excision margin width or the size of DCIS.[14]

Another option, which was not included in the VNPI, was the use of anti-oestrogens. Several studies have explored this[15] and found that tamoxifen may provide some protection, but it is not as potent as RT. Modern management now includes anti-oestrogens in selected cases.

Other predictive tools in DCIS

The Memorial Sloan Kettering Cancer Center (MSKCC) nomogram and other predictors of local recurrence

Similar to the VNPI, the MSKCC in the USA proposed a graphical nomogram to individualise the risk estimates of invasive breast tumour recurrence (IBTR) in women with DCIS treated with BCS.[16] The model incorporated 10 variables (age, family history, screen/clinical detection, adjuvant RT, adjuvant endocrine therapy, nuclear grade, presence of necrosis, margin status, number of excisions and year of surgery); it has been shown to assist in individual decision making regarding various treatment options.

Multigene expression to predict local recurrence risk

Solin and colleagues[17] performed a multigene breast cancer assay on surgically excised DCIS ($n = 327$) with no RT from the Eastern Cooperative

Oncology Group (ECOG) E5194 study to predict local recurrence. Based on DCIS scores (derived from seven cancer-related and five reference genes) for low-, intermediate- and high-risk groups, the 10-year risks were 10.6%, 26.7% and 25.09% ($p < 0.006$) for any recurrence, respectively, whilst for invasive recurrence they were 3.7%, 12.3% and 19.2% ($p < 0.006$). A recent meta-analysis of 3,478 women from five articles evaluated two molecular signatures: Oncotype Dx[18] DCIS (prognostic of local recurrence) and DCISionRT (prognostic of local recurrence and predictive of RT benefit). In the low-risk group, the pooled hazard ratio (HR) of BCS plus RT versus BCS alone was 0.62 (95% CI = 0.39–0.99) for any breast event; however, it was not significant for invasive recurrence (HR = 0.58, 95% CI = 0.25–1.32). In the high-risk group, the pooled HR for BCS plus RT was 0.39 (95% CI = 0.20–0.77) for invasive and 0.34 (95% CI = 0.22–0.52) for any breast recurrence. The authors concluded that risk prediction of molecular signatures was independent of other risk stratification tools in DCIS, with a tendency towards RT de-escalation.

Conclusions

The VNPI was one of the first prognostic and management algorithms for DCIS and achieved widespread global use after its publication. In modern practice, a more nuanced approach is now seen, with greater use of MRI, oncoplastic surgery, gene arrays and biological markers and use of anti-oestrogens. However, in medical facilities where these are not available, the VNPI score may still serve as a valuable guideline for shared decision making with patients.

REFERENCES

1. Fisher B, et al. Lumpectomy compared with lumpectomy and radiation therapy for the treatment of intraductal breast cancer. *N Engl J Med*. 1993;328(22):1581–6.
2. Silverstein MJ. The University of Southern California/Van Nuys prognostic index for ductal carcinoma *in situ* of the breast. *Am J Surg*. 2003;186(4):337–43.
3. Silverstein MJ. Ductal carcinoma *in situ* of the breast: 11 reasons to consider treatment with excision alone. *Womens Health*. 2008;4(6):565–77.
4. Silverstein MJ, Lagios MD. Choosing treatment for patients with ductal carcinoma *in situ*: fine tuning the University of Southern California/Van Nuys Prognostic Index. *J Natl Cancer Inst Monogr*. 2010;2010(41):193–6.
5. Silverstein MJ. Radical mastectomy to radical conservation (Extreme Oncoplasty): a revolutionary change. *J Am Coll Surg*. 2016;222(1):1–9.
6. Bali R, et al. Wide local excision versus oncoplastic breast surgery: differences in surgical outcome for an assumed margin (0, 1, or 2 mm) distance. *Clin Breast Cancer*. 2018;18(5):e1053–7.
7. Francis A, Fallowfield L, Rea D. The LORIS trial: addressing overtreatment of ductal carcinoma *in situ*. *Clin Oncol*. 2015;27(1):6–8.
8. Elshof LE, et al. Feasibility of a prospective, randomised, open-label, international multicentre, phase III, non-inferiority trial to assess the safety of active surveillance for low risk ductal carcinoma *in situ*—The LORD study. *Eur J Cancer*. 2015;51(12):1497–510.

9. Hwang ES, et al. The COMET (Comparison of Operative versus Monitoring and Endocrine Therapy) trial: a phase III randomised controlled clinical trial for low-risk ductal carcinoma *in situ* (DCIS). *BMJ Open*. 2019;9(3):e026797.

10. Bartram A, et al., Breast MRI in DCIS size estimation, breast-conserving surgery and oncoplastic breast surgery. *Cancer Treat Rev*. 2021;94:102158.

11. Healy NA, et al. Does pre-operative breast MRI have an impact on surgical outcomes in high-grade DCIS? *Br J Radiol*. 2022:20220306.

12. Marinovich ML, et al. The association of surgical margins and local recurrence in women with ductal carcinoma *in situ* treated with breast-conserving therapy: a meta-analysis. *Ann Surg Oncol*. 2016;23(12):3811–21.

13. Correa C, et al. Overview of the randomized trials of radiotherapy in ductal carcinoma *in situ* of the breast. *J Natl Cancer Inst Monogr*. 2010;2010(41):162–77.

14. Thompson AM, et al. Management and 5-year outcomes in 9938 women with screen-detected ductal carcinoma *in situ*: the UK Sloane Project. *Eur J Cancer*. 2018;101:210–9.

15. Houghton J, et al. Radiotherapy and tamoxifen in women with completely excised ductal carcinoma *in situ* of the breast in the UK, Australia, and New Zealand: randomised controlled trial. *Lancet*. 2003;362(9378):95–102.

16. Rudloff U, et al. Nomogram for predicting the risk of local recurrence after breast-conserving surgery for ductal carcinoma *in situ*. *J Clin Oncol*. 2010;28(23):3762–9.

17. Solin LJ, et al. A multigene expression assay to predict local recurrence risk for ductal carcinoma *in situ* of the breast. *J Natl Cancer Inst*. 2013;105(10):701–10.

18. Ouattara D, et al. Molecular signatures in ductal carcinoma *in situ* (DCIS): a systematic review and meta-analysis. *J Clin Med*. 2023;12(5).

CHAPTER 29

Comparisons between Different Polychemotherapy Regimens for Early Breast Cancer: Meta-Analyses of Long-Term Outcome among 100,000 Women in 123 Randomised Trials

Peto R, Davies C, Godwin J, Gray, R, Pan, HC, Clarke, M, et al.
Lancet 379(9814):432–444, 2012

Chemotherapy has been a standard treatment for women with a high risk of breast cancer recurrence for decades. As each new chemotherapy regimen has been trialled, incremental benefits have been demonstrated, initially between CMF (cyclophosphamide, methotrexate and 5-fluorouracil) chemotherapy and placebo, and more recently when compared to the previous standard chemotherapy. Numerous clinical trials have been conducted over several decades, each with slightly different criteria. This research involved collection and meta-analysis of individual patient data from all of the primary trials of adjuvant chemotherapy, giving a unique and powerful insight into the efficacy of different regimens and the subgroups where effects are more notable.

PAPER DESCRIPTION

- **Objective**: This meta-analysis was undertaken to identify differences in efficacy between adjuvant polychemotherapy regimens for breast cancer.

- **Design**: Individual patient-level data assessed in a meta-analysis of all randomised trials comparing adjuvant polychemotherapy regimens for breast cancer.

- **Sample Size**: 100,000 women from 123 trials:
  1. Thirty-two thousand patients from 64 trials comparing polychemotherapy versus no chemotherapy
  2. Eighteen thousand patients from 20 trials comparing any anthracycline-based regimen versus standard or near-standard CMF

DOI: 10.1201/b23352-29

3. Seven thousand patients from six trials comparing higher versus lower anthracycline dosages
4. Forty-four thousand patients from 33 trials comparing taxane-based versus non-taxane-based regimens

- **Follow-Up**: Variation between original studies. Results for recurrence, breast cancer mortality and overall mortality reported as 0–4 years, 5–9 years and 10-plus years.

- **Inclusion Criteria**: All randomised trials from 1973 to 2003 comparing polychemotherapy regimens for early breast cancer, comprising:
  1. Taxane-based versus non-taxane-based regimens
  2. Anthracycline-based regimen versus standard or near-standard CMF regimens
  3. Higher versus lower anthracycline dosages
  4. Polychemotherapy versus no adjuvant chemotherapy

- **Exclusion Criteria**:
  1. Trials of intensive chemotherapy with stem cell rescue
  2. Trials only comparing variations in dose density

- **Interventions or Treatments Compared**:
  1. Taxane-plus-anthracycline-based regimens versus non-taxane-based chemotherapy. Non-taxane-based groups (control group) either gave chemotherapy at standard frequencies and doses, or in some studies higher cumulative doses were given in the non-taxane/control group in an attempt to balance for the additional doses being given in the taxane group.
  2. Anthracycline-based regimen versus standard or near-standard CMF.
  3. Chemotherapy (anthracycline-based regimen or standard/near-standard CMF) versus no adjuvant chemotherapy.

- **Results**: These meta-analyses identified several important findings. First is that standard CMF and standard 4AC (four cycles of Adriamycin and cyclophosphamide) regimens were roughly equivalent, halving recurrence rates at 2 years, and reducing recurrence rates at 8 years by a third. The absolute reduction in breast cancer mortality at 10 years was 6.2% for the CMF regimen and 6.5% for the anthracycline-based regimen.
  With regard to dose-related response, chemotherapy regimens with lower doses per cycle were noted to be less effective. Regimens with substantially more chemotherapy than standard 4AC or CMF, such as CAF (cyclophosphamide, Adriamycin and fluorouracil) and CEF (cyclophosphamide, epirubicin and fluorouracil) regimens, could confer a further reduction of 15–20% in breast cancer mortality rates.

There was great variation between studies on the benefit of adding a taxane to anthracycline regimens; however, the study concluded that a taxane-plus-anthracycline-based regimen slightly, but nonetheless significantly, improved outcomes compared to anthracycline-based controls.

The reductions in early recurrence (0–4 years), any recurrence and breast cancer mortality observed in the trials included in this meta-analysis for both taxane-based and anthracycline-based regimens appeared largely independent of age, nodal status, tumour diameter, tumour differentiation or oestrogen receptor (ER) status on subgroup analyses.

EXPERT COMMENTARY BY JESSICA BANKS, LYNDA WYLD AND JANET BROWN

Paper significance

The Early Breast Cancer Trialists' Collaborative Group (EBCTCG) was set up in 1984–1985 to coordinate quinquennial worldwide meta-analyses, bringing together individual patient data from all randomised trials of the treatment of early breast cancer. This meta-analysis comes 35 years after the first report of the benefit of adjuvant chemotherapy for breast cancer and is an update of a previous meta-analysis, on chemotherapy and hormonal therapy for early breast cancer, published in 2005.[1] This update includes the preliminary taxane trial results in addition to updated outcomes on previously reported chemotherapy trials.

For 'early' breast cancer—cancer confined to the breast and locoregional lymph nodes—macroscopic disease is removed surgically. However, local or distant microscopic deposits can lead to recurrence. The introduction of effective cyto-toxic agents in treating breast cancer both neoadjuvantly (prior to surgery) and adjuvantly (post surgery) has been instrumental in reducing breast cancer recurrence and mortality by eradicating micro-metastases.

The early (25-year-old) chemotherapy trials reported in this meta-analysis, which compared CMF or anthracycline-based regimens (4AC) to no chemotherapy, demonstrated a significant reduction in both breast cancer mortality and overall mortality with chemotherapy. These early trials underpin the rationale for adjuvant chemotherapy following breast surgery to improve overall survival.

In this meta-analysis, the inclusion of the taxane trial results, where taxane–anthracycline regimens were compared to standard anthracycline regimens, demonstrated that taxane–anthracycline-based regimens lead to a further reduction in breast cancer mortality. However, the scale of the benefit varied, depending on the chemotherapy regimen used. For trials using a standard anthracycline-based regimen in both arms, with the addition of four separate cycles of a taxane in the taxane–anthracycline arm, a further 15–20% improvement in breast cancer mortality (2.8% absolute gain at 8 years) was observed. Other studies added more anthracycline to the control group to 'balance' the additional chemotherapy the taxane group were receiving; the results from these trials are more difficult to interpret. There was still a significant reduction in breast cancer mortality of 1.4% at 5 years across all studies; however, when the control group received double the anthracycline cycles of the taxane group, no significant benefit in favour of taxanes is observed. Despite this variation in results, this meta-analysis highlights that either adding a taxane to a 4AC regimen or increasing the cycles and cumulative dose of anthracycline further reduces breast cancer mortality compared to standard chemotherapy.

For modern chemotherapy regimens, the priorities are to balance efficacy with short- and long-term toxicity and avoid overtreatment in groups where chemotherapy offers little benefit. To this end, modern treatment algorithms are often supported by the use of multigene arrays such as Oncotype Dx and MammaPrint. With regard to toxicity, anthracyclines have harmful dose-dependent effects on the myocardium[2] and latent haematological effects that can lead to acute myeloid leukaemia. A further consideration for women with *HER2*-positive breast cancer is that trastuzumab is also cardiotoxic, and increasing the cumulative dose of anthracyclines may lead to higher rates of cardiac damage and restrict the use of trastuzumab.

This meta-analysis demonstrated that chemotherapy is beneficial in both ER-positive and ER-negative disease. Chemo-endocrine therapy produced a substantially greater proportional reduction in breast cancer mortality than endocrine therapy alone in both younger and older women with ER-positive breast cancer. This is important, as previous studies have suggested that a pathological complete response to neoadjuvant chemotherapy is more likely with ER-negative disease and consequently ER status may affect the proportional risk reduction with adjuvant chemotherapy.[3]

Paper limitations

Since the publication of this meta-analysis, several techniques have been developed to further categorise patients with breast cancer into high or low risk. Multigene expression signatures based on tumour RNA profile identify a patient's genomic risk, which can be used alongside clinical risk scores to better inform the use of chemotherapy and reduce overtreatment. ER-positive disease can be broadly divided into luminal A (*HER2*-negative, not highly proliferative and well differentiated) and luminal B (highly proliferative). This meta-analysis did not have access to luminal type or multigene expression signatures, and therefore cannot comment on the role of molecular heterogeneity and its possible effects on the risks and benefits of chemotherapy.

Another limitation is from the trials included in this meta-analysis: Very few women older than 70 years of age were recruited, yet a third of all breast cancers occur in women over 70. Although the proportional risk reductions with chemotherapy noted in this paper were not affected by age, the gain in life expectancy is less in older women due to competing causes of death. Higher toxicity rates in older women must also be considered before commencing chemotherapy.

In addition, there is increasing complexity of systemic therapy regimens, often with the addition of newer agents such as platinum derivatives and molecular targeting agents such as poly (ADP-ribose) polymerase (PARP) inhibitors, *HER2*-targeting agents, immunotherapy and CDK4/6 inhibitors as well as extended endocrine regimes and bisphosphonates. There is also now the added complexity of neoadjuvant therapy and post-neoadjuvant therapy for poor responders. Therefore, as valuable as the paper is, the outcomes reported are likely to be less beneficial given current regimens in place with modern practice.

Conclusions

This meta-analysis demonstrates the benefit of adjuvant chemotherapy in reducing mortality in early breast cancer. However, challenges still exist in identifying the patients who are less likely to benefit from adjuvant chemotherapy and avoiding overtreatment in this group.

Additional papers of interest

Publications exploring the value of gene arrays in tailoring chemotherapy to patients who will benefit the most include the following (see also Chapters __ and __, respectively, for the MINDACT and TailorX trials):

MonarchE: Abemaciclib Combined With Endocrine Therapy for the Adjuvant Treatment of HR+, HER2-, Node-Positive, High-Risk, Early Breast Cancer (MonarchE). Stephen R. D. Johnston, et al. *J Clin Oncol.* 38:3987–3998.

Keynote 522: Pembrolizumab for Early Triple-Negative Breast Cancer. P. Schmid, et al. *N Engl J Med.* 2020;382:810–21.

OlympiA: Adjuvant Olaparib for Patients with *BRCA1-* or *BRCA2*-Mutated Breast Cancer A.N.J. Tutt, et al, *N Engl J Med.* 2021 June 24; 384(25): 2394–2405.

REFERENCES

1. Early Breast Cancer Trialists' Collaborative Group (EBCTCG). Effects of chemotherapy and hormonal therapy for early breast cancer on recurrence and 15-year survival: an overview of the randomised trials. *Lancet.* 2005;365(9472):1687–717.
2. Volkova M, Russell R 3rd. Anthracycline cardiotoxicity: prevalence, pathogenesis and treatment. *Curr Cardiol Rev.* 2011;7(4):214–20.
3. Berry DA, Cirrincione C, Henderson IC, Citron ML, Budman DR, Goldstein LJ, et al. Estrogen-receptor status and outcomes of modern chemotherapy for patients with node-positive breast cancer. *JAMA.* 2006;295(14):1658–67.

Adjuvant Capecitabine for Breast Cancer after Preoperative Chemotherapy: CREATE-X

Masuda N, Lee S-J, Ohtani S, Im Y-H, Lee E-S, Yokota I, et al.
N Engl J Med 376:2147–2159, 2017

Residual disease following neoadjuvant chemotherapy (NACT) is considered a prognostic indicator for disease recurrence and reduced survival rates, when compared to achieving a pathological complete response (pCR), which is associated with a favourable outcome. In patients with *HER2*-negative disease, options for additional systemic therapy are limited, particularly in cases of triple-negative breast cancer (TNBC) where endocrine therapy is ineffective. Capecitabine, an oral prodrug of fluorouracil, has been utilised in the treatment of metastatic breast cancer and various other solid cancers. Previous trials investigating adjuvant therapy involving capecitabine, in combination with other chemotherapeutic agents for breast cancer, failed to demonstrate significant survival benefits. The Capecitabine for Residual Cancer as Adjuvant Therapy (CREATE X) trial has re-established capecitabine as a valuable tool for managing patients with residual breast cancer after previous NACT for women who have not had a pCR.[1] The study is one of several practice-changing trials showing that biological response to NACT can be used to tailor therapy to target resistant disease and so improve outcomes.

PAPER DESCRIPTION

- **Objective**: The objective of this study was to assess the effectiveness and safety of adjuvant capecitabine monotherapy in patients with *HER2*-negative primary breast cancer who have residual invasive disease after NACT.

- **Design**: The CREATE X trial was a multicentre, open-label, Phase III randomised controlled trial. The participants were randomly allocated with a 1:1 ratio to either capecitabine in combination with standard therapy or standard therapy alone. Standard therapy included endocrine therapy in oestrogen receptor (ER)-positive patients and adjuvant radiotherapy. Balancing factors considered during randomisation included ER status, nodal status, age (≤ 50 or > 50), taxane use, 5-fluorouracil (5-FU) use and trial site. Follow-up was conducted at 6 months, and annual mammograms were performed at 12-monthly intervals. The primary end point of the study was disease-free survival (DFS), while secondary end points included overall survival (OS) and the incidence of adverse effects. The analysis was conducted based on an intention-to-treat approach for evaluating efficacy and a per-protocol analysis for sensitivity. Adverse effects were graded according to the National Cancer Institute Common Terminology Criteria for Adverse Events (NCICTCAE).[2]

- **Sample Size**: The study specified a sample size of 427 participants in each arm. A hazard ratio (HR) of 0.74 was determined, with a two-sided *p*-value of 0.05.

- **Inclusion Criteria**: The study included patients with *HER2*-negative primary breast cancer who had residual invasive disease (in the breast or nodes) after NACT containing anthracycline and/or a taxane. The inclusion criteria encompassed stage I to IIIB breast cancer, an Eastern Cooperative Oncology Group (ECOG) performance status of 0–1 and an age range of 20 to 74.

- **Exclusion Criteria**: Exclusion criteria consisted of bilateral breast cancer, multiple synchronous cancers and previous therapy involving 5-FU.

- **Intervention or Treatment Received**: Following surgery, the treatment group received oral capecitabine (1250 mg per square meter of body surface area, twice per day, on days 1 to 14) every 3 weeks for six or eight cycles. Concomitant postsurgical endocrine therapy and radiation therapy were permitted.

- **Results**: Between 2007 and 2012, a total of 910 patients were enrolled across centres in Japan and South Korea. Among them, 887 patients were included in the intention-to-treat analysis (443 patients in the capecitabine group and 444 in the control group).

    There were 844 patients included in the per-protocol analysis of drug safety.

    The demographic characteristics of the two groups were similar. The median age of the participants was 48 years (range = 25–74 years). Among the study population, 68% had ER-positive tumours, and 32% had TNBC. Endocrine therapy was used in 67%, and 70% received radiotherapy. A pre-specified interim efficacy analysis conducted in 2015 demonstrated that the primary end point was achieved, leading to the early termination of the trial. The median follow-up period was 3.6 years.

    The rate of DFS at 5 years was 74.1% in the capecitabine group versus 67.6% in the control group (HR = 0.70, 95% confidence interval

[CI] = 0.53–0.92, p = 0.01). The OS rate at 5 years was also higher in the capecitabine group than in the control group (89.2% vs. 83.9%, HR = 0.59, 95% CI = 0.39–0.90, p = 0.01). The survival benefits of capecitabine were greater in women with TNBC (DFS HR = 0.58, 95% CI = 0.39–0.87; OS HR = 0.52, 95% CI = 0.30–0.90).

Hand–foot syndrome was observed in 73.4% of the patients in the capecitabine group, primarily at grade 1–2 severity. Grade 3 hand–foot syndrome was seen in 11% of patients. Other adverse effects included diarrhoea, vomiting, fatigue, neutropenia and elevated liver enzymes. Overall, grade 3 toxicities were observed in 25.5% of patients in the capecitabine group, compared to 1.8% in the control group.

EXPERT COMMENTARY BY SOUDAMINI NAYAK, LYNDA WYLD AND JANET BROWN

Paper significance

The results of the CREATE X trial have generated high-quality evidence supporting the use of post-NACT adjuvant capecitabine monotherapy, demonstrating significant survival benefits for patients with stage II and III *HER2*-negative breast cancer. This finding holds particular value in the context of TNBC, where limited adjuvant systemic therapy options currently exist. Importantly, the trial design itself has highlighted the importance of identifying precise subgroups of breast cancer patients who are likely to benefit from specific treatments in future clinical trials. These findings contribute to the growing body of knowledge aimed at improving personalised treatment strategies and enhancing outcomes for breast cancer patients.

Paper limitations

Generalisability: The study population was predominantly Asian. Asian populations may have pharmacogenetics and pharmacokinetics different from other populations. This may limit generalisability to other populations and regions. There was a lack of clarity about the use of platinum-based chemotherapy.

Lack of blinding: The trial was an open-label study, meaning that both the participants and the investigators were aware of the treatment assignments. This lack of blinding could introduce potential bias in assessing outcomes and adverse effects.

Long-term outcomes and adverse effects: Long-term outcomes and potential late adverse effects of capecitabine therapy are awaited. Adverse effects like hand–foot syndrome are more frequent and may adversely affect the quality of life of patients who have already been exposed to NACT-related side effects.

Concerns about failure to declare financial conflicts of interest: Payments received from pharmaceutical companies in relation to this trial were allegedly not fully disclosed, even after the post-publication corrections.[3]

Applicability: This study was carried out before adjuvant/neoadjuvant immunotherapy and CDK4/6 inhibitors became the standard of care in TNBC and ER-positive breast cancer, respectively.

In context of the relevant current literature

Previous trials assessing adjuvant capecitabine have failed to demonstrate statistically significant survival benefits. One such randomised controlled trial, sponsored by Hoffmann-La Roche, compared the addition of capecitabine (X) to a standard regimen of doxorubicin (A) plus cyclophosphamide followed by docetaxel (T). This study included low-risk, slow-growing early breast cancer patients, and although it did not show an improvement in DFS due to low event rates, a positive trend in DFS (HR = 0.84) and OS (HR = 0.68) was observed at 5 years. Subgroup analysis focussing on TNBCs indicated better OS.[4]

In the FinXX trial, which enrolled 1,500 patients with high-risk/node-positive disease, participants were randomly assigned to receive standard chemotherapy with or without capecitabine.[5] While the results demonstrated a trend towards improved survival (HR = 0.70, 95% CI = 0.60–1.04, $p = 0.087$), the trial did not reach its primary end point. However, the 10-year results showed significant benefits in DFS (HR = 0.43, 95% CI = 0.24–0.79, $p = 0.007$) and OS (HR = 0.55, 95% CI = 0.32–0.96, $p = 0.037$), specifically in the TNBC subgroup receiving capecitabine.

The GEICAM/2003-10 trial conducted by the GEICAM Spanish Breast Cancer Group compared a postsurgical standard chemotherapy regimen with and without sequential capecitabine in node-positive operable breast cancers.[6] The results of this study demonstrated contrasting outcomes, with favourable DFS observed in the control arm (HR = 1.03). In other words, the addition of sequential capecitabine did not show significant improvement in DFS compared to the control group.

The GEICAM/2003-11_CIBOMA/2004-01 trial investigated the use of extended adjuvant capecitabine following standard chemotherapy in patients with early TNBC.[7] The study did not demonstrate a statistically significant improvement in DFS when adding extended capecitabine to standard chemotherapy for patients with early TNBC. However, in a preplanned subset analysis, patients with a non-basal phenotype appeared to derive benefit from capecitabine.

Although the aforementioned trials did not meet their primary end points, they suggested the potential benefits of adjuvant capecitabine in TNBC. However, the proportion of TNBC patients included in these trials was less than 15%, making them underpowered for analysis. In contrast, the CREATE X trial had a more enriched sample population, including only patients with nonpathological complete response (non-pCR) after NACT, with 32% TNBC patients.

In contrast to these trials, which had broader inclusion criteria encompassing various pathological staging and tumour biology, the CREATE X trial had more focussed inclusion criteria, specifically targeting high-risk non-pCR patients.

Conclusions

In patients with residual *HER2*-negative invasive disease in the breast or nodes after NACT, additional therapy with capecitabine may offer survival benefits. This is particularly true in women with TNCB.

REFERENCES

1. Masuda N, Lee S-J, Ohtani S, Im Y-H, Lee E-S, Yokota I, et al. Adjuvant Capecitabine for breast cancer after preoperative chemotherapy. *New Engl J Med*. 2017;376(22):2147–59. doi:10.1056/nejmoa1612645

2. Common terminology criteria for adverse events v3.0 (CTCAE) August 9, 2003. Available at: https://ctep.cancer.gov/protocoldevelopment/electronic_applications/docs/ctcaev3.pdf (Accessed: 19 May 2023).

3. Ozaki A, Saito H, Sawano T, ShimadaY, Tanimoto T., et al. Accuracy of post-publication Financial Conflict of Interest corrections in medical research: a secondary analysis of pharmaceutical company payments to the authors of the CREATE-X trial report in the *New England Journal of Medicine*. *Bioethics*. 2021;35(7):704–13. doi:10.1111/bioe.12854

4. O'Shaughnessy J, Koeppen H, Xiao Y, Lackner MR, Paul D, Stokoe C, et al. Patients with slowly proliferative early breast cancer have low five-year recurrence rates in a phase III adjuvant trial of Capecitabine. *Clin Cancer Res*. 2015;21(19):4305–11. doi:10.1158/1078-0432.ccr-15-0636

5. Joensuu H, Kellokumpu-Lehtinen PL, Huovinen R, Jukkola A, Tanner M, Ahlgren J, et al. Adjuvant Capecitabine, docetaxel, cyclophosphamide, and epirubicin for early breast cancer: final analysis of the randomized FINXX trial. *J Clin Oncol*. 2012;30(1):11–8. doi:10.1200/jco.2011.35.4639

6. Martín M, Ruiz Simón A, Borrego MR, N, Rodríguez-Lescure Á, Muñoz-Mateu M, et al. Epirubicin plus cyclophosphamide followed by docetaxel versus epirubicin plus docetaxel followed by Capecitabine as adjuvant therapy for node-positive early breast cancer: results from the GEICAM/2003-10 study. *J Clin Oncol*. 2015;33(32):3788–95. doi:10.1200/jco.2015.61.9510

7. Lluch A, Barrios CH, Torrecillas L, Ruiz-Borrego M, Bines J, Segalla J, et al. Phase III trial of Adjuvant Capecitabine after standard Neo-/adjuvant chemotherapy in patients with early triple-negative breast cancer (GEICAM/2003-11_CIBOMA/2004-01). *J Clin Oncol*. 2020;38(3):203–13. doi:10.1200/jco.19.00904

CHAPTER 31

Relevance of Breast Cancer Hormone Receptors and Other Factors to the Efficacy of Adjuvant Tamoxifen: Patient-Level Meta-Analysis of Randomised Trials

Early Breast Cancer Trialists' Collaborative Group (EBCTCG).
Lancet 378:771–784, 2011

PAPER DESCRIPTION

- **Objective**: This paper is a collaborative meta-analysis assessing the impact of adjuvant tamoxifen on disease recurrence and death rates in early breast cancer.

- **Design**: The Early Breast Cancer Trialists' Collaborative Group (EBCTCG) was founded in 1985 and is based in Oxford. It involves almost every major international triallist who has undertaken randomised trials in breast cancer treatment. Triallists send patient-level data to the group periodically to allow the most definitive analysis of treatment effects. This publication is a meta-analysis of individual patient data from 20 trials in early breast cancer assessing the impact of adjuvant tamoxifen on disease recurrence and death rates.

- **Sample Size**: Data are included on 21,457 individual patients from 20 different trials.

- **Inclusion Criteria**: Women with early breast cancer treated with definitive surgery were included from trials of adjuvant tamoxifen versus no endocrine treatment, in which only the use of tamoxifen differed. Only trials with treatment duration longer than 2 years were included. Women were classified as oestrogen receptor (ER)-positive (≥10 fmol/mg of cytosol protein) or ER-negative (<10 fmol/mg).

- **Exclusion Criteria**: Trials in women with ductal carcinoma in situ were excluded.

DOI: 10.1201/b23352-31

- **Intervention or Treatment Received**: All women were randomly assigned evenly between adjuvant tamoxifen and the control group (no endocrine therapy).

- **Results**: Compliance with tamoxifen therapy was 69–86%, with a weighted mean of 82%. In ER-positive disease, the use of tamoxifen reduced the recurrence rate by half during years 0–4 and reduced the recurrence rate by a third during years 5–9. There was no difference after 10 years in recurrence rate. This equates to a total recurrence rate reduction of 39% (relative risk [RR] = 0.61, $p < 0.00001$). Analysis for breast cancer mortality showed a substantial mortality reduction in the tamoxifen group continuing beyond 10 years (RR during ≥10 years = 0.73, $p < 0.00001$). Interestingly, this mortality reduction had significant extra benefit throughout each of the time period categories, with an absolute mortality difference of 3% at 5 years (mortality 9% in the tamoxifen group vs. 12% in the control group) but increasing with time to triple that by 15 years (24% vs. 33%). Thus, the recurrence reduction in years 0–9 caused a highly significant reduction in breast cancer mortality during and after years 0–9. In ER-negative disease, the use of tamoxifen had no effect on recurrence.

  ER status and progesterone receptor (PR) status were strongly associated (PR was positive in 76% of ER-positive cases and only 21% of ER-negative disease). However, PR status was not predictive of response to tamoxifen in total or for ER-positive or ER-negative subgroups, and was not further investigated.

  Importantly, the level of ER positivity did not affect the strength of the protective effect. Even for weakly positive ER (ER = 10–19 fmol/mg), there was a substantial benefit (RR = 0.67), and the proportional effect at the highest levels of ER-positive (≥200 fmol/mg) was only marginally better (RR = 0.52).

  This work demonstrated that tamoxifen was of further substantial benefit even if chemotherapy had been given, producing a further reduction of a quarter in the 10-year recurrence risk. For patients receiving chemotherapy, the benefit of tamoxifen was slightly higher if it was started concurrently with chemotherapy rather than after; however, this was not statistically significant, and these trials did not randomise for tamoxifen timing.

  The risk of recurrence was reduced in a small but significant way in higher tamoxifen doses ($p = 0.02$ for the trend of RRs for 20 mg, 30 mg and 40 mg daily doses), but there was no dose effect found for breast cancer mortality or endometrial cancer incidence.

  In terms of length of tamoxifen treatment, reductions in recurrence and mortality in years 0–4 were similar between tamoxifen for 1–2 years and for 5 years. However, the reduction in recurrence during years 5–9 was greater in trials of tamoxifen with a duration of 5 years.

From these studies, the main life-threatening side effects of tamoxifen were uterine cancer and thromboembolic disease. There were nine deaths in the tamoxifen group from uterine cancer, compared to one in the control group. There were six deaths from pulmonary embolus (PE) in the tamoxifen group versus zero in the control group. There were no other differences in the 'mortality without recurrence' group. Tamoxifen increased uterine cancer incidence (RR = 2.4, p = 0.00002). It also reduced contralateral breast cancer incidence. There was no effect on other types of cancer. These protective and adverse effects persisted for some years after treatment ended. Of note, the uterine cancer risk and excess risk of fatal PE were strongly correlated with age, with little absolute risk for the age category <54 years old. By contrast, the reduction in contralateral breast cancers was independent of age.

EXPERT COMMENTARY BY FIONA JAMES AND TOM HUBBARD

Paper significance

Although the aims were to investigate all patients who had received 5 years of adjuvant tamoxifen, this was not precisely the case. Some patients from the control arm will have been switched to receive tamoxifen as evidence for its superiority arose in later trials, and so the finding that there was a significantly greater mortality reduction with 5 years of tamoxifen compared to only 2 years may truly be stronger than suggested. In addition, the treatment effects of receiving 5 years of tamoxifen may be underestimated, as one-sixth of the treated patients in the trials were only allocated 2–3 years of tamoxifen, and of those allocated to 5 years of tamoxifen, 18% had discontinued treatment within 2 years.

Age was not correlated with recurrence risk or tamoxifen efficacy, but being young is a major determinant of gain in life expectancy from avoidance of recurrence. Half of patients diagnosed with breast cancer were under 55 years at diagnosis, and for these women with ER-positive disease, tamoxifen is a major hormonal treatment option,[1] and there is little excess risk of uterine cancer or fatal PE in this age category. By contrast, in older women, the risk of excess death from uterine cancer or PE is around 1%, although in modern practice these older women will largely be postmenopausal and therefore be treated with aromatase inhibitors in modern treatment protocols.

This study evidenced the substantial benefit of tamoxifen in weakly ER-positive disease and confirmed no benefit of tamoxifen in ER-negative disease. The ER status was the only tumour or patient characteristic that strongly predicted tamoxifen efficacy. Reassuringly, the cutoff used in most guidelines and trials is that used in this analysis to determine ER positivity (10 fmol/mg, equivalent to an Allred immunohistochemistry [IHC] score of ≥2/8).[2,3]

Paper limitations

One of the main limitations of the study is its applicability to current prescribing practices. Around half of the women included in the study were <55 years of age, with no subgroup analysis according to menopausal status. Tamoxifen is the main endocrine therapy for premenopausal women, but aromatase inhibitors are the mainstay of treatment for postmenopausal women. Therefore, around half of the women (older, postmenopausal women with less to gain in life expectancy) analysed in the study would likely have not been given tamoxifen in current treatment regimes. Treatment options for endocrine therapy are increasingly nuanced and guided by tumour biology, with options for endocrine therapy switching[4] and extended therapy,[5] so the proportion of patients to whom the study outcomes apply is diminishing.

Conclusions

This longer follow-up of trials of tamoxifen use has added to the previous evidence that adjuvant tamoxifen use substantially reduces recurrence and mortality rates for ER-positive breast cancer and that this effect continues well beyond 10 years. This effect is also independent of age, nodal status, tumour grade, tumour size and chemotherapy use. Due to this strong evidence base, tamoxifen is currently recommended for adjuvant endocrine therapy for premenopausal women with ER-positive breast cancer in UK[6] and US guidelines.[7]

REFERENCES

1. Fisher B, Costantino JP, Wickerham DL, Cecchini RS, Cronin WM, Robidoux A, et al. Tamoxifen for the prevention of breast cancer: current status of the National Surgical Adjuvant Breast and Bowel Project P-1 study. *J Natl Cancer Inst.* 2005;97:1652–62.
2. Harvey JM, Clark GM, Osborne CK, Allred DC. Estrogen receptor status by immunohistochemistry is superior to the ligand-binding assay for predicting response to adjuvant endocrine therapy in breast cancer. *J Clin Oncol.* 1999;17:1474–81.
3. Early Breast Cancer Trialists' Collaborative Group. Effects of chemotherapy and hormonal therapy for early breast cancer on recurrence and 15-year survival: an overview of the randomised trials. *Lancet.* 2005;365:1687–717.
4. Coombes R, Kilburn L, Snowdon C, Paridaens R, Coleman R, Jones S, et al. Survival and safety of exemestane versus tamoxifen after 2–3 years' tamoxifen treatment (Intergroup Exemestane Study): a randomised controlled trial. *Lancet.* 2007;369:559–70.
5. Davies C, Pan H, Godwin J, Gray R, Arriagada R, Raina V, et al. Long-term effects of continuing adjuvant tamoxifen to 10 years versus stopping at 5 years after diagnosis of oestrogen receptor-positive breast cancer: ATLAS, a randomised trial. *Lancet.* 2013;381:805–16.

6. National Institute for Health and Care Excellence (NICE). Early and locally advanced breast cancer: diagnosis and management [NG101] [Internet]. NICE; 2018 [Accessed 08/07/2023]. Available from: https://www.nice.org.uk/guidance/ng101.

7. Burstein HJ, Temin S, Anderson H, Buchholz TA, Davidson NE, Gelmon KE, et al. Adjuvant endocrine therapy for women with hormone receptor–positive breast cancer: American Society of Clinical Oncology clinical practice guideline focused update. *J Clin Oncol.* 2014;32:2255.

CHAPTER 32

Long-Term Effects of Continuing Adjuvant Tamoxifen to 10 Years versus Stopping at 5 Years after Diagnosis of Oestrogen Receptor–Positive Breast Cancer: ATLAS, a Randomised Trial

Davies C, Pan H, Godwin J, et al.
Lancet 9869:805–816, 2013

PAPER DESCRIPTION

- **Objective/Research Question**: Does 10 years of adjuvant tamoxifen have superior outcomes (breast cancer recurrence and mortality) compared to 5 years of adjuvant tamoxifen?

- **Design**: International trial from 36 countries recruited between 1996 and 2005. Software allocated eligible women randomly 1:1 to treatment arms of 5 years versus 10 years of tamoxifen. There was no placebo arm. Randomisation was minimised 1:1 to balance allocation by country or region and major prognostic factors (age, nodal status, tumour diameter and oestrogen receptor [ER] status).

- **Sample Size**: A total of 15,244 women were randomly allocated to continue tamoxifen for another 5 years or stop immediately. However, not all were included in the analysis: 2,350 were excluded completely, as the tamoxifen duration before allocation was <4 years, and 6,048 had unknown or negative ER status. Ultimately, 6,846 patients with ER-positive disease were included for analysis; 3,428 continued on tamoxifen to 10 years (intervention), and 3,418 stopped tamoxifen at 5 years (control).

  There were 12,894 women included in the analysis of side effects.

- **Inclusion Criteria**:
  1. Women with early breast cancer (where all detected disease could be removed)
  2. Taking adjuvant tamoxifen for between 4 and 5 years (or had stopped in the past year and could resume treatment)

DOI: 10.1201/b23352-32

3. Clinically disease free (any local recurrence removed)
4. No restrictions on age, initial surgery or histology, hormone receptor status, nodal status or other treatments

- **Exclusion Criteria**: Tamoxifen contraindicated (clinician assessed).

- **Intervention or Treatment Received**: Tamoxifen 20 mg per day for either 5 years (control group) or 10 years (intervention group). All other treatment was at clinicians' discretion. There was no additional follow-up, but clinicians were sent a form asking about endocrine therapy compliance, recurrence, new primary, hospital admissions and, if death, cause of death. Completeness of follow-up was similar for both treatment arms, which was 77% at 15 years since diagnosis.

- **Results**: In all the main outcomes, continuing tamoxifen for 10 years (intervention) had better outcomes than stopping tamoxifen at 5 years (control). The intervention group had a lower risk of recurrence (617/3,428 [18%] intervention vs. 711/3,418 [21%] control, relative risk [RR] = 0.84, 95% confidence interval [CI] = 0.76–0.94, $p = 0.002$), reduced breast cancer mortality (331/3,428 [9.66%] intervention vs. 397/3,418 [11.6%] control, $p = 0.01$) and reduced overall mortality (deaths: 639/3,428 [18.6%] intervention vs. 722/3,418 [21.1%] control, $p = 0.01$). When comparing the intervention with the control group, there was an absolute reduction in risk of recurrence of 3.7% and breast cancer mortality of 2.8%.

  The main effects on recurrence and breast cancer mortality became apparent in the second decade, in keeping with the previous trials of tamoxifen which showed that much of the benefit is derived after completion of the endocrine treatment course.[1] Subgroup analysis of factors affecting recurrence showed that risk reduction was similar across patients, tumour characteristics and sites of first recurrence.

  Side effects can be significant with endocrine treatment and lead to early discontinuation. At year 7 after diagnosis, 84% of those in the intervention group (i.e., allocated to 10 years of tamoxifen) were still taking tamoxifen, and 4% of the control group (who should have stopped treatment after 5 years) were still on tamoxifen. The compliance in the intervention group reduced to around 60% by year 10.

  The risk of serious side effects was significantly increased in the intervention arm for pulmonary embolus (RR = 1.87, 95% CI = 1.13–3.07, $p = 0.01$) and endometrial cancer (RR = 1.74, 95% CI = 1.30–2.34, $p < 0.01$). The cumulative risk of endometrial cancer was 3.1% intervention versus 1.6% control, but there was no statistically significant difference in mortality. The risk of ischaemic heart disease was significantly lower in the intervention arm (RR = 0.75, 95% CI = 0.60–0.95, $p = 0.02$). However, the authors concluded this may be a chance finding since the apparent protection was seen beyond the treatment period and no significant protection against heart disease was seen in trials of tamoxifen versus no tamoxifen.[1]

EXPERT COMMENTARY BY FIONA JAMES AND TOM HUBBARD

Paper significance

This trial demonstrated that continuing tamoxifen beyond 5 years to 10 years provides further protection against breast cancer recurrence and breast cancer mortality.

Paper limitations

The main limitation is its applicability to current practice of patients receiving tamoxifen. The Adjuvant Tamoxifen: Longer Against Shorter (ATLAS) trial suggested that extended tamoxifen was beneficial regardless of age and menopausal status. However, around 50% of women in the trial were over 55, and over 90% were postmenopausal. Given that premenopausal women are more likely to receive tamoxifen, it is possible that the treatment effects reported may not directly relate to this patient group since they make up such a small proportion in this study.

There were some limitations in the design of the trial, particularly that their planned recruitment was 20,000 women but only 15,000 were recruited (due to the publication of the MA.17 trial), and of these, only 6,000 ended up being suitable for analysis. At the time of recruitment, over 2,000 patients had taken tamoxifen for less than 4 years and would have been randomised to stop, so these were excluded. There were also over 6,000 who had an unknown ER status. This resulted in a large number of patients being recruited to the trial but not analysed.

Similar to other endocrine treatment studies, adherence was around 80%, and meta-analysis suggests that 'real-life' (i.e., outside of clinical trial) adherence with endocrine therapy is much lower (41–72%) at 5 years,[2] and is likely to further decrease with a 10-year course. Analysis was done on an intention-to-treat basis, so the true benefits of tamoxifen for people actually taking the treatment may be greater than reported, though this is also true for any adverse effects.

In context of the relevant current literature

It had been established through multiple randomised controlled trials and the Early Breast Cancer Trialists' Collaborative Group (EBCTCG) meta-analysis that for women with ER-positive breast cancer, adjuvant treatment with tamoxifen for 5 years reduced breast cancer mortality by about a third,[1] with benefit at 15 years of follow-up. Some trials had investigated shorter courses of tamoxifen (1–2 years) which were shown to be inferior to a 5-year course, so the question was therefore whether a longer course of treatment (10 years) would have a greater effect on breast cancer recurrence and mortality. Earlier trials examining extended tamoxifen therapy recruited relatively few patients and had insufficient follow-up,[3] particularly given that adjuvant tamoxifen had been shown to have a prolonged carryover effect after treatment cessation.

The UK-based multicentre Adjuvant Tamoxifen—To Offer More? (aTTom) trial[4] had randomised 7,000 women to continue tamoxifen to 10 years versus stopping at 5 years; however, at the time of publishing ATLAS, the long-term data were not mature. The aTTOm trial included a third (2,755 of 6,953) of women confirmed as ER-positive, with the remainder untested. This differs from ATLAS, since the ER-untested women were not included in the analysis. The aTTOm trial had broadly similar results to ATLAS: 10 years of tamoxifen was shown to reduce breast cancer recurrence, breast cancer mortality and overall mortality which was time dependent (i.e., the effect was seen in years 5–9). Subsequently, aTTom has reported trans-aTTom[5] (looking at histological predictors of those who may benefit from extended endocrine therapy) and is undertaking further tissue analysis in trans-aTTom which is yet to report.

Another highly relevant trial of extended adjuvant endocrine therapy was the MA.17 trial.[6] This was a randomised, double-blind, placebo-controlled trial of over 5,000 women investigating whether treatment with letrozole for 5 years, after patients had already received 5 years of tamoxifen, benefited postmenopausal women with ER-positive or unknown breast cancer. This study demonstrated that treatment with letrozole after 5 years of tamoxifen resulted in improvement in disease-free survival and that the rate of death due to breast cancer was almost halved. This interim analysis of the MA.17 trial halted the trial and stopped further recruitment to ATLAS, which posed difficulties in interpretation of results for both trials.

Within ATLAS, the increased risks of pulmonary embolus and endometrial cancer were significant in the intervention arm, but this must be considered in the context that the majority of patients within the trial were postmenopausal with a higher natural risk of these conditions. Aromatase Inhibitors are now the standard adjuvant endocrine treatment for postmenopausal women, who are most at risk of these tamoxifen-related side effects. Therefore, premenopausal women who are at higher risk of breast cancer recurrence have the most to gain from 10 years of tamoxifen, but with a lower risk of these side effects.

Conclusions

The ATLAS trial was a significant trial demonstrating that extending adjuvant tamoxifen to 10 years decreased both the risk of breast cancer recurrence and mortality. It did not identify if any subgroups of patients may benefit more than others from such extended therapy. The study influenced treatment and guidelines internationally, with consideration for recommending extended therapy (beyond 5 years) with tamoxifen being recommended in current UK[7] and US[8] guidelines, for those patients already on tamoxifen therapy.

Relevant additional papers

Abstract of an EBCTCG meta-analysis of extended endocrine therapy:

Gray, Richard, and Early Breast Cancer Trialists' Collaborative Group. "Abstract GS3-03: Effects of prolonging adjuvant aromatase inhibitor therapy beyond five years on recurrence and cause-specific mortality: An EBCTCG meta-analysis of individual patient data from 12 randomised trials including 24,912 women." *Cancer Research* 79, no. 4_Supplement (2019): GS3-03.

Association of Breast Surgery guidelines for endocrine treatment for breast cancer:

Association of Breast Surgery. Best Practice Guidelines: Endocrine treatment for breast cancer. 2020. Accessed 24/05/2023. (Internet) https://associationof-breastsurgery.org.uk/media/332034/abs-endocrine-guidance-2021-v1.pdf

REFERENCES

1. Early Breast Cancer Trialists' Collaborative Group. Relevance of breast cancer hormone receptors and other factors to the efficacy of adjuvant tamoxifen: patient-level meta-analysis of randomised trials. *Lancet.* 2011;378:771–784.
2. Murphy CC, Bartholomew LK, Carpentier MY, Bluethmann SM, Vernon SW. Adherence to adjuvant hormonal therapy among breast cancer survivors in clinical practice: a systematic review. *Breast Cancer Res Treat.* 2012;134:459–78.
3. Fisher B, Dignam J, Bryant J, DeCillis A, Wickerham DL, Wolmark N, et al. Five versus more than five years of tamoxifen therapy for breast cancer patients with negative lymph nodes and estrogen receptor-positive tumors. *J Natl Cancer Inst.* 1996;88:1529–42.
4. Gray RG, Rea D, Handley K, Bowden SJ, Perry P, Earl HM, et al. aTTom: Long-term effects of continuing adjuvant tamoxifen to 10 years versus stopping at 5 years in 6,953 women with early breast cancer. *American Society of Clinical Oncology.* 2013.
5. Bartlett J, Sgroi D, Treuner K, Zhang Y, Ahmed I, Piper T, et al. Breast Cancer Index and prediction of benefit from extended endocrine therapy in breast cancer patients treated in the Adjuvant Tamoxifen—To Offer More?(aTTom) trial. *Ann Oncol.* 2019;30:1776–83.
6. Goss PE, Ingle JN, Martino S, Robert NJ, Muss HB, Piccart MJ, et al. A randomized trial of letrozole in postmenopausal women after five years of tamoxifen therapy for early-stage breast cancer. *New Engl J Med.* 2003;349:1793–802.
7. National Institute for Health and Care Excellence (NICE). Early and locally advanced breast cancer: diagnosis and management [NG101] [Internet]. NICE; 2018 [Accessed 24/01/2019]. Available from: https://www.nice.org.uk/guidance/ng101.
8. Burstein HJ, Temin S, Anderson H, Buchholz TA, Davidson NE, Gelmon KE, et al. Adjuvant endocrine therapy for women with hormone receptor–positive breast cancer: American Society of Clinical Oncology clinical practice guideline focused update. *J Clin Oncol.* 2014;32:2255.

CHAPTER 33

Tailoring Adjuvant Endocrine Therapy for Premenopausal Breast Cancer

Francis PA, Pagani O, Fleming GF, et al.
N Engl J Med 379:122–137, 2018

PAPER DESCRIPTION

- **Objective/Research Question**: This paper reports the updated results from two landmark trials investigating the difference in recurrence rates between the use of tamoxifen alone, tamoxifen plus ovarian suppression or the aromatase inhibitor exemestane plus ovarian suppression in premenopausal women undergoing definitive treatment for early breast cancer. These studies are the Suppression of Ovarian Function Trial (SOFT) and Tamoxifen and Exemestane Trial (TEXT).[1] These were initiated by the International Breast Cancer Study Group in 2003 to address the value of adding ovarian suppression or using an aromatase inhibitor, to build on the evidence that adjuvant treatment with tamoxifen reduces the recurrence of premenopausal oestrogen receptor (ER)-positive breast cancer, with increasing benefits of extending treatment duration.[2]

- **Design**: This paper reports on two large, multicentre, randomised controlled trials.

- **Sample Size**: After exclusions, 3,047 were included in SOFT and 2,660 in TEXT, making a combined intention-to-treat population of 4,690.

- **Inclusion Criteria**: Both trials included women with operable breast cancer positive for ERs (in at least 10% of cells). In SOFT, these women had to be premenopausal after chemotherapy; in TEXT, they included anyone who was premenopausal at diagnosis, including those who were rendered postmenopausal after chemotherapy. The use of chemotherapy, radiotherapy and *HER2*-targeted treatment was not mandated and was according to accepted guidelines.

- **Exclusion Criteria:** Pre-menopausal after surgery or chemotherapy (whichever was the later). Either distant metastases, involved margins, residual axillary disease, prior breast cancer or other cancers (save BCC, SCC or in-situ breast/cervical), bilateral breast cancers and either locally advanced or inflammatory cancers. Prior bilateral ovarian radiotherapy or oophrectomy (or anticpiating having that within 5 years). Either lactating or pregnant, on HRT or already taking endocrine therapy.

- **Intervention or Treatment Received**: In SOFT, women were randomised to receive tamoxifen 20 mg per day, tamoxifen 20 mg per day plus ovarian suppression, or exemestane 25 mg per day plus ovarian suppression in a 1:1:1 ratio for 5 years. Randomisation was stratified according to chemotherapy use, lymph node status, institution and intended method of ovarian suppression (triptorelin, bilateral oophorectomy or ovarian irradiation). In TEXT, women were randomised to receive exemestane plus ovarian suppression by triptorelin or tamoxifen with triptorelin in a 1:1 ratio for a duration of 5 years.

- **Results**: These results are a pre-specified update analysis of SOFT and TEXT after a median follow-up of 8 and 9 years, respectively. From SOFT, the 8-year rate of disease-free survival for tamoxifen plus ovarian suppression was 83.2%, which is significantly better than the 78.9% rate for tamoxifen alone (hazard ratio [HR] = 0.76, 95% confidence interval [CI] = 0.62–0.93, $p = 0.009$). The 8-year rate of disease-free survival for exemestane plus ovarian suppression was 85.9%, a 7% improvement compared to tamoxifen alone (HR = 0.65, 95% CI = 0.53–0.81). In the combined analysis, the disease-free survival rate was significantly higher in the exemestane plus ovarian suppression group at 86.8%, compared to the tamoxifen plus ovarian suppression group at 82.8% (HR = 0.77, 95% CI = 0.67–0.90, $p < 0.001$).

  Within the specified outcome of disease-free recurrence, it can be argued that the most clinically relevant in terms of morbidity and mortality is distant recurrence, compared to local recurrence, locoregional recurrence, contralateral breast cancer or death by any cause, at this early time point. Considering this, the risk of distant recurrence was significantly lower in those receiving exemestane plus ovarian suppression, with a distant recurrence–free survival rate of 91.8% in comparison with tamoxifen plus ovarian suppression at 89.7% (HR = 0.8, 95% CI = 0.66–0.96, $p = 0.02$). Distant recurrence occurred in 433 women (9.2%), and the majority of these cases were in those who received chemotherapy (87.8%).

  In subgroup analysis, the only treatment heterogeneity was according to *HER2* status, where the improvement in disease-free survival with exemestane plus ovarian suppression compared to tamoxifen plus ovarian suppression was much bigger in *HER2*-negative disease than in other groups.

  In terms of treatment toxicity, early discontinuation of endocrine treatment occurred in 22.5% of the tamoxifen-alone group, 19.3% of the tamoxifen plus ovarian suppression group and 23.7% of the exemestane plus ovarian suppression group. Adverse events of grade 3 toxicity (which usually requires hospitalisation) or higher occurred in 24.6% of the tamoxifen group, 31.0% of the tamoxifen plus ovarian suppression group and 32.3% of the exemestane plus ovarian suppression group. The adverse events overrepresented in the ovarian suppression groups were musculoskeletal symptoms, osteoporosis, hypertension and glucose control problems.

EXPERT COMMENTARY BY FIONA JAMES
AND DOUGLAS FERGUSON

Paper significance

Prior to this paper, the best evidence available on the subject was the 5-year SOFT report showing that the addition of ovarian suppression to tamoxifen did not result in a significant improvement in disease-free survival.[3] This updated analysis of SOFT showed that after a longer follow-up period, tamoxifen plus ovarian suppression resulted in an absolute difference of 4.2% lower risk of recurrence, a second invasive cancer or death than tamoxifen alone. Exemestane plus ovarian suppression resulted in even higher rates of disease-free survival, with an absolute difference of 7.0% compared to tamoxifen alone. The combined trial analysis update showed that exemestane plus ovarian suppression resulted in sustained and higher rates of disease-free survival than tamoxifen and ovarian suppression. The longer follow-up period (pre-planned) enabled the identification of the known persisting endocrine treatment benefit after the active treatment period had finished, and it enabled the outcome differences between the treatment regimens to become clear. The rates of adverse events with ovarian suppression were much higher than for tamoxifen alone.

Paper limitations

Participants were analysed in an intention-to-treat analysis, so with the high, but consistent, rates of endocrine therapy discontinuation (19–24%), both the impact on disease-free survival and the toxicities are likely to be underestimated. Another limitation was that some women received subtherapeutic ovarian suppression in the SOFT trial, with the SOFT-EST sub-study revealing that in the first year of the study, at each time point analysed, at least 17% of patients had levels greater than the oestradiol threshold set for successful ovarian oestrogen suppression.[4]

Weighing these data, the potential benefits from ovarian suppression and exemestane must be balanced with the increased rates of toxicity, and an individual personalised decision must be made for each patient. Some groups will gain more benefit than others from intensifying adjuvant endocrine therapy; these include women younger than 35 years, women deemed to have a high enough risk of recurrence to receive adjuvant chemotherapy and women with higher risk HER2-negative disease. Longer follow-up data will be needed to robustly confirm these findings and assess their impact on survival and late adverse events.

In context of the relevant current literature

Conclusions

This paper concluded that adding ovarian suppression to tamoxifen resulted in significantly higher rates of disease-free survival, with further improvement seen with exemestane plus ovarian suppression. For patients who have high-risk *HER2*-negative cancer, the absolute benefits of exemestane plus ovarian suppression in reduction in recurrence (particularly distant) make this combination worthy of use in clinical practice. In women who are deemed to be at sufficient risk for recurrence to receive adjuvant chemotherapy, and who remained premenopausal after chemotherapy, ovarian suppression results in clinically meaningful benefits in disease-free survival. This conclusion has been translated into clinical guidelines (National Institute for Health and Care Excellence [NICE][5] and European Society for Medical Oncology [ESMO][6]) and confirmed in a further large meta-analysis which included two other important trials (Austrian Breast Cancer Study Group [ABCSG] XII[7] and Hormonal Bone Effects [HOBOE][8]).[9] The further planned late follow-up analysis should add further weight to these findings.

REFERENCES

1. Regan, et al. Adjuvant treatment of premenopausal women with endocrine-responsive early breast cancer: design of the TEXT and SOFT trials. *Breast*. 2013;22:1094–100.
2. Goldhirsch A, et al. Meeting highlights: International Consensus Panel on the Treatment of Primary Breast Cancer. *J Clin Oncol*. 2001;19:3817–27.
3. Francis PA, et al. Adjuvant ovarian suppression in premenopausal breast cancer. *N Engl J Med*. 2015;372:436–46.
4. Bellet, et al. Twelve-month estrogen levels in premenopausal women with hormone receptor-positive breast cancer receiving adjuvant triptorelin plus exemestane or tamoxifen in the suppression of ovarian function trial (SOFT): the SOFT-EST substudy. *J Clin Oncol*. 2016; 34(14):1584–93.
5. https://www.nice.org.uk/guidance/ng101/evidence/evidence-review-d-endocrine-therapy-pdf-4904666609
6. Paluch-Shimon, et al. ESOeESMO 4th International Consensus Guidelines for Breast Cancer in Young Women (BCY4). *Ann Oncol*. 2020.
7. Gnant, et al. Adjuvant endocrine therapy plus zoledronic acid in premenopausal women with early-stage breast cancer: 62-month follow-up from the ABCSG-12 randomised trial. *Lancet Oncol*. 2011;12(7):631–41.
8. Perrone, et al. Adjuvant zoledronic acid and letrozole plus ovarian function suppression in premenopausal breast cancer: HOBOE phase 3 randomised trial. *Eur J Cancer*. 2019;118:178–86.
9. Early Breast Cancer Trialists' Collaborative Group (EBCTCG). Aromatase inhibitors versus tamoxifen in premenopausal women with oestrogen receptor-positive early-stage breast cancer treated with ovarian suppression: a patient-level meta-analysis of 7030 women from four randomised trials. *Lancet Oncol*. 2022;23:382–92.

CHAPTER 34

Anastrozole Alone or in Combination with Tamoxifen versus Tamoxifen Alone for Adjuvant Treatment of Postmenopausal Women with Early Breast Cancer: First Results of the ATAC Randomised Trial

Arimidex, Tamoxifen, Alone or in Combination; ATAC Trialists' Group.
Lancet 359(9324):2131–2139, 2002

PAPER DESCRIPTION

- **Objective/Research Question**: To compare the safety and efficacy of an aromatase inhibitor (AI), anastrozole, with those of tamoxifen alone and the combination of anastrozole plus tamoxifen for 5 years, as adjuvant treatment in postmenopausal women with early, operable, hormone receptor–positive breast cancer.

  Safety outcomes were adverse side effects from anastrozole and tamoxifen either alone or in combination.

  The efficacy measure was disease-free survival (DFS) at 5 years.

- **Design**: This was a multicentre randomised controlled trial across 23 countries. Block randomisation (size 6) was utilised (**Figure 34.1**), with patients being randomised in a 1:1:1 ratio. Standard dosing of tamoxifen (20 mg) and anastrozole (1 mg) was utilised.

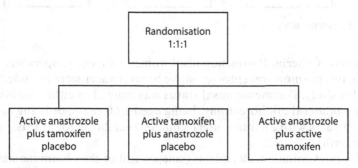

Figure 34.1 Randomisation.

DOI: 10.1201/b23352-34

Assessments were made at 3 months, at 6 months, then 6-monthly for 5 years and then annually for up to 10 years.

Baseline characteristics of patients, tumours and primary treatment were similar across all three arms. Patients with N2 disease (across three arms 10.4%, 9.1% and 9.2%) and T3 tumours (across three arms 2.7%, 2.2% and 2.3%) were included with early breast cancer patients.

Hormone positivity was defined as positivity for either oestrogen or progesterone receptors according to local cutoff values, but hormone receptor–negative tumours were also included in the analysis, although there was equal spread across the three arms (8.3%, 8.7% and 7.6%).

The study was powered to 90%, and the necessary sample size was achieved. Statistical analysis was on an intention-to-treat basis using a log-rank test, and Cox's proportional hazards were used for baseline characteristics, with a nominal p-value of 0.048 used to ensure a true 5% significance level.

- **Sample Size**: The primary end point of DFS was used to calculate the sample size. The study was powered to 90%, and for non-inferiority to be concluded between anastrozole and tamoxifen, 352 events per group were required from 9,000 patients, and this was achieved (**Figure 34.2**).

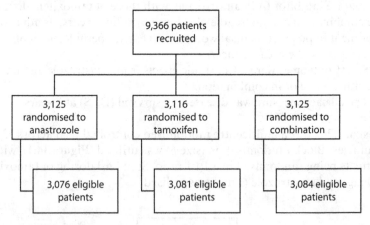

Figure 34.2 Sample size.

- **Inclusion Criteria**: Postmenopausal women with early, operable, invasive, hormone receptor–positive breast cancer were included in this study. Postmenopausal status was defined as either having had a bilateral oophorectomy, being aged ≥ 60 years, or being aged 45–59 years with an intact uterus but amenorrhoeic for at least 12 months.

On randomisation, all patients (independent of their hormone status) were included since, at the time, hormone receptor–negative patients were felt to derive some benefit from adjuvant treatment. Some tumours were later found to be hormone receptor–negative.

- **Exclusion Criteria**: Patients were excluded if they had metastatic disease or received neoadjuvant chemotherapy. They were also excluded if adjuvant chemotherapy was started more than 8 weeks after surgery or if chemotherapy was completed more than 8 weeks before starting randomised treatment. Further exclusions included those having already received hormonal therapy for breast cancer prevention, having already received adjuvant hormonal therapy, or refusing to stop hormone replacement therapy (HRT).

- **Intervention or Treatment Received**: Patients were randomised to receive either anastrozole alone, tamoxifen alone or anastrozole and tamoxifen in combination.

- **Primary and Secondary End Points**: Primary end points were DFS (defined as the earliest occurrence of local or distant recurrence, new primary breast cancer or death from any cause) and occurrence of adverse events. Secondary end points were time to recurrence (including contralateral tumours) and incidence of new contralateral primary breast tumours.

- **Results**: DFS survival was significantly longer for patients on anastrozole alone than for those who received either tamoxifen alone (hazard ratio [HR] = 0.83, 95% confidence interval [CI] = 0.71–0.96, p = 0.013) or the anastrozole–tamoxifen combination (HR = 0.81, 95% CI = 0.70–0.94, p = 0.006).

  DFS estimates at 3 years were 89.4%, 87.4% and 87.2% on anastrozole, tamoxifen and the combination, respectively. DFS estimates in the hormone receptor–positive population at 3 years were 91.2%, 89.3% and 88.9% for anastrozole, tamoxifen and the combination, respectively.

  Time to recurrence was also improved in the anastrozole group compared to tamoxifen (HR = 0.79, 95% CI = 0.67–0.94, p = 0.008). There was no difference in the annual recurrence rates between patients treated with tamoxifen alone and anastrozole alone in the first year of follow-up, but a difference emerged in the second and third years of follow-up.

  Because of the sample size, the standard prognostic factors (tumour size, tumour grade, oestrogen receptor status and age) predicted recurrence as expected. The recurrence rate was more than three times higher in women with hormone receptor–negative tumours than in those who were hormone receptor–positive.

  A significant reduction in primary contralateral breast cancers was found in the anastrozole group; the odds were reduced by 58% (odds ratio = 0.42, 95% CI = 0.22–0.79, p = 0.007).

With regard to adverse events, anastrozole was associated with a reduction in menopausal-type side effects, ischaemic cerebrovascular events, venous thromboembolic events and endometrial cancer.

By contrast, musculoskeletal disorders and fractures were significantly more common with anastrozole than with tamoxifen. However, all three treatment regimens were well tolerated by most patients, with 73–78% compliance across all three arms.

The finding that the combination of anastrozole plus tamoxifen was no better than tamoxifen and worse than an AI alone was unexpected and may relate to changes in tumour proliferation (as indicated by changes in Ki67), and it has led to further research trials such as the Peri-Operative Endocrine Therapy: Individualising Care (POETIC) trial.

EXPERT COMMENTARY BY ALEX HUMPHREYS AND DOUGLAS FERGUSON

Paper significance

This was the first paper to show that anastrozole had greater efficacy than tamoxifen, and because of the rapid accrual rate and the sample size, they were able to achieve excellent interim results even at 2–3 years after recruitment.

In its first analysis published in 2002, it showed anastrozole had a superior efficacy to tamoxifen (89.4% vs. 87.4% DFS rate at 3 years), and the relative risk reduction in recurrence rates for anastrozole against tamoxifen increased to 27%.

Paper limitations

Although they represented only small numbers, hormone receptor–negative patients were included in the analysis; however, the spread across all three arms was similar. Disclosures identified that the trial was sponsored by AstraZeneca, which had representation (in the minority) on steering committees.

In context of the relevant current literature

Anastrozole is superior to tamoxifen as first-line therapy for advanced breast cancer in postmenopausal women: results of a North American multicentre randomized trial. Arimidex Study Group. *J Clin Oncol* 2000; 18: 3758–76.

Published in 2000, this randomised, double-blind multicentre study evaluated anastrozole versus tamoxifen as a first-line therapy for hormone receptor–positive tumours in postmenopausal women. The study group's primary end points included response to treatment, time to progression and tolerability.

They reported similar findings to the Arimidex, Tamoxifen, Alone or in Combination (ATAC) trial, demonstrating that anastrozole was as effective as tamoxifen in disease response, but anastrozole had an advantage over tamoxifen in terms of time to progression (median time to progression of 11.1 months vs. 5.6 months for anastrozole and tamoxifen, respectively). Both treatments were well tolerated; however, thromboembolic events and vaginal bleeding were reported in fewer patients who received anastrozole.

The importance of oestrogen receptor status with regard to prognosis is well established,[1] as is the clear benefit in adjuvant endocrine treatment for hormone receptor–positive early breast cancers.[2] ATAC was the first trial to show a benefit in DFS of an AI compared with tamoxifen in postmenopausal women with early hormone receptor–positive breast cancer. This benefit was further identified in the Breast International Group (BIG) 1-98 trial[3] randomising patients to tamoxifen and another AI, letrozole, in isolation or combination, and similar effects to the ATAC findings were also seen in longer-term follow-up.[4]

Anastrozole lacks the partial agonist effects of tamoxifen that result in tamoxifen having an increased risk of side effects (hot flushes and vaginal discharge or bleeding) and the less common, but more serious, risks of endometrial cancer and thromboembolic events.[5] Anastrozole is better tolerated, with less toxicity than tamoxifen; however, the side effect profiles differ between the two different classes of drugs, with polyarthralgia being seen much more commonly with anastrozole, as is an increased incidence of fractures. Anastrozole also showed a striking 58% reduction in the incidence of contralateral cancers.[6]

The International Exemestane Study (IES) was published soon after ATAC, and it showed a 4.7% greater DFS after switch to an AI (exemestane) after 2 to 3 years of tamoxifen, compared to 5 years of tamoxifen.[7] Another switch trial, the Austrian Breast and Colorectal Cancer Study Group/Arimidex-Nolvadex (ABCSG/ARNO) trial, using anastrozole after 2 years of tamoxifen against 5 years of tamoxifen, showed a 3% better event-free survival.[8] These studies added to the evidence of benefit of AI over tamoxifen for women with oestrogen receptor–positive breast cancer.

Conclusions

The findings from the ATAC study significantly influenced endocrine treatment protocols for newly diagnosed postmenopausal patients with early, hormone receptor–positive, operable breast cancer, and the recommendation of an AI as first-line adjuvant treatment for this population is clear in the St Gallen guidelines, the National Institute for Health and Care Excellence (NICE) guidelines[9] and the American Society of Clinical Oncology.[10]

REFERENCES

1. Cooke T, George D, Shields R, Maynard P, Griffiths, K. Oestrogen receptors and prognosis in early breast cancer. *Lancet.* 1979;1:995–7.
2. Nolvadex Adjuvant Trial Organisation (NATO). Controlled trial of tamoxifen as adjuvant agent in management of early breast cancer. Interim analysis at four years. *Lancet.* 1983;1:257–61.
3. BIG 1-98 Collaborative Group, Mouridsen, H., Giobbie-Hurder, A., Goldhirsch, A., et al. Letrozole therapy alone or in sequence with tamoxifen in women with breast cancer. *New Engl J Med.* 2009;361:766–76.
4. Regan MM, Neven P, Giobbie-Hurder A, et al. Assessment of letrozole and tamoxifen alone and in sequence for postmenopausal women with steroid hormone receptor-positive breast cancer: the BIG 1-98 randomised clinical trial at 8.1 years median follow up. *Lancet Oncol.* 2011;12(12):1101–8.
5. Forbes JF, Cuzick J, Buzdar A, et al. Effect of anastrozole and tamoxifen as adjuvant treatment for early-stage breast cancer: 100-month analysis of the ATAC trial. *Lancet Oncol,* 2008;9:45–53.
6. Cuzick J, Sestak I, Baum M, et al. Effect of anastrozole and tamoxifen as adjuvant treatment for early-stage breast cancer: 10-year analysis of the ATAC trial. *Lancet Oncol.* 2010;11:1135–41.
7. Charles Coombes R, Hall E,Gibson LJ, Paridaens R, et al., for the Intergroup Exemestane Study. A randomized trial of exemestane after two to three years of tamoxifen therapy in postmenopausal women with primary breast cancer. *N Engl J Med.* 2004;350:1081–92. doi:10.1056/NEJMoa040331
8. Jakesz R, Jonat W, Gnant M, Mittlboeck M, et al., ABCSG and the GABG. Switching of postmenopausal women with endocrine-responsive early breast cancer to anastrozole after 2 years' adjuvant tamoxifen: combined results of ABCSG trial 8 and ARNO 95 trial. *Lancet.* 2005;366:455–62. doi:10.1016/S0140-6736(05)67059-6
9. National Institute for Health and Care Excellence (NICE). Early and locally advanced breast cancer: diagnosis and management [NG101] [Internet]. NICE; 2018 [Accessed 24/01/2019]. Available from: https://www.nice.org.uk/guidance/ng101.
10. Burstein HJ, Temin S, Anderson H, Buchholz TA, Davidson NE, Gelmon KE, et al. Adjuvant endocrine therapy for women with hormone receptor–positive breast cancer: American Society of Clinical Oncology clinical practice guideline focused update. *J Clin Oncol.* 2014;32:2255.

CHAPTER 35

11 Years' Follow-Up of Trastuzumab after Adjuvant Chemotherapy in HER2-Positive Early Breast Cancer: Final Analysis of the HERceptin Adjuvant (HERA) Trial

Cameron D, Piccart-Gebhart MJ, Gelber RD, Procter M, Goldhirsch A, de Azambuja E, et al. and Herceptin Adjuvant (HERA) Trial Study Team.
Lancet 389(10075):1195–1205, 2017

Overexpression of the *HER2* protein is exhibited by 20%–25% of breast cancers and is associated with an aggressive phenotype and increased risk of disease recurrence. Trastuzumab is a humanised monoclonal antibody which targets the fourth domain of the *HER2* extracellular structure. Binding of trastuzumab to the *HER2* protein reduces cell proliferation via interruption of cell-signalling pathways and induces antibody-dependent cell-mediated cytotoxicity. The HERceptin Adjuvant (HERA) study investigated whether addition of adjuvant trastuzumab treatment to standard neoadjuvant or adjuvant (neo/adjuvant) chemotherapy improved clinical outcomes in women with *HER2*-positive early breast cancer.

PAPER DESCRIPTION

- **Objective/Research Question**: To evaluate long-term outcomes (>5 years) of adjuvant trastuzumab in patients with early breast cancer confirmed as *HER2*-positive. The primary end point was disease-free survival. Secondary end points included cardiac safety, overall survival (OS), site of first disease-free survival event and time to distant recurrence.

- **Design**: The HERA trial was an international, open-label, Phase III, randomised controlled trial involving women with *HER2*-positive (overexpressing or amplified) early-stage invasive breast cancer. Patients must have completed locoregional therapy (surgery with or without radiotherapy) and a minimum of four courses of chemotherapy (adjuvant, neoadjuvant or both). Patients were recruited between 2001 and 2005 and randomly assigned (1:1:1) to observation, 1 year of trastuzumab or 2 years of trastuzumab. In this long-term follow-up study, the median

DOI: 10.1201/b23352-35

follow-up was 11 years. Individual patients were followed up with clinical and laboratory assessments every 6 months for years 3–5, and then once per year up to year 10. Annual chest radiography was required up to year 6, and annual mammography up to year 10. Hazard ratios (HRs) were estimated from Cox models, and survival curves were estimated by the Kaplan–Meier method.

- **Sample Size**: Of the 5,102 patients recruited to the HERA trial, 5,052 were included in the final safety analysis: 1,697 were randomised to observation, 1,682 to 1 year of trastuzumab and 1,673 to 2 years of trastuzumab. Eight hundred and eighty-four observation group patients crossed over to trastuzumab after the release of interim analysis results in 2005.

- **Inclusion Criteria**:
  - Histologically confirmed, completely excised invasive breast cancer with *HER2* overexpression (3+) or *HER2* amplification (+ on FISH) locally assessed and centrally verified
  - Determined hormone receptor status with tumour tissue available for central review
  - All pathological tumour sizes in node-positive disease
  - >1 cm pathological tumour size in node-negative disease
  - At least four cycles of neo/adjuvant chemotherapy (approved regimens included anthracyclines with no taxanes, anthracyclines and taxanes, non-anthracyclines and other regimens approved by the HERA Committee)
  - All oestrogen receptor (ER)-positive tumours to be treated with endocrine therapy unless contraindicated
  - Adequate baseline hepatic, renal and bone marrow function
  - Normal left ventricular ejection fraction (LVEF), ≥55 percent after completion of radiotherapy and chemotherapy

- **Exclusion Criteria**:
  - Presence of distant metastases
  - Previous invasive breast carcinoma
  - Previous non-breast neoplasm, except for curatively treated basal-cell or squamous cell carcinoma of the skin or in situ carcinoma of the cervix
  - Clinical stage T4 tumours
  - Inflammatory breast cancers
  - Involvement of supraclavicular nodes
  - Suspicious internal mammary nodes, unless subjected to radiotherapy
  - Prior mediastinal irradiation (except internal mammary-node irradiation for the present breast cancer)

- Cumulative doses of anthracycline exceeding 360 mg/m^2 for doxorubicin or 720 mg/m^2 for epirubicin, or stem cell support for chemotherapy
- Cardiac exclusion criteria: History of documented congestive cardiac failure, coronary artery disease with previous myocardial infarction, angina pectoris requiring medication, uncontrolled hypertension, clinically significant valvular disease and unstable arrhythmias

- **Intervention or Treatment Received**: Patients assigned to receive trastuzumab were administered a single loading dose of 8 mg/kg intravenously, and then maintenance doses of 6 mg/kg every 3 weeks for either 1 or 2 years depending on group assignment.

- **Results**: Overall, 2,642 (52%) patients were aged 49 years or younger at study entry. Patients started trastuzumab at a median of 8.4 months after initial diagnosis. The HR for the 1-year trastuzumab group versus observation was 0.76 (95% confidence interval [CI] = 0.68–0.86), and the HR for the 2-year trastuzumab group versus observation was 0.77 (95% CI = 0.69–0.87). Ten-year disease-free survival was 63% in the observation group, 69% in the 1-year trastuzumab group and 69% in the 2-year trastuzumab group. At 12 years, the OS was 73% in the observation group, 79% in the 1-year trastuzumab group and 80% in the 2-year trastuzumab group. OS was higher in the hormone receptor–positive cohort than the hormone receptor–negative cohort: 76% versus 70% (observation), 81% versus 78% (1-year trastuzumab) and 81% versus 79% (2-year trastuzumab) at 12 years. There were two (0.1%) primary cardiac end points (defined as New York Heart Association [NYHA] Class III or IV toxicity and a clinically significant LVEF drop of at least 10% from baseline and to an absolute LVEF <50% or cardiac death) in the observation group, 18 (1%) in the 1-year trastuzumab group and 17 (1%) in the 2-year trastuzumab group. There were 15 (0.9%) secondary cardiac end points (defined as NYHA class I or II with a LVEF drop of at least 10% from baseline and to an absolute LVEF <50%) in the observation group, 74 (4.4%) in the 1-year trastuzumab group and 122 (7.3%) in the 2-year trastuzumab group.

EXPERT COMMENTARY BY WILSON CHEAH PUI FUI AND ELLEN COPSON

Paper significance

This 11-year follow-up of the HERA trial provides the longest survival data of any trial assessing the addition of anti-*HER2* therapy to standard neo/adjuvant chemotherapy for *HER2*-positive early breast cancer. Following National Institute for Health and Care Excellence (NICE) approval in 2005 (NG101) based on the initial HERA findings, adjuvant trastuzumab for a 1-year period remains a standard treatment for selected (lower risk) cases of early *HER2*-positive breast cancer. The success of the HERA trial also provided a model for subsequent adjuvant clinical trials of newer anti-*HER2* therapies. This unique study provides more complete long-term cardiac safety data than other trials, and indicated that trastuzumab is safer than data from the original trials in the metastatic setting had suggested.

Paper limitations

The main limitation of this publication is the fact that 52% of the observation group patients subsequently crossed over to receive trastuzumab following publication of data at the first interim analysis point in 2005. It would be anticipated that this intention-to-treat analysis is likely to provide an underestimate of the long-term efficacy of trastuzumab. In addition, use of anthracycline–taxane chemotherapy was much lower in the HERA study (26% of patients) than in current practice, and therefore, again, current real-world efficacy may be greater than the results published in this study.

In the trial, 52% of the patients had hormone receptor–positive disease, whereas the true proportion in an incident breast cancer population is nearer to/upwards of 60%. Therefore, the true benefit in the majority population which have hormone receptor–positive tumours may need a more cautious analysis.

In context of the relevant current literature

Numerous studies have confirmed the efficacy of adding adjuvant trastuzumab to chemotherapy in early operable *HER2*-positive breast cancer. A recent meta-analysis of seven randomised trials, including the HERA trial, demonstrated the reduction of recurrence and mortality during the first 10 years of follow-up by about a third, with an absolute reduction of 6.4% in breast cancer mortality, consistent with this follow-up HERA study.[1] The proportional reduction appears to be unaffected by any tumour or patient characteristics.

Cardiotoxicity outcomes remain an essential decision point for oncologists and patients. A systematic review and meta-analysis of eight randomised trials showed that trastuzumab use increased risk of congestive cardiac failure by 2.17 times, with a 3.71-fold increased risk of reduced LVEF; these findings corresponded with previous meta-analyses and this study.[2] The UK National Cancer Research Institute (NCRI) have produced key recommendations which emphasised the importance of a proactive approach to managing cardiac health in breast cancer patients treated with trastuzumab.[3] The UK Persephone trial has additionally demonstrated that a 6-month duration of adjuvant trastuzumab is non-inferior to 12 months of treatment in terms of 4-year disease-free survival but is associated with less cardiotoxicity and fewer severe adverse events; this is therefore an alternative treatment option for patients recommended to receive adjuvant trastuzumab.[4]

While the introduction of trastuzumab dramatically improved outcomes for *HER2*-positive breast cancer, progression during trastuzumab therapy remained a significant challenge in the metastatic setting. Pertuzumab, a monoclonal antibody *HER* heterodimer inhibitor which provides a more comprehensive *HER* pathway blockade, is superior when used in combination with trastuzumab, compared to single-agent trastuzumab in metastatic *HER2*-positive patients. The Clinical Evaluation of Pertuzumab and Trastuzumab (CLEOPATRA) trial reported that median progression-free survival was improved by 6.3 months in the pertuzumab–trastuzumab group compared to the placebo–trastuzumab group.[5]

The results of CLEOPATRA rapidly led to clinical trials of pertuzumab in the early breast cancer setting. The NeoSphere trial investigated the use of pertuzumab in the neoadjuvant setting and showed a significantly improved pathological complete response rate with pertuzumab and trastuzumab plus docetaxel (45.8%) compared to trastuzumab plus docetaxel (29.0%).[6] Further analysis of patients from the trial demonstrated an improvement in 5-year progression-free survival rates with pertuzumab and trastuzumab plus docetaxel (86%) compared to trastuzumab plus docetaxel (81%).[7]

In addition, the APHINITY trial investigated the addition of adjuvant pertuzumab to trastuzumab in the early breast cancer setting and demonstrated significantly improved 3-year invasive disease–free survival with pertuzumab (94.1% vs. 93.2%), especially in node-positive disease (92.0% vs. 90.2%) when compared to a placebo.[8]

Pertuzumab plus trastuzumab is now regarded as the gold standard treatment for *HER2*-positive breast cancers in the neoadjuvant setting, whilst in the adjuvant setting, pertuzumab approval in the UK is limited to node-positive disease. Patients with node-negative disease continue to receive adjuvant trastuzumab monotherapy.

Current strategies also include adapting treatment according to tumour response to neoadjuvant chemotherapy plus trastuzumab/pertuzumab. The KATHERINE trial demonstrated the benefit of switching to trastuzumab emtansine (T-DM1), an antibody–drug conjugate of trastuzumab and the cytotoxic agent emtansine, as adjuvant therapy in patients with residual disease post neoadjuvant trastuzumab/pertuzumab.[9] This trial is discussed in detail in Chapter 38. Trials are currently in progress to study the use of Enhertu (trastuzumab–deruxtecan), another antibody–drug conjugate in the early breast cancer setting.

Conclusions

One year of adjuvant trastuzumab significantly increases disease-free survival and OS in *HER2*-positive early breast cancer with no additional benefit of 2 years of trastuzumab. There is no evidence of late emergent side effects, including no evidence of long-term cardiac deterioration up to 10 years after treatment.

REFERENCES

1. Early Breast Cancer Trialists' Collaborative group (EBCTCG). Trastuzumab for early-stage, HER2-positive breast cancer: a meta-analysis of 13 864 women in seven randomised trials. *Lancet Oncol.* 2021;22(8):1139–50. doi:10.1016/S1470-2045(21)00288-6
2. Genuino AJ, Chaikledkaew U, The DO, Reungwetwattana T, Thakkinstian A. Adjuvant trastuzumab regimen for HER2-positive early-stage breast cancer: a systematic review and meta-analysis. *Expert Rev Clin Pharmacol.* 2019;12(8):815–24. doi:10.1080/17512433.2019.1637252
3. Jones AL, Barlow M, Barrett-Lee PJ, et al. Management of cardiac health in trastuzumab-treated patients with breast cancer: updated United Kingdom National Cancer Research Institute recommendations for monitoring. *Br J Cancer.* 2009;100(5):684–92. doi:10.1038/sj.bjc.6604909
4. Earl HM, Hiller L, Vallier AL, et al. 6 versus 12 months of adjuvant trastuzumab for HER2-positive early breast cancer (PERSEPHONE): 4-year disease-free survival results of a randomised phase 3 non-inferiority trial. *Lancet.* 2019;393(10191):2599–612. doi:10.1016/S0140-6736(19)30650-6
5. Swain SM, Baselga J, Kim SB, et al. Pertuzumab, Trastuzumab, and Docetaxel in HER2-Positive Metastatic Breast Cancer. *New Engl J Med.* 2015;372(8):724–34. doi:10.1056/NEJMoa1413513
6. Gianni L, Pienkowski T, Im YH, et al. Efficacy and safety of neoadjuvant pertuzumab and trastuzumab in women with locally advanced, inflammatory, or early HER2-positive breast cancer (NeoSphere): a randomised multicentre, open-label, phase 2 trial. *Lancet Oncol.* 2012;13(1):25–32. doi:10.1016/S1470-2045(11)70336-9
7. Gianni L, Pienkowski T, Im YH, et al. 5-year analysis of neoadjuvant pertuzumab and trastuzumab in patients with locally advanced, inflammatory, or early-stage HER2-positive breast cancer (NeoSphere): a multicentre, open-label, phase 2 randomised trial. *Lancet Oncol.* 2016;17(6):791–800. doi:10.1016/S1470-2045(16)00163-7
8. von Minckwitz G, Procter M, de Azambuja E, et al. Adjuvant Pertuzumab and Trastuzumab in Early HER2-Positive Breast Cancer. *New Engl J Med.* 2017;377(2):122–31. doi:10.1056/NEJMoa1703643
9. von Minckwitz G, Huang CS, Mano MS, et al. Trastuzumab Emtansine for Residual Invasive HER2-Positive Breast Cancer. *New Engl J Med.* 2019;380(7):617–28. doi:10.1056/NEJMoa1814017

CHAPTER 36

Adjuvant Olaparib for Patients with BRCA1- or BRCA2-Mutated Breast Cancer

Tutt ANJ, Garber JE, Kaufman B, et al.

N Engl J Med 384(25):2394–2405, 2021

Poly (ADP ribose) polymerase (PARP) inhibitors are a class of systemic anti-cancer therapies which target the impaired DNA repair mechanisms found in some cancer cells. Cells normally utilise two main methods of DNA repair: homologous recombination of double-strand breaks involving BRCA1 and BRCA2 proteins, and single-strand break repair via PARP. PARP inhibitors trap PARP at sites of DNA damage. The resulting accumulation of unrepaired DNA single-strand breaks causes replication fork collapse during DNA replication and double-strand breaks. Impairment of one DNA repair pathway alone is not lethal and can be compensated for by the other pathway, allowing cell survival. PARP inhibitors were designed specifically to exploit the homologous recombination DNA repair deficiency associated with a constitutional pathogenic mutation in the *BRCA1* and *BRCA* 2 genes; in this setting, PARP inhibition causes synthetic lethality and cell death. The OlympiA study aimed to investigate the efficacy of the PARP inhibitor olaparib in the adjuvant treatment of early breast cancer patients with confirmed germline *BRCA1* or *BRCA2* pathogenic mutations.

PAPER DESCRIPTION

- **Objective/Research Question**: To assess if adjuvant therapy with olaparib after completion of standard neoadjuvant or adjuvant chemotherapy improved invasive disease–free survival for high-risk *HER2*-negative early breast cancer patients with confirmed germline *BRCA1* or *BRCA2* pathogenic mutations.

- **Design**: This multicentre study was a Phase III, double-blinded randomised control trial. High-risk, *HER2*-negative, germline *BRCA*-mutated breast cancer patients who had completed local treatment and chemotherapy (either adjuvant or neoadjuvant) were randomised to receive either olaparib or placebo twice daily for 1 year.

    The primary end point was invasive disease-free survival, defined as time from randomisation until one of the following events occurs: ipsilateral invasive breast tumour, locoregional invasive disease, distant recurrence, contralateral invasive breast cancer, second primary invasive cancer or death

DOI: 10.1201/b23352-36

from any cause. Secondary end points included distant disease–free survival, overall survival and safety. An intention-to-treat analysis was performed.

- **Sample Size**: A total of 1,836 patients (including six men) were recruited from 420 centres across 23 different countries and randomised in a 1:1 ratio to receive either olaparib or placebo.

- **Inclusion Criteria**:
  - Confirmed *BRCA1* or *BRCA2* pathogenic or likely pathogenic variant
  - High-risk, *HER2*-negative primary breast cancer
  - At least six cycles of definitive neoadjuvant or adjuvant chemotherapy containing anthracyclines, taxanes or both (platinum and endocrine therapies also permitted)

- **Exclusion Criteria**:
  - Received local therapy <2 *or* >12 weeks before trial entry.
  - Chemotherapy after surgery in those who had already undergone neoadjuvant chemotherapy.
  - Axillary node–negative disease *or* an invasive primary tumour measuring <2 cm in triple-negative breast cancer patients who received adjuvant chemotherapy.
  - Fewer than four positive lymph nodes in oestrogen receptor (ER)-positive or progesterone receptor (PR)-positive disease treated with adjuvant chemotherapy.
  - Pathological complete response to neoadjuvant therapy. 'Pathological complete response' was defined as an absence of breast cancer in breast or resected lymph nodes in triple-negative disease and as a clinical and pathologic staging plus ER status and tumour grade (CPS+EG) score >2 in ER/PR-positive disease.

- **Intervention or Treatment Received**: Patients randomised to the olaparib arm received 300 mg oral olaparib twice daily for 1 year. The placebo arm received an oral placebo twice daily for 1 year. Patients were stratified according to hormone receptor status, timing of previous chemotherapy (neoadjuvant or adjuvant) and use of platinum chemotherapy for current breast cancer. After randomisation, medical assessment was performed every 4 weeks for 24 weeks and then every 3 months through year 2, every 6 months in years 3 to 5 and annually thereafter. All patients underwent mammography, breast magnetic resonance imaging (MRI) or both on at least an annual basis. Additional imaging was done as deemed necessary where disease recurrence was suspected.

- **Results**:
  - **Efficacy**: At 3 years, invasive disease–free survival (primary end point) was significantly higher in patients randomised to olaparib (85.9%) than

placebo (77.1%), with a hazard ratio of 0.58 (99.5% confidence interval [CI] = 0.41–0.82) and a p-value of <0.001, an 8.8% difference (95% CI = 4.5–13.0). These findings were preserved on subgroup analysis across all the pre-specified stratification groups (including *BRCA1* or *BRCA2* mutation, hormone receptor status and chemotherapy timing). When looking at overall survival specifically, 92% of those in the olaparib group were alive at the 3-year timepoint (59 deaths) compared to 88.3% in the placebo group (89 deaths), with a hazard ratio of 0.68 (99% CI = 0.44–1.05). However, this between-group difference of 3.7% did not meet the predetermined threshold for significance of $p < 0.01$.

Distant disease–free survival (secondary end point) was also significantly higher amongst patients in the olaparib arm than the placebo arm at the 3-year mark, with a hazard ratio of 0.57 (99.5% CI = 0.39–0.83) and a p-value of <0.001. This corresponded to 87.5% of those in the olaparib group and 80.4% of those in the control group being alive and free of distant disease—a 7.1% difference (95% CI = 3.0–11.1).

- **Safety**: Early discontinuation of the trial regimen (including due to recurrence) occurred in 236 patients (25.9%) in the olaparib group compared with 187 (20.7%) in the placebo group. Frequency of permanent discontinuation of the trial regimen due to adverse events was higher, at 9.9% (90 patients), in the olaparib group compared with 4.2% (38 patients) of the placebo group. The most common adverse events leading to discontinuation of olaparib were nausea (2.0%), anaemia (1.8%), fatigue (1.3%) and decreased neutrophil count (1.0%). Despite this, the overall frequency of serious adverse events was similar in both groups at 8.7% (79 patients) and 8.4% (76 patients), respectively. Similarly, there was no excess of 'adverse events of special interest' (namely, pneumonitis, myelodysplastic syndromes or new primary cancers) in the olaparib group (3.3% vs. 5.1% in the control group).

The most salient adverse event reported in the olaparib group was anaemia, affecting 23.5% of patients compared to 3.9% in the placebo group, with 8.4% experiencing grade 3 or higher anaemia compared to 0.3% in the placebo group. Nausea and fatigue were more common in the investigational arm (56.9% and 40.1%, respectively, compared to 23.3% and 27.1% in the placebo group). There were no statistically significant differences observed in quality of life between the groups as measured by the European Organization for Research and Treatment of Cancer's scale.

EXPERT COMMENTARY BY ANTHONY MARK MONAGHAN AND ELLEN COPSON

Paper significance

The OlympiA study was the first clinical trial to demonstrate the benefit of a PARP inhibitor as an adjuvant treatment for breast cancer. Publication of these data led directly to the National Institute for Health and Care Excellence's

(NICE) recommendation of olaparib 'as an option for the adjuvant treatment of HER2-negative high-risk early breast cancer that has been treated with neoadjuvant or adjuvant chemotherapy in adults with germline BRCA1 or 2 mutations' in May 2023.[2]

In order to ensure that all early breast cancer patients who would potentially benefit from adjuvant olaparib therapy can be identified, publication of this NICE recommendation has been rapidly followed by an update of the National Genomic Test Directory[3] to permit high-risk breast cancer patients (as defined by OlympiA trial inclusion criteria) to access germline *BRCA* testing via a new test code (R444), even if not eligible under the conventional R208 test criteria for familial breast cancer susceptibility gene testing. Given its demonstration of *BRCA* status impact on systemic treatment choice, the Olympia study implicitly highlights the importance of earlier and faster access to germline CSG testing. This has been described as a shifting paradigm from 'who to test' to 'who not to test' and is currently accelerating implementation of 'mainstreaming' of genetic testing in breast cancer. This system allows surgeons or oncologists to request *BRCA* testing themselves to obviate the need for referrals to dedicated genetics specialists, thus improving efficiency and speed of testing.[4] The latest National Genomic Test Directory lists both surgery and oncology as permitted requesting specialties for germline testing in breast cancer patients.[3]

Paper limitations

The strengths of this study include sound methodology with a large, demographically diverse population and double-blinded design, and inclusion of patients who had received both neoadjuvant and adjuvant chemotherapy of varying regimen types (including platinum-containing agents).

Limitations include restriction of recruitment to patients with *BRCA1* and *BRCA2* pathogenic variants. Whilst these are the most prevalent high-penetrance breast cancer predisposition genes (CPGs), epidemiological data suggest they account for only around 15% of familial breast cancer cases in total.[5] *PALB2, CHEK2, ATM, RAD51C* and *RAD51D* have also been identified as CPGs which increase breast cancer risk by affecting homologous recombination DNA repair,[6] and these genes are now included in the National Health Service (NHS) familial breast cancer gene test panel.[3] It remains unclear whether patients with pathogenic germline mutations in these other breast CPGs would also benefit from adjuvant PARP inhibitor therapy. There is also currently no consensus regarding the use of PARP inhibitors in the treatment of breast tumours with somatic *BRCA1* or *BRCA2* mutations in the absence of underlying germline mutations; clinical trials are in progress to investigate this further.[7]

Recruitment into the OlympiA trial occurred prior to publication of the KEYNOTE-522 trial data (see Chapter 37), and therefore no patients in this study received immunotherapy which has now been adopted by many countries as a routine neoadjuvant treatment option for triple-negative breast cancer. The role of adjuvant PARP inhibitors in patients treated with immunotherapy or receiving adjuvant capecitabine is not yet proven. Further follow-up of the OlympiA cohort is required to understand the long-term safety risks associated with adjuvant PARP inhibitor therapy.

In context of the relevant current literature

Approximately 20% of breast cancer cases are familial, and 5%–10% are associated with an underlying mutation in a high-penetrance CPG, of which *BRCA1* and *BRCA2* are the most common.[5] Breast cancer patients with underlying *BRCA1 or BRCA2* mutations have a high lifetime risk of second breast cancers and other primary tumours, particularly ovarian cancer. A UK-based prospective cohort study of young-onset breast cancer (Prospective Study of Outcomes in Sporadic versus Hereditary Breast Cancer [POSH study]) has, however, demonstrated that *BRCA* status does not independently affect breast cancer prognosis.[8]

Prior to the advent of targeted therapies for this patient group, clinical trials focussed on the hypothesis that cancer patients with germline (g)*BRCA1/2* mutations would exhibit enhanced responses to platinum chemotherapies due to intrinsic vulnerability to DNA crosslinking agents. The Triple Negative Trial (TNT), a randomised clinical trial, compared carboplatin with docetaxel as first-line therapy in patients with triple-negative breast cancer and demonstrated conclusively that the *gBRCA*-mutated patients had significantly greater responses to carboplatin than *BRCA* wild-type patients.[9] Subsequent investigations of carboplatin benefit and *BRCA* status in the neoadjuvant setting have now been superseded by trial evidence that all patients with triple-negative breast cancer benefit from platinum adjuvant or neoadjuvant chemotherapy regardless of *BRCA* status.[10] There is currently no consensus on use of platinum chemotherapy in the adjuvant or neoadjuvant treatment of non-triple-negative breast tumours in *gBRCA* carriers.

Prior to OlympiA, the clinical benefit of PARP inhibitors in metastatic breast cancer had been demonstrated in two Phase III clinical trials. The OlympiAD and EMBRACA trials compared PARP inhibitor monotherapy (olaparib in OlympiAD and talozaparib in EMBRACA) with chemotherapy of the physician's choice in pretreated *HER2*-negative metastatic breast cancer patients with *gBRCA* mutations. Both studies reported significant improvements in progression-free survival with PARP inhibitors and improved tolerability compared to chemotherapy. Studies in the metastatic setting have not yet shown an overall survival benefit.

Conclusions

The OlympiA study was a large-scale, rigorously designed, randomised controlled trial which yielded novel and well-founded data on the efficacy of PARP inhibitors in early, high-risk breast cancer associated with *BRCA1/2* pathogenic variants. Its findings have already facilitated major changes to international guidance for early breast cancer management and led to adjuvant olaparib receiving NICE approval in the UK. It is likely this paper will prove to be seminal in this field, especially as cancer management continues evolving to become more targeted with respect to genetic susceptibility.

REFERENCES

1. Tutt ANJ, Garber JE, Kaufman B, et al. Adjuvant Olaparib for Patients with BRCA1- or BRCA2-Mutated Breast Cancer. *N Engl J Med*. 2021;384(25):2394–405.
2. NICE Guidance: Olaparib for adjuvant treatment of BRCA mutation-positive HER2-negative high-risk early breast cancer after chemotherapy. Recommendations [Internet]. [cited 2023 Jun 12]. Available from: https://www.nice.org.uk/guidance/ta886/evidence
3. National Genomic Test Directory – NHS England [Internet]. [cited 2023 Jun 8]. Available from: https://www.england.nhs.uk/wp-content/uploads/2018/08/Rare-and-inherited-disease-eligibility-criteria-version-6-January-2024.pdf
4. Rahman N. Mainstreaming genetic testing of cancer predisposition genes. *Clin Med*. 2014;14(4):436–9. doi:10.7861/clinmedicine.14-4-436
5. Stratton MR, Rahman N. The emerging landscape of breast cancer susceptibility. *Nat Genet*. 2008;40(1):17–22. doi:10.1038/ng.2007.53
6. Breast Cancer Association Consortium, Dorling L, Carvalho S, et al. Breast cancer risk genes—association analysis in more than 113,000 women. *N Engl J Med*. 2021;384(5): 428–39. doi:10.1056/NEJMoa1913948
7. Balic M, Thomssen C, Gnant M, Harbeck N. St. Gallen/Vienna 2023: optimization of treatment for patients with primary breast cancer – a brief summary of the consensus discussion. *Breast Care*. 2023. doi:10.1159/000530584
8. Copson ER, Maishman TC, Tapper WJ, et al. Germline BRCA mutation and outcome in young-onset breast cancer (POSH): a prospective cohort study. *Lancet Oncol*. 2018;19(2):169–80. doi:10.1016/S1470-2045(17)30891-4
9. Tutt A, Tovey H, Cheang MCU, et al. Carboplatin in BRCA1/2-mutated and triple-negative breast cancer BRCAness subgroups: the TNT Trial. *Nat Med*. 2018;24(5):628–37. doi:10.1038/s41591-018-0009-7
10. Geyer CE, Sikov WM, Huober J, et al. Long-term efficacy and safety of addition of carboplatin with or without veliparib to standard neoadjuvant chemotherapy in triple-negative breast cancer: 4-year follow-up data from BrighTNess, a randomized phase III trial. *Ann Oncol*. 2022;33(4):384–94. doi: 10.1016/j.annonc.2022.01.009. Epub 2022 Jan 31. PMID: 35093516.
11. Robson M, Seock-Ah I, Senkus E, et al. Olaparib for metastatic breast cancer in patients with a germline BRCA mutation. *N Engl J Med*. 2017;377:523–33. doi:10.1056/NEJMoa1706450
12. Litton JK, Rugo HS, Ettl J, et al. Talazoparib in patients with advanced breast cancer and a germline BRCA mutation. *N Engl J Med*. 2018;379(8):753–63. doi:10.1056/NEJMoa1802905. Epub 2018 Aug 15. PMID: 30110579.

CHAPTER 37

Pembrolizumab for Early Triple-Negative Breast Cancer

Schmid P, Cortes J, Dent R, et al.

New Engl J Med 386(6):556–567, 2022

Pembrolizumab is an immune checkpoint inhibitor (ICPI), a type of immuno-therapy that blocks the programmed death 1 (PD1) receptor expressed on T cells. In cancer, PD1 binds to its ligand, programmed death ligand 1 (PDL1), which is expressed by both innate immune cells and tumour cells and prevents T cells from killing cancer cells. Triple-negative breast cancer (TNBC) is char-acterised by a higher density of immune cell infiltrates, a higher expression of PDL1 and a higher tumour mutational burden than other breast cancer sub-types, making ICPI a promising treatment option in TNBC.[1] Furthermore, the use of anthracyclines, taxanes and platinum-based neoadjuvant chemo-therapy is associated not only with improved pathological complete responses (pCRs) but also with increased PDL1 expression in tumour cells in TNBC.[2] The KEYNOTE-522 study investigated whether the combination of chemotherapy and ICPI improves clinical outcomes in this group of patients.

PAPER DESCRIPTION

- **Objective/Research Question**: To assess if the addition of pembrolizumab to standard neoadjuvant chemotherapy for oestrogen receptor (ER)-negative, progesterone receptor (PR)-negative and *HER2*-negative breast cancer increases pCR and event-free survival (EFS).

- **Design**: This study was an international, multicentre, Phase III, double-blind randomised controlled trial. Patients were randomly allocated, in a 2:1 ratio, to either pembrolizumab or placebo in combination with the backbone chemotherapy.

  Patients were stratified by lymph node status, tumour size and adminis-tration schedule of carboplatin prior to randomisation. No crossover was permitted between the neoadjuvant and adjuvant phases.

  pCR was defined as ypT0/Tis ypN0 at the time of surgery and was determined by a local pathologist blinded to the treatment arms. EFS was defined as time from randomisation to disease progression and was determined by an investigator who was blind to the treatment arms. An intention-to-treat analysis was performed.

DOI: 10.1201/b23352-37

- **Sample Size**: A total of 1,174 patients were randomly allocated to either the pembrolizumab–chemotherapy (n = 784) or placebo–chemotherapy arm (n = 390).

- **Inclusion Criteria**: Patients with newly diagnosed, previously untreated, stage II or III and centrally histologically confirmed ER-negative, PR-negative and *HER2*-negative invasive breast carcinoma, regardless of PDL1 status, with an Eastern Cooperative Oncology Group (ECOG) performance status of 0–1 were eligible for inclusion.

- **Exclusion Criteria**:
  1. Patients with active autoimmune disease that had been treated with systemic treatment within the previous 2 years
  2. Immunodeficiency or use of immunosuppressive treatment within the previous week
  3. A history of human immunodeficiency virus (HIV) infection
  4. A history of non-infectious pneumonitis that was treated with corticosteroids
  5. Current pneumonitis, active tuberculosis, hepatitis B or C virus infection or any active other infection
  6. Clinically significant cardiovascular disease

- **Intervention or Treatment Received**: Patients were randomly allocated to either pembrolizumab or placebo. Patients received four cycles of neoadjuvant pembrolizumab or placebo once every 3 weeks plus weekly paclitaxel plus carboplatin (three or once-weekly regimen), followed by four cycles of pembrolizumab or placebo plus doxorubicin or epirubicin plus cyclophosphamide.

  Patients underwent definitive surgery 3 to 6 weeks after the last cycle of the neoadjuvant treatment. Patients received postoperative radiotherapy as per the standard of care and adjuvant pembrolizumab or placebo once every 3 weeks for up to nine cycles. Adjuvant capecitabine was not permitted according to the protocol.

- **Results**: At the primary analysis in September 2018, pembrolizumab was associated with a 13.5% (95% confidence interval [CI] = 5.4–21.8) higher pCR compared to the control group, a difference that was statistically significant. Specifically, 64.8% (260/401 patients) in the pembrolizumab and 51.2% (103/201 patients) in the placebo arm had pCR. The pCR improvement in the pembrolizumab arm was independent of the PDL1 status (PDL1-positive: 68.9% [230/334 patients] vs. 54.9% [90/164 patients]; PDL1-negative: 45.3% [29/64 patients] vs. 30.3% [10/33 patients]) and was generally consistent across the different subgroups.

At the first interim analysis at 18 months, 91.3% (95% CI = 88.8–93.3) in the pembrolizumab arm and 85.3% (95% CI = 80.3–89.1) in the placebo arm were alive without disease progression. Pembrolizumab was associated with a 37% improvement in disease progression compared to placebo (hazard ratio [HR] = 0.63, 95% CI = 0.43–0.93). The frequency of grade 3 or higher treatment-related toxicity was 78.0% in the pembrolizumab arm and 73.0% in the placebo arm, with a mortality rate of 0.4% ($n = 3$) and 0.3% ($n = 1$), respectively. Safety was consistent with previously reported toxicity profiles of immunotherapy with no safety concerns. The use of pembrolizumab did not compromise exposure to chemotherapy or increase the frequency of common chemotherapy-related side effects.

EXPERT COMMENTARY BY CONSTANTINOS SAVVA AND ELLEN COPSON

Paper significance

TNBC is the most aggressive biological subtype of breast cancer, with high rates of recurrence and poor survival in the metastatic setting.[3] pCR has been proven to be predictive of long-term survival, and it is therefore accepted as a surrogate marker of treatment benefit in patients with TNBC.[4] Increased pCR rates should also result in increased rates of breast-conserving surgery, which is associated with better quality of life.[5] In the KEYNOTE-522 trial, broad eligibility criteria and a standard platinum, anthracycline and taxane chemotherapy regimen were used, meaning that the study findings are generalisable to most newly diagnosed stage II–III TNBC patients. For these reasons, pembrolizumab is now recommended as an option, in combination with chemotherapy, for neoadjuvant treatment and then as a single agent as adjuvant treatment after surgery by the UK National Institute for Health and Care Excellence (NICE; approved in December 2022), the European Medicines Agency (EMA) and the US Food and Drug Administration (FDA).

Paper limitations

The key strengths of this double-blind trial are the large sample size and use of platinum-based chemotherapy in both treatment arms, permitting a direct comparison of the pembrolizumab–chemotherapy combination with the neoadjuvant chemotherapy regimen associated with the highest pCR rate in early TNBC.

The main limitation of this paper is the short follow-up period preventing evaluation of long-term overall survival and toxicity profile. In addition, the study design does not allow assessment of the relative contributions of neoadjuvant or adjuvant treatment to clinical outcomes, as adjuvant pembrolizumab was given regardless of pCR status. The optimal duration of backbone chemotherapy and adjuvant pembrolizumab remains to be defined. Furthermore, adjuvant pembrolizumab may not offer additional benefit in patients who achieved pCR. De-escalation of adjuvant treatment in patients with TNBC with pCR will be evaluated in the OptimICE-pCR trial.[6]

Adjuvant capecitabine was not incorporated into the trial design, and the germline *BRCA1* and *BRCA2* mutation status was not considered in this study. Prospective studies and biomarker research are required to improve tailoring of post-neoadjuvant treatment to the individual patient.

In context of the relevant current literature

The 3-year clinical outcomes of KEYNOTE-522 were presented at the European Society for Medical Oncology (ESMO) congress in 2021.[7] EFS at 36 months was 84.5% in the pembrolizumab arm and 76.8% in the placebo arm (HR = 0.63, 95% CI = 0.48–0.82). EFS by pCR response was 94.4% versus 92.5% in patients with pCR and 67.4% versus 56.8% in patients without pCR. Stratified analysis of pCR by nodal status showed a greater benefit in patients with nodal disease (64.8% vs. 44.1%) compared to patients with node-negative disease (64.9% vs. 58.6%). Nevertheless, this trial was not powered to detect a statistically significant difference among the different patient subgroups, and hence these findings should be interpreted with caution. Despite the larger benefit of pembrolizumab in node-positive patients, the EFS was similar across all subgroups.

The results of KEYNOTE-522 are supported by other clinical trials that investigated the combination of ICPI and chemotherapy in early TNBC, as shown in **Table 37.1**. The Impassion130 and Neo-TRIP trials showed that the atezolizumab–chemotherapy combination was associated with a higher pCR rate compared to the placebo–chemotherapy arm in PDL1-positive patients.[3,8] The GeparNuevo trial showed that neoadjuvant durvalumab was associated with improved clinical outcomes compared to the placebo group, independently of the presence of pCR.[9] Invasive disease-free survival was longer in node-positive patients that received durvalumab.[9] The Neo-PACT trial, which evaluated the efficacy of anthracycline-free neoadjuvant chemotherapy in combination with pembrolizumab, showed that immune hot tumours defined by the presence of tumour-infiltrating T cells or DetermaIO immune-related gene signatures are associated with a higher pCR rate.[10] Although the findings of I-SPY2 in relation to pCR were consistent with other immuno-oncology studies, this trial was not powered enough to detect a statistically significant difference in EFS between pembrolizumab and the control group.[11]

The differences in the clinical outcomes in the different studies may be attributed to the different sample sizes, patient characteristics such as PDL1 expression and stage, different backbone chemotherapies and the type and duration of ICPI.

Table 37.1 Randomised clinical trials that investigated the addition of immune checkpoint inhibitors (ICPIs) to chemotherapy in early breast cancer

	IMpassion031[3]	NeoTRIP[8]	GeparNuevo[9]	I-SPY2[11]	Neo-PACT[10]
Phase	III	III	II	II	II
Population	Untreated stage II–III, TNBC	Untreated stage II–III, TNBC	Untreated stage II–III, TNBC	Untreated stage II–III TNBC and HR+/HER2–	Untreated stage I–III TNBC
N	333	280	174	107	117
Immunotherapy	Atezolizumab	Atezolizumab	Durvalumab	Pembrolizumab	Pembrolizumab
Neoadjuvant CT	nabT followed by AC	nabT and Cb	nabT followed by AC	T followed by AC	Cb and T
Adjuvant Tx	Atezolizumab	Anthracyclines	Physician's choice CT	Physician's choice CT	Not applicable
Primary end point	pCR in ITT and in PDL1+ patients	EFS	pCR in ITT	pCR in ITT	pCR
PDL1+	46%	56%	86.8%	NR	46%
pCR	58% vs. 41%, $p = 0.0044$	48.6% vs. 44.4%, $p = 0.48$	53.4% vs. 44.2%, $p = 0.287$	60% (44–75) vs. 22% (13–20) (TNBC)	60% (51–70)
EFS: HR (95% CI)	0.76 (0.40–1.40)	NR	0.54 (0.27–1.09)	0.60 (TNBC)	2-year EFS 80%; 98% in pCR group and 82% in no pCR group
DFS: HR (95% CI)	0.74 (0.32–1.70)	NR	0.37 (0.15–0.87)	—	NR
OS: HR (95% CI)	0.69 (0.25–1.87)	NR	0.26 (0.09–0.79)	—	NR

Abbreviations: AC: Anthracycline and cyclophosphamide chemotherapy; Cb: carboplatin; CT: chemotherapy; DDFS: distant disease–free survival; DFS: disease–free survival; EFS: event-free survival; HR: hazard ratio; HR+: hormone receptor–positive; IDFS: invasive disease–free survival; ITT: intention to treat; nabT: nab-paclitaxel; NR: not reported; OS: overall survival; pCR: pathological complete response; PDL1+: programmed death ligand 1–positive; T: docetaxel; TNBC: triple-negative breast cancer; Tx: therapy.

Conclusions

Publication of data from the KEYNOTE-522 study has directly resulted in the use of preoperative and adjuvant pembrolizumab becoming the standard of care for early-stage, high-risk TNBC regardless of the PDL1 status. Nevertheless, further prospective studies are required to identify predictive biomarkers of immunotherapy sensitivity,[12] determine the optimal duration of adjuvant immunotherapy and evaluate the role of other adjuvant therapies in nonresponders.

REFERENCES

1. Abdou, Y., et al. Immunotherapy in triple negative breast cancer: beyond checkpoint inhibitors. *NPJ Breast Cancer*. 2022;8(1):121.
2. Kim R, Kin T. Current and future therapies for immunogenic cell death and related molecules to potentially cure primary breast cancer. *Cancers*. 2021;13(19).
3. Mittendorf EA, et al. Neoadjuvant atezolizumab in combination with sequential nab-paclitaxel and anthracycline-based chemotherapy versus placebo and chemotherapy in patients with early-stage triple-negative breast cancer (IMpassion031): a randomised, double-blind, phase 3 trial. *Lancet*. 2020;396(10257):1090–100.
4. Spring LM, et al. Pathologic complete response after neoadjuvant chemotherapy and impact on breast cancer recurrence and survival: a comprehensive meta-analysis. *Clin Cancer Res*. 2020;26(12):2838–48.
5. Hanson SE, et al. Long-term quality of life in patients with breast cancer after breast conservation vs mastectomy and reconstruction. *JAMA Surgery*. 2022;157(6):e220631.
6. Hirsch, I, et al. Optimizing the dose and schedule of immune checkpoint inhibitors in cancer to allow global access. *Nat Med*. 2022;28(11):2236–7.
7. Schmid P, et al. VP7-2021: KEYNOTE-522: Phase III study of neoadjuvant pembrolizumab + chemotherapy vs. placebo + chemotherapy, followed by adjuvant pembrolizumab vs. placebo for early-stage TNBC. *Ann Oncol*. 2021;32(9):1198–200.
8. Gianni, L, et al. Pathologic complete response (pCR) to neoadjuvant treatment with or without atezolizumab in triple-negative, early high-risk and locally advanced breast cancer: NeoTRIP Michelangelo randomized study. *Ann Oncol*. 2022;33(5): 534–43.
9. Loibl S, et al. Neoadjuvant durvalumab improves survival in early triple-negative breast cancer independent of pathological complete response. *Ann Oncol*. 2022;33(11): 1149–58.
10. Sharma P, et al. Clinical and biomarker results of neoadjuvant phase II study of pembrolizumab and carboplatin plus docetaxel in triple-negative breast cancer (TNBC) (NeoPACT). *J Clin Oncol*. 2022;40(16_suppl):513.
11. Nanda R, et al. Effect of pembrolizumab plus neoadjuvant chemotherapy on pathologic complete response in women with early-stage breast cancer: an analysis of the ongoing phase 2 adaptively randomized I-SPY2 trial. *JAMA Oncol*. 2020;6(5):676–84.
12. Santa-Maria CA. Optimizing and refining immunotherapy in breast cancer. *JCO Oncol Pract*. 2023;19(4):190–1.

CHAPTER 38

Trastuzumab Emtansine for Residual Invasive HER2-Positive Breast Cancer

von Minckwitz G, Huang C-S, Mano MS, et al. for the KATHERINE Investigators.
N Engl J Med 380:617–628, 2019

T-DM1 (ado-trastuzumab emtansine; Kadcyla) is an antibody–drug conjugate (ADC) consisting of an anti-HER2 antibody linked to a microtubule inhibitor chemotherapy drugs, by combining the targeting ability of an antibody with a cytotoxic, ADCs can potentially deliver higher doses of chemotherapy into cancer cells whilst avoiding intolerable systemic toxicities. The KATHERINE study investigated whether the use of T-DM1 in the adjuvant setting improved oncological outcomes for women with early HER2-positive breast cancer with residual disease after neoadjuvant chemotherapy (NACT).

PAPER DESCRIPTION

- **Objective/Research Question**: To determine whether adjuvant treatment with T-DM1 compared with standard adjuvant therapy improves oncological outcomes in HER2-positive early breast cancer patients with residual disease at surgery post NACT with trastuzumab and a taxane.

- **Design**: This was a multicentre, Phase III, open-label, randomised controlled trial. Patients were randomised in a 1:1 ratio to receive adjuvant treatment with T-DM1 or trastuzumab.
  Randomisation was stratified according to tumour stage, oestrogen receptor status, preoperative anti-HER2 therapy and nodal status at surgery.
  The primary outcome was invasive disease–free survival (IDFS). Secondary outcomes included disease-free survival, overall survival, distant recurrence–free survival and safety.
  The primary analysis was based on the intention-to-treat population.

- **Sample Size**: A total of 1,486 patients were included in the KATHERINE trial, with 743 patients randomised to the T-DM1 arm and 743 patients randomised to receive trastuzumab.

- **Inclusion Criteria**: Patients were eligible for inclusion if they had histologically confirmed, HER2-positive, nonmetastatic, invasive primary breast cancer at presentation, and if residual disease was present

DOI: 10.1201/b23352-38

following surgery after completing NACT with taxane-based chemotherapy and trastuzumab. HER2 status was confirmed centrally prior to
enrolment.

- **Exclusion Criteria**: Gross residual disease after mastectomy or positive
  margins after breast-conserving surgery; progressive disease during
  NACT; symptomatic heart failure or a history of left ventricular ejection
  fraction (LVEF) of < 40%.

- **Intervention Received**: Patients received 14 cycles of either adjuvant
  T-DM1 at a dose of 3.6 mg/kg intravenously every 3 weeks or trastuzumab at a dose of 6 mg/kg intravenously every 3 weeks.
  Assessments for disease recurrence were performed every 3 months
  from the date of randomisation until year 2, then every 6 months until
  year 5 and annually until year 10. The LVEF was also assessed at intervals
  up to year 5.

- **Results**: Median follow-up was 41.4 months (range = 0.1 to 62.7) in the
  T-DM1 group and 40.9 months (range = 0.1 to 62.6) in the trastuzumab
  group.
  IDFS was higher in the T-DM1 group than in the trastuzumab group
  (hazard ratio for invasive disease or death [HR] = 0.50, 95% confidence
  interval [CI] = 0.39–0.64, $P < 0.001$). The risk of distant recurrence was
  lower in the T-DM1 group than in the trastuzumab group (HR = 0.60,
  95% CI = 0.45 to 0.79). Estimated 3-year IDFS percentages were 88.3% in
  the T-DM1 group and 77.0% in the trastuzumab group.
  Grade 3 or higher adverse events occurred in 25.7% of patients in
  the T-DM1 group and 15.4% of those in the trastuzumab group, whilst
  adverse events leading to discontinuation of trial therapy occurred in 18%
  of patients in the T-DM1 group and 2.1% of patients in the trastuzumab
  group. The most common of these were thrombocytopenia, deranged liver
  function tests, peripheral neuropathy and reduced LVEF. Importantly,
  among those who suffered peripheral neuropathy in the T-DM1 group,
  this had resolved by the time of data cutoff in most patients (74.6%).

EXPERT COMMENTARY BY MACLYN AUGUSTINE AND ELLEN COPSON

Paper significance

The KATHERINE trial was the first clinical trial to provide an alternative
adjuvant treatment option for patients who had not achieved pathological
complete response with standard neoadjuvant treatment for HER2-positive
early breast cancer. Results indicate that T-DM1 significantly improves outcomes in this patient group (50% lower risk of invasive disease or death).

Importantly, T-DM1 was superior to standard trastuzumab adjuvant treatment, regardless of hormone receptor status, number of neoadjuvant agents received or type of neoadjuvant agents received. The results of the KATHERINE trial resulted in the recommendation of T-DM1 as an option for the adjuvant treatment of HER2-positive early breast cancer in adults who have residual invasive disease in the breast or lymph nodes after neoadjuvant taxane-based and HER2-targeted therapy by the UK National Institute for Health and Care Excellence (NICE),[1] European Society of Medical Oncology (ESMO) and US National Comprehensive Cancer Network guidelines.

Prior to the KATHERINE trial, the main purpose of NACT had been seen as providing a means of downstaging the tumour prior to surgery. The results of this trial highlighted the benefit of the neoadjuvant treatment approach in terms of additionally providing valuable information regarding tumour sensitivity to treatment and permitting a more individualised approach to postsurgical therapy. This treatment approach has subsequently been extended to triple-negative breast cancer.

Paper limitations

The main strengths of this study are the large sample size, central confirmation of HER2 status and intention-to-treat analysis. The study arms were well matched regarding patient characteristics and tumour pathology.

Limitations include the open-label trial design, and variable use of anti-HER2 therapies in the neoadjuvant treatment period; 80.2% of the trastuzumab arm and 80.8% of the T-DM1 arm received trastuzumab as neoadjuvant anti-HER2 therapy, with most of the remaining patients receiving trastuzumab–pertuzumab (18.7% vs. 17.9%) and a very small number receiving other anti-HER2 antibodies. Subgroup analysis indicated slightly greater benefit from T-DM1 in those who received neoadjuvant trastuzumab only, compared with neoadjuvant pertuzumab–trastuzumab (HR = 0.49 vs. HR = 0.54), but the analysis was not adequately powered for this comparison.

The authors acknowledge that some patients lose HER2 overexpression status during neoadjuvant treatment, and as KATHERINE only used the pre-treatment biopsy to define HER2 status, this phenomenon may have affected the results.

Finally, the impact of T-DM1 on overall survival did not meet the pre-specified criteria for significance; this may be important when counselling patients on their overall prognosis.

In context of the relevant current literature

Twenty to twenty-five percent of early breast cancers overexpress the HER2 protein, and this feature is associated with higher disease recurrence and a more aggressive disease phenotype than HER2-negative tumours. The benefit of a 1-year course of adjuvant HER2-targeted treatment was first demonstrated by the HERA trial[2] (see Chapter 35). The Neoadjuvant Herceptin (NOAH) trial subsequently reported enhanced complete pathological response rates with the addition of trastuzumab to chemotherapy in the neoadjuvant setting.[3] Based on the results of these trials, completion of 1 year of adjuvant trastuzumab became standard practice for HER2-positive patients who had received neoadjuvant therapy, irrespective of pathological response status.

Following the Phase II Neosphere study,[4] which showed a further improvement in complete pathological response rates with the addition of a second anti-HER2 antibody, pertuzumab, to neoadjuvant treatment with chemotherapy plus trastuzumab, dual anti-HER2 antibody treatment in the neoadjuvant setting received rapid approval. The APHINITY trial[5] subsequently randomised patients to receive either pertuzumab or placebo added to standard adjuvant chemotherapy plus 1 year of treatment with trastuzumab for resected, operable, HER2-positive breast cancer. Results showed that after 3 years, the rate of IDFS was 92.0% in the pertuzumab group, compared with 90.2% in the placebo group (HR for an invasive-disease event = 0.77, 95% CI = 0.62–0.96, $P = 0.02$). Adjuvant pertuzumab subsequently received approval by NICE for use in patients with node-positive breast cancer.[6]

Follow-up of both the NOAH[7] and Neosphere[8] cohorts highlighted the concept that pathological complete response could be an early indicator of long-term outcome in early-stage HER2-positive breast cancer. There was therefore a clear need to identify alternative treatment strategies for patients with residual disease after NACT.

T-DM1 is composed of the HER2 receptor–specific antibody trastuzumab and a cytotoxic agent, emtansine (DM1), which is a microtubule inhibitor. This combination aims to combine the effect of trastuzumab with directly delivering a cytotoxic agent into the intracellular compartment of tumour cells that overexpress HER2. The safety and survival benefit of T-DM1 in the metastatic setting were confirmed by the EMILIA trial,[9] which showed that T-DM1 improved overall survival compared with lapatinib plus capecitabine in patients with HER2-positive advanced breast cancer previously treated with trastuzumab and a taxane (HR = 0.68, 95% CI = 0.55–0.85, $P < 0.001$).

Following the success of the KATHERINE trial, further studies are now underway to investigate the impact of novel anti-HER2 therapies in patients with residual disease post standard pertuzumab–trastuzumab NACT. CompassHER2 RD (Comprehensive Use of Pathologic Response Assessment to Optimize Therapy in HER2-Positive Breast Cancer Residual Disease) is randomising patients with residual disease to either standard-of-care T-DM1 adjuvant therapy or T-DM1 plus the oral anti-HER2 small-molecule drug tuca-tinib. The conjugated chemotherapy anti-HER2 antibody drug Enhertu (fam-trastuzumab deruxtecan-nxki) has produced exciting results in the metastatic setting, including superiority to T-DM1 in a head-to-head study.[10] Clinical trials of this drug in neoadjuvant and adjuvant settings are now in progress.

The ExteNET trial[11] investigated whether 1 year of extended adjuvant therapy with neratinib, compared with placebo, after completion of 1 year of trastu-zumab improved outcomes. Results showed that after a median follow-up of 5.2 years, patients in the neratinib group had significantly lower relapse rates than those in the placebo group (116 vs. 163 events; stratified HR = 0.73, 95% CI = 0.57–0.92, p = 0.0083). This treatment is now approved for patients who received only trastuzumab in the adjuvant setting and had residual disease if treated in the neoadjuvant setting.

Conclusions

The KATHERINE trial has shown that outcomes for patients with HER2-positive early breast cancer can be improved with the use of additional adjuvant T-DM1 in those with residual disease following neoadjuvant taxane-based chemotherapy with trastuzumab. The risk of side effects is greater than with anti-HER2 antibodies alone therapy, however, and patients must be appropri-ately counselled and monitored when this agent is used clinically.

REFERENCES

1. Trastuzumab emtansine for adjuvant treatment of HER2-positive early breast cancer. NICE technology appraisal guidance 632. Published: 10 June 2020.
2. Cameron D, Piccart-Gebhart MJ, Gelber RD, Procter M, Goldhirsch A, de Azambuja E, et al., Herceptin Adjuvant (HERA) Trial Study Team. 11 years' follow-up of trastu-zumab after adjuvant chemotherapy in HER2-positive early breast cancer: final analysis of the HERceptin Adjuvant (HERA) trial. *Lancet.* 2017;389(10075):1195–205. doi:10.1016/S0140-6736(16)32616-2. Epub 2017 Feb 17. Erratum in: *Lancet.* 2019 Mar 16;393(10176):1100. PMID: 28215665; PMCID: PMC5465633.
3. Gianni L, Eiermann W, Semiglazov V, Manikhas A, Lluch A, Tjulandin S, et al. Neoadjuvant chemotherapy with trastuzumab followed by adjuvant trastuzumab versus neoadjuvant che-motherapy alone, in patients with HER2-positive locally advanced breast cancer (the NOAH trial): a randomised controlled superiority trial with a parallel HER2-negative cohort. *Lancet.* 2010;375(9712):377–84. doi:10.1016/S0140-6736(09)61964-4. PMID: 20113825.
4. Gianni L, Pienkowski T, Im YH, Roman L, Tseng LM, Liu MC, et al. Efficacy and safety of neoadjuvant pertuzumab and trastuzumab in women with locally advanced, inflammatory, or early HER2-positive breast cancer (NeoSphere): a randomised multicentre, open-label, phase 2 trial. *Lancet Oncol.* 2012;13(1):25–32. doi:10.1016/S1470-2045(11)70336-9. Epub 2011 Dec 6. PMID: 22153890.
5. von Minckwitz G, Procter M, de Azambuja E, Zardavas D, Benyunes M, Viale G, et al., APHINITY Steering Committee and Investigators. Adjuvant pertuzumab and trastuzumab in early HER2-positive breast cancer. *N Engl J Med.* 2017;377(2):122–31. doi: 10.1056/

NEJMoa1703643. Epub 2017 Jun 5. Erratum in: N Engl J Med. 2017 Aug 17;377(7):702. Erratum in: N Engl J Med. 2018 Oct 18;379(16):1585. PMID: 28581356; PMCID: PMC5538020.

6. Pertuzumab for adjuvant treatment of HER2-positive early stage breast cancer. NICE technology appraisal guidance 569. Published: 20 March 2019.

7. Gianni L, Eiermann W, Semiglazov V, Lluch A, Tjulandin S, Zambetti M, et al. Neoadjuvant and adjuvant trastuzumab in patients with HER2-positive locally advanced breast cancer (NOAH): follow-up of a randomised controlled superiority trial with a parallel HER2-negative cohort. *Lancet Oncol.* 2014;15(6):640–7. doi:10.1016/S1470-2045(14)70080-4. Epub 2014 Mar 20. Erratum in: Lancet Oncol. 2018 Dec;19(12):e667. PMID: 24657003.

8. Gianni L, Pienkowski T, Im YH, Tseng LM, Liu MC, Lluch A, et al. 5-year analysis of neoadjuvant pertuzumab and trastuzumab in patients with locally advanced, inflammatory, or early-stage HER2-positive breast cancer (NeoSphere): a multicentre, open-label, phase 2 randomised trial. *Lancet Oncol.* 2016;17(6):791–800. doi:10.1016/S1470-2045(16)00163-7. Epub 2016 May 11. PMID: 27179402.

9. Verma S, Miles D, Gianni L, Krop IE, Welslau M, Baselga J, et al., EMILIA Study Group. Trastuzumab emtansine for HER2-positive advanced breast cancer. *N Engl J Med.* 2012;367(19):1783–91. doi:10.1056/NEJMoa1209124. Epub 2012 Oct 1. Erratum in: N Engl J Med. 2013 Jun 20;368(25):2442. PMID: 23020162; PMCID: PMC5125250.

10. Cortés J, Kim SB, Chung WP, Im SA, Park YH, Hegg R, et al., DESTINY-Breast03 Trial Investigators. Trastuzumab deruxtecan versus trastuzumab emtansine for breast cancer. *N Engl J Med.* 2022;386(12):1143–54. doi:10.1056/NEJMoa2115022. PMID: 35320644.

11. Martin M, Holmes FA, Ejlertsen B, Delaloge S, Moy B, Iwata H,et al., ExteNET Study Group. Neratinib after trastuzumab-based adjuvant therapy in HER2-positive breast cancer (ExteNET): 5-year analysis of a randomised, double-blind, placebo-controlled, phase 3 trial. *Lancet Oncol.* 2017;18(12):1688–700. doi:10.1016/S1470-2045(17)30717-9. Epub 2017 Nov 13. PMID: 29146401.

CHAPTER 39

Breast-Conserving Surgery with or without Irradiation in Early Breast Cancer (PRIME II)

Kunkler IH, Williams LJ, Jack WJL, Cameron DA, Dixon JM
Breast-conserving surgery with or without irradiation in early breast cancer.
New England Journal of Medicine. 16;388(7):585–94, 2023

For most older women with early breast cancer, standard treatment after breast-conserving surgery is whole-breast radiotherapy and endocrine treatment. Numerous randomised trials have confirmed that radiotherapy after breast conservation reduces the rate of local recurrence substantially and may have a small long-term (15-year) benefit on survival on meta-analysis of these trials.[1] The PRIME II trial aimed to assess the effect of omission of radiotherapy on local control in older women at low risk of local recurrence.

PAPER DESCRIPTION

- **Objective/Research Question**: The study aimed to answer the question of whether there is a group of older women on adjuvant endocrine therapy with low-risk breast cancer for whom adjuvant radiotherapy can be safely omitted after breast-conserving surgery.

- **Design**: Phase III randomised controlled trial conducted between 2003 and 2009 in 76 hospitals in four countries.

- **Sample Size**: One thousand three hundred and twenty-six patients were randomly allocated to either whole-breast radiotherapy (40–50 Gy in 15–25 fractions +/– boost) ($n = 658$) or no radiotherapy ($n = 668$).

- **Inclusion Criteria**:
  - Age ≥65 years
  - Excision margin ≥1 mm in all directions
  - Primary tumour size ≤3 cm
  - Oestrogen receptor (ER)-positive, progesterone receptor (PR)-positive and treated with adjuvant endocrine therapy
  - Axillary node negative
  - Tumour grade 1–2

DOI: 10.1201/b23352-39

- **Exclusion Criteria**: Age ≥ 65 years of age. A history of in situ or invasive carcinoma of either breast. Malignant disease within the previous 5 years (except non-melanomatous skin cancer or carcinoma in situ of the cervix).

- **Results**: At 9.1 years median follow-up, ipsilateral tumour recurrence was higher in the no-radiotherapy arm (9.5%) compared to the radiotherapy arm (0.9%; hazard ratio (HR) = 10.4, 95% confidence interval [CI] = 4.1–26.1, $p < 0.001$). However, patients in the no-radiotherapy arm had similar rates of distant recurrence (no radiotherapy: 1.6% vs. radiotherapy: 3.0%), breast cancer–specific survival (no radiotherapy: 97.4% vs. radiotherapy: 97.9%) and overall survival (no radiotherapy: 80.8% vs. radiotherapy: 80.7%) as in the radiotherapy arm, with only 13% of deaths due to breast cancer. There were no substantial differences in cumulative incidence of regional recurrence, contralateral breast cancer or new cancers.

EXPERT COMMENTARY BY PUTERI ABDUL HARIS AND DAVID DODWELL

Paper significance

In women aged ≥65 years with node-negative, hormone receptor–positive breast cancer of less than 3 cm size, radiotherapy significantly reduced the risk of locoregional recurrence, with no difference in distant metastases and breast cancer mortality. Radiotherapy can be safely omitted in these patients, provided they receive 5 years of adjuvant endocrine therapy.

Paper limitations

Data on comorbidities and endocrine treatment compliance were not collected. Age in isolation does not correlate with life expectancy, and there is no international consensus on an acceptable rate of local recurrence with radiotherapy omission.

Selection of patients for radiotherapy omission could be aided by a biomarker profile, which the PRIMETIME study is investigating (https://doi.org/10.1186/ISRCTN41579286).

In context of the relevant current literature

There are now several trials which support the possible approach of radiotherapy omission in older patients with low-risk disease. Decision making is not, however, always straightforward.

The improved life expectancy, and generally better fitness, of older patients compared to the calendar period when it was felt that the approach of radiotherapy omission should be investigated means that long-term freedom from recurrence is important. This is particularly the case if one considers that salvage surgical treatment for within-breast recurrence may need to be performed in much older and less fit patients.

Furthermore, the approach of radiotherapy omission is dependent on the need for patients to receive and adhere to endocrine therapy for 5 years, and it is recognised that 30%–40% of patients are unable to achieve this. This is unsurprising, given the recognised and often underappreciated toxicity of aromatase inhibitors.

The greater convenience of a five-fraction course, rather than the 15–25 fractions used in PRIME II, may reduce the attractiveness of radiotherapy omission. Five-fraction radiotherapy was shown to be safe and effective in the FAST-Forward trial.[2] In addition, there is increasing evidence of the safety and reduced toxicity of accelerated partial-breast irradiation[3] instead of whole-breast irradiation, which is another reason why radiotherapy omission is potentially less attractive than it was in the past. Many women, given the choice, may opt for a 1-week course of radiotherapy in preference to the need to take endocrine therapy for 5 years, and it would seem appropriate to offer this option.

Additional relevant studies

Hughes KS, et al. Lumpectomy plus tamoxifen with or without irradiation in women age 70 years or older with early breast cancer: long-term follow-up of CALGB 9343. *J Clin Oncol.* 2013;31:2382–7.

Blamey RW, et al. Radiotherapy or tamoxifen after conserving surgery for breast cancer of excellent prognosis: British Association of Surgical Oncology (BASO) II trial. *Eur J Cancer.* 2013;49:2294–302.

Conclusions

Radiotherapy omission is an option for women aged ≥65 years with early-stage, hormone receptor–positive breast cancer after breast-conserving surgery on endocrine treatment. However, treatment decisions should be individualised by weighing the potential benefits and risks of treatment.

REFERENCES

1. Early Breast Cancer Trialists' Collaborative Group. Effect of radiotherapy after breast-conserving surgery on 10-year recurrence and 15-year breast cancer death: meta-analysis of individual patient data for 10 801 women in 17 randomised trials. *The Lancet.* 2011 Nov 12;378(9804):1707–16.

2. Brunt AM, Haviland JS, Wheatley DA, Sydenham MA, Alhasso A, Bloomfield DJ, Chan C, Churn M, Cleator S, Coles CE, Goodman A. Hypofractionated breast radiotherapy for 1 week versus 3 weeks (FAST-Forward): 5-year efficacy and late normal tissue effects results from a multicentre, non-inferiority, randomised, phase 3 trial. *The Lancet*. 2020 May 23;395(10237):1613–26.

3. Coles CE, Griffin CL, Kirby AM, Titley J, Agrawal RK, Alhasso A, Bhattacharya IS, Brunt AM, Ciurlionis L, Chan C, Donovan EM. Partial-breast radiotherapy after breast conservation surgery for patients with early breast cancer (UK IMPORT LOW trial): 5-year results from a multicentre, randomised, controlled, phase 3, non-inferiority trial. *The Lancet*. 2017 Sep 9;390(10099):1048–60.

Effect of Radiotherapy after Breast-Conserving Surgery on 10-Year Recurrence and 15-Year Breast Cancer Death: Meta-Analysis of Individual Patient Data for 10,801 Women in 17 Randomised Trials

Early Breast Cancer Trialists' Collaborative Group (EBCTCG)
Darby S, McGale P, Correa C, et al.

Lancet 378(9804):1707–1716, 2011

Breast-conserving surgery (BCS) is traditionally followed by radiotherapy to the breast because of historic trials, such as the National Surgical Adjuvant Breast and Bowel Project (NSABP) B-06,[1] which demonstrated that BCS is safe if combined with radiotherapy. The beneficial effect of radiotherapy was mainly felt to be reduction in rates of locoregional disease only. After BCS, radiotherapy reduces recurrence and breast cancer death, but it may do so more for some groups of women than for others. This paper describes the absolute magnitude of these reductions according to various prognostic and other patient characteristics, and relates the absolute reduction in 15-year risk of breast cancer death to the absolute reduction in 10-year recurrence risk.

PAPER DESCRIPTION

- **Objective/Research Question**: To assess the effect of radiotherapy after BCS on the risk of recurrence and breast cancer mortality.

- **Design**: Meta-analysis of individual patient data in 17 randomised trials, conducted between 1976 and 1999, of radiotherapy versus no radiotherapy after BCS.

- **Sample Size**: Information was available for 10,801 women. Eight thousand three hundred and thirty-seven of the patients had pathologically confirmed axillary nodal status. Of these, 7,287 had pN0 disease, and 1,050 had pN+ disease.

- **Inclusion Criteria**: Trials beginning before the year 2000 of adjuvant radiotherapy versus no radiotherapy after BCS were included.

- **Intervention or Treatment Received**: In most of the trials, radiotherapy was given to the conserved breast only.

- **Results**: Median follow-up was 9.5 years, and 25% of women were followed up for > 10 years.

  Radiotherapy halved the average annual rate of any (locoregional or distant) recurrence (risk reduction [RR] = 0.52, 95% confidence interval [CI] = 0.48–0.56) and reduced the annual breast cancer death rate by one-sixth (RR = 0.82, 95% CI = 0.75–0.90).

  The proportional reduction in any first recurrence was greatest in the first year (RR = 0.31, 95% CI = 0.26–0.37) but was still present during years 5–9 (RR = 0.59, 95% CI = 0.50–0.70). Beyond 10 years, information about recurrence was incomplete. In comparison, there were substantial numbers of breast cancer deaths after 10 years, with few events in the first few years.

  The absolute RR for any recurrence in the radiotherapy arm versus BCS-alone arm was 15.7% (95% CI = 13.7–17.7, $p < 0.00001$).

  The 15-year absolute RR in breast cancer death was 3.8% (95% CI = 1.6–6.0, $p = 0.00005$), suggesting that about one breast cancer death was prevented for every four recurrences avoided by radiotherapy.

  In pN0 disease, the absolute reduction in recurrence risk varied significantly with age, grade, oestrogen receptor (ER) status, tamoxifen use and extent of surgery (lumpectomy or quadrantectomy).

  This could not be reliably explored in pN+ disease due to fewer patients in this group.

  The 15-year absolute reduction in breast cancer death in pN+ disease with radiotherapy was 8.5% (95% CI = 1.8–15.2).

EXPERT COMMENTARY BY PUTERI ABDUL HARIS AND DAVID DODWELL

Paper significance

This study showed that radiotherapy after BCS not only reduces the risk of locoregional recurrence but also reduces mortality from breast cancer.

Study limitations

There have been improvements in the multidisciplinary management of breast cancer which would not be reflected by the trials included in this meta-analysis.

Thus, the absolute benefit to be gained from radiotherapy might be less pronounced due to the generally lower risk of recurrence. However, the proportional benefit is likely to be similar.

In context of the relevant current literature

Radiotherapy after BCS halves the risk of any recurrence and reduces the breast cancer death rate by one-sixth in all groups of women, and this varies little depending on available prognostic factors. The absolute benefit varies depending on baseline risk factors.

The dominance of breast-conserving therapy, comprising wide excision and breast irradiation, in the management of early breast cancer owes its place in modern care because of the efforts of pioneering clinical triallists who, in a sceptical and sometimes hostile environment, dared to question the prevailing orthodoxy prevalent in the 1960s and 1970s that mastectomy was mandatory in all patients.[1,2]

The first Early Breast Cancer Trialists' Collaborative Group (EBCTCG) meta-analysis addressing this issue brought together all the available trials and brought the authority and legitimacy of individual patient data meta-analysis to the conclusion that breast-conserving therapy was as effective and as safe as mastectomy. This is now embedded into routine care, and it is easy to forget that the introduction of breast-conserving therapy was one of the most, if not the most, important development in the management of early breast cancer. In contemporary care, developments in oncoplastic breast surgery and neoadjuvant systemic therapy, to effect pre-surgical downstaging, have since extended the scope of breast conservation.

Many have suggested more recently that there may even be a survival improvement associated with breast conservation compared to mastectomy,[3,4] but this belief is based on observational data, and causality cannot be confirmed. This is because in observational studies, despite attempts to adjust for bias, it is inevitable that some residual imbalance will persist which will tend to favour women treated with conservation surgery (e.g., larger tumours are more likely to be treated with mastectomy). This issue was reviewed in an editorial recently.[5]

Conclusions

This meta-analysis confirms the need for breast irradiation after BCS in the great majority of cases. Not only did radiotherapy improve locoregional control, but in patients with node-positive disease, it also improved survival to an extent which was similar to that of systemic adjuvant therapies.

REFERENCES

1. Fisher B, Anderson S, Bryant J, Margolese RG, Deutsch M, Fisher ER, et al. Twenty-year follow-up of a randomized trial comparing total mastectomy, lumpectomy, and lumpectomy plus irradiation for the treatment of invasive breast cancer. *N Engl J Med.* 2002;347(16):1233–41.
2. Veronesi U, Banfi A, Salvadori B, Luini A, Saccozzi R, Zucali R, et al. Breast conservation is the treatment of choice in small breast cancer: long-term results of a randomized trial. *Eur J Cancer.* 1990;26(6):668–70.
3. Hartmann-Johnsen OJ, Karesen R, Schlichting E, Nygard JF. Survival is better after breast conserving therapy than mastectomy for early stage breast cancer: a registry-based follow-up study of norwegian women primary operated between 1998 and 2008. *Ann Surg Oncol.* 2015;22(12):3836–45.
4. van Maaren MC, Strobbe LJA, Koppert LB, Poortmans PMP, Siesling S. Nationwide population-based study of trends and regional variation in breast-conserving treatment for breast cancer. *Br J Surg.* 2018;105(13):1768–77.
5. Dodwell, D., Wheatley D. Counterpoint: Does mastectomy reduce overall survival in early stage breast cancer? *Clin Oncol.* 2021;33 (7):448–50.

CHAPTER 41

Whole-Breast Irradiation with or without a Boost for Patients Treated with Breast-Conserving Surgery for Early Breast Cancer: 20-Year Follow-Up of a Randomised Phase 3 Trial

Bartelink H, Maingon P, Poortmans P, et al. On behalf of the European Organisation for Research and Treatment of Cancer Radiation Oncology and Breast Cancer Groups.

Lancet 16:47–56, 2015

Since the introduction of breast-conserving treatment, various radiation doses after lumpectomy have been used. This randomised trial compared standard whole-breast radiotherapy (WBRT) versus WBRT plus a boost of 16 Gray (Gy) to the tumour bed. Outcomes included overall survival, local control and fibrosis. All patients had stage I and II breast cancer treated with breast-conserving treatment. Here, 20-year follow-up results are presented. This is the key study to demonstrate the value of boost radiotherapy for high local recurrence risk breast cancer.

PAPER DESCRIPTION

- **Objective/Research Question**: To assess the oncological outcomes and adverse events (in particular, fibrosis of the breast) in patients who had a boost dose after breast-conserving surgery alongside WBRT compared to WBRT alone.

- **Design**: Phase III randomised controlled trial, conducted between 1989 and 1996, involving 31 hospitals internationally.

- **Sample Size**: Five thousand three hundred and eighteen patients were randomly assigned to the no-boost ($n = 2,657$) and boost groups ($n = 2,661$).

- **Follow-Up**: Median follow-up was 17.2 years.

- **Inclusion Criteria**: Patients with early-stage breast cancer (T1–2, N0–1, M0) who underwent complete macroscopic excision of breast tumour plus axillary dissection were included.

DOI: 10.1201/b23352-41

- **Exclusion Criteria**:
  - > 70 years old
  - Pure carcinoma *in situ*
  - Multiple tumour foci in > 1 quadrant
  - Previous history of other malignancy
  - Performance status of over 2
  - Residual microcalcifications on mammography
  - Concurrent pregnancy or lactation
  - Radiotherapy started > 9 weeks after surgery, or > 6 months if chemo-therapy given

- **Intervention or Treatment Received**: Patients were randomised to receive 16 Gy in an eight-fraction boost dose to the tumour bed, or no boost dose after 50 Gy in 25 fractions of adjuvant WBRT.

- **Primary and Secondary End Points**: The primary end point was overall survival, and secondary end points were local control, cosmesis and fibrosis.

- **Results**: Survival was equivalent in both arms, with a 20-year overall survival rate of 61.1% in the no-boost group and 57.9% in the boost group (hazard ratio [HR] = 1.05, 99% confidence interval [CI] = 0.92–1.19, $p = 0.323$) with a risk of distant relapse of 24.8% and 26%, respectively (HR = 1.06, 99% CI = 0.92–1.24, $p = 0.29$).

  Thirteen percent of patients in the no-boost group had ipsilateral breast tumour recurrence (IBTR) as first failure versus 9% of patients in the boost group (HR = 0.65, 99% CI = 0.52–0.81, $p < 0.0001$), with younger age associated with higher risk. The absolute risk reduction was largest in patients ≤40 years old. The benefit of the boost dose was independent of tumour characteristics, type of boost and adjuvant systemic treatment.

  Late radiation side effects were increased in the boost group, with a cumulative incidence of severe fibrosis of 5.2% versus 1.8% in the no-boost group ($p < 0.0001$). Cumulative incidence of any degree of fibrosis was 71.4% in the boost group versus 57.2% in the no-boost group ($p < 0.0001$).

EXPERT COMMENTARY BY PUTERI ABDUL HARIS AND DAVID DODWELL

As a result of these findings, a boost dose should be considered in all women aged ≤50 years old.

With increasing age, the risk of developing severe fibrosis with a boost dose increases, while the absolute benefit in terms of IBTR decreased to about 3% in patients over 50 years old. For women > 50 years old, a boost dose can be considered in patients with additional risk factors (e.g., high-grade disease), and the potential side effects would need to be balanced with the potential benefit when counselling patients.

Study limitations

Central pathology review was only done for one-third of patients, but only a few were discordant. Although all patients included had 50 Gy in 25 fractions of adjuvant radiotherapy, the benefit of a boost dose is likely to be applicable after routine 15-fraction radiotherapy, as the UK Standardisation of Breast Radiotherapy (START) trial showed non-inferiority between these two doses. Fibrosis was also difficult to measure objectively.

The role of a boost in young women, in low-grade disease or after neoadjuvant chemotherapy remains unclear. Defining a target volume for boost irradiation can be challenging after oncoplastic breast surgery, and there is a recommendation that clips should be placed in the tumour bed at the time of surgery to permit boost dose localisation.

In context of the relevant current literature

Boost dose reduces the risk of within-breast recurrence but does not improve overall survival. This benefit was independent of age, although the absolute largest benefit was seen in younger patients. However, a boost dose was associated with a higher rate of fibrosis and poorer cosmesis.

The concept of a tumour bed boost after adjuvant breast radiotherapy is based on the observation that the majority of ipsilateral breast cancer recurrences occur in the vicinity of the original primary tumour. Based on the histopathological examination of mastectomy specimens, Holland and colleagues described that 60% of patients had cancer cells within 2 cm of the original primary tumour, and only 11% of patients had cancer cells within 4 cm of the index lesion.[1] This led to the design of randomised trials investigating the addition of 10–25 Gy to the tumour bed after 45–50 Gy of WBRT.[2–4]

Observation of poor cosmetic outcomes related to radiation dose in the European Organisation for Research and Treatment of Cancer (EORTC) 10801 trial[5] led to the design of EORTC 22881-10882 (Bartelink et al.; see chapter title for trial name), delivering an additional dose of 16 Gy to the tumour bed instead of 25 Gy as delivered in the previous trial (due to the poor cosmetic outcome associated with the latter). Although the largest absolute benefit was seen in younger women, this trial suggests the possible role of boost in some women who are aged > 50 years old and have histological characteristics that are likely to be predictive of high IBTR rates in this cohort, namely, hormone receptor negativity and high grade.[6] The association of increased local control with higher radiation dose is consistent with a smaller trial by Romestaing and colleagues.[2]

Several prognostic factors have been associated with an increased risk of local relapse, and these include young age, the presence of DCIS, positive margins, lymphovascular invasion and high grade. Apart from age, there is variation in the published guidelines by collaborative groups and national agencies on boost recommendations. There is also variation in boost dose, radiation modality and planning technique. Through defined inclusion criteria and radiotherapy quality assurance protocols in ongoing and future trials, consistency in boost practices can be improved in the future.

Additional relevant studies

Romestaing P, et al. Role of a 10-Gy boost in the conservative treatment of early breast cancer: results of a randomized clinical trial in Lyon, France. *J Clin Oncol.* 1997;15:963–68.

Schaverien, et al. Use of boost radiotherapy in oncoplastic breast-conserving surgery–a systematic review. *Eur J Surg Oncol.* 2013;39(11):1179–85.

Conclusions

There is a valid clinicopathological basis for delivering a tumour bed boost. However, as there is no survival benefit, and due to poorer cosmesis associated with the tumour bed boost, it is important to discuss this choice with patients who would derive the most benefit to enable informed, shared decision making.

REFERENCES

1. Holland R, et al. The presence of an extensive intraductal component following a limited excision correlates with prominent residual disease in the remainder of the breast. *J Clin Oncol.* 1990;8(1):113–8.
2. Romestaing P, Lehingue Y, Carrie C, Coquard R, Montbarbon X, Ardiet JM, et al. Role of a 10-Gy boost in the conservative treatment of early breast cancer: results of a randomized clinical trial in Lyon, France. *J Clin Oncol.* 1997;15(3):963–8
3. Teissier E, Henry M, Ramaioli A, Lagrange JL, Courdi A, Bensadoun RJ, et al. Boost in conservative treatment: 6 years results of randomized trial. *Breast Cancer Res Treat* 1998;50:287
4. Polgar C, Fodor J, Orosz Z, Major T, Takacsi-Nagy Z, Mangel LC, et al. Electron and high-dose-rate brachytherapy boost in the conservative treatment of stage I-II breast cancer first results of the randomized Budapest boost trial. *Strahlenther Onkol.* 2002;178(11):615–23.
5. Van Dongen JA, Bartelink H, Fentiman IS, et al. Randomized clinical trial to assess the value of breast-conserving therapy in stage I and II breast cancer, EORTC 10801 trial 992. *J Natl Cancer Inst Monogr.* 11:15–18, 1992.
6. Vrieling C, et al. Prognostic factors for local control in breast cancer after long-term follow-up in the EORTC boost vs no boost trial: a randomized clinical trial. *JAMA Oncol.* 2017;3(1):42–48.

CHAPTER 42

Effect of Radiotherapy after Mastectomy and Axillary Surgery on 10-Year Recurrence and 20-Year Breast Cancer Mortality: Meta-Analysis of Individual Patient Data for 8135 Women in 22 Randomised Trials

Early Breast Cancer Trialists' Collaborative Group.
Lancet 383(9935):2127–2135, 2014

Postmastectomy radiotherapy is usually recommended for women with high-recurrence-risk breast cancer, with guidelines suggesting that women with disease greater than 5 cm, locally advanced (T3 or T4), with involved margins or with nodal disease should be offered treatment. Postmastectomy radiotherapy has been shown in previous meta-analyses to reduce the risks of both recurrence and breast cancer mortality in all women with node-positive disease considered together. However, the benefit in women with only one to three positive lymph nodes has been an area of uncertainty. The benefit must be weighed against the risks, with evidence of negative quality-of-life impacts[1] and long-term adverse events. This study aimed to assess the effect of postmastectomy radiotherapy in women stratified by nodal burden, after mastectomy and axillary surgery.

PAPER DESCRIPTION

- **Objective/Research Question**: To assess the benefit of radiotherapy after mastectomy and axillary surgery in women with breast cancer.

- **Design**: Meta-analysis of individual data for 8,135 women randomly assigned to treatment groups during 1964–1986 in 22 trials of radiotherapy to the chest wall and regional lymph nodes versus no radiotherapy after mastectomy and axillary surgery. Outcomes investigated were recurrence and breast cancer mortality.

- **Sample Size**: Four thousand and sixty-five patients had mastectomy with axillary sampling, 183 with unknown axillary surgery extent, and 3,887 with axillary dissection. Pathological nodal status was known for 3,786 of women who had mastectomy and axillary dissection, and they were categorised into three groups: no positive nodes ($n = 700$), 1–3 positive nodes ($n = 1,314$) and ≥4 positive nodes ($n = 1,772$).

- **Follow-Up**: Median follow-up was 9.8 years.

- **Inclusion Criteria**: Trials beginning before 2000 of patients who had radiotherapy or not after mastectomy and axillary surgery for breast cancer.

- **Exclusion Criteria**: EBCTCG meta-analyses have inclusion criteria for trials (not patients) and thus don't have exclusion criteria.

- **Intervention Received**: Radiotherapy included the chest wall, the supraclavicular fossa ± axilla and the internal mammary chain.

- **Results**: In women with negative lymph nodes, radiotherapy had no significant effect on recurrence or breast cancer mortality, but overall mortality was increased (relative risk [RR] = 1.23, 95% confidence interval [CI] = 1.02–1.49, $p = 0.03$).

  Among women with 1–3 positive nodes, radiotherapy reduced locoregional recurrence ($p < 0.00001$), overall recurrence (RR = 0.68, 95% CI = 0.57–0.82, $p = 0.00006$) and breast cancer mortality (RR = 0.80, 95% CI = 0.67–0.95, $p = 0.01$).

  In women with ≥4 positive nodes, radiotherapy reduced locoregional recurrence ($p < 0.00001$), overall recurrence (RR = 0.79, 95% CI = 0.69–0.90, $p = 0.0003$) and breast cancer mortality (RR = 0.87, 95% CI = 0.77–0.99, $p = 0.04$).

  Proportional reductions in recurrence and breast cancer mortality in the node-positive patients were not affected by the use of systemic therapy.

EXPERT COMMENTARY BY PUTERI ABDUL HARIS AND DAVID DODWELL

Paper significance

This study demonstrated that the benefit of postmastectomy radiotherapy extended to women with 1–3 positive lymph nodes, regardless of systemic therapy. The chest wall was an important radiotherapy target.

The absolute gain from radiotherapy is now likely to be smaller due to improvements in systemic treatment, but proportional gains are likely larger due to improvements in radiotherapy technique.

Paper limitations

The quality of included studies and heterogeneity were not reported, but all were randomised trials, and individual patient data were analysed. The effect of radiotherapy after primary systemic therapy is uncertain.

In context of the relevant current literature

One of the main findings throughout the Early Breast Cancer Trialists' Collaborative Group's (EBCTCG) analyses of locoregional radiotherapy was the reduction in breast cancer mortality that accompanied the improvements in locoregional control.

Durable reductions in the risk of local recurrence were seen within 5 years, but improvements in breast cancer mortality were not evident until between 5 and 10 years. These findings are now well-known, but at the time they provided the first evidence that locoregional control of breast could reduce both distant disease recurrence and mortality.

The obvious implication is that persistence of undetectable cancer in the chest wall and regional lymph nodes can cause symptomatic distant disease and subsequent death.

The 'four-to-one' ratio (one breast cancer death prevented for each locoregional recurrence prevented) came to be a common way to describe this effect, although recently there has been a realisation that this relationship is somewhat simplistic and varies according to the type of surgery (e.g., mastectomy recurrence with a ratio of nearer 2:1).

This meta-analysis led to a greater use of postmastectomy radiotherapy in intermediate-risk disease.

The results of the Selective Use of Postoperative Radiotherapy after Mastectomy (SUPREMO) trial[2] (https://www.supremo-trial.com), where patients with intermediate-risk disease were randomised to have locoregional irradiation or not, following mastectomy, are awaited and will help in appreciating the effect of postmastectomy radiotherapy in more recently treated patients.

This is important, as locoregional recurrence rates have fallen in more recently treated patients, and so the absolute benefits of postmastectomy radiotherapy may well be smaller than that seen in the trials included within this meta-analysis. From a surgical perspective, the data from this study have significant implications for breast reconstruction decision making. Now women with any degree of nodal disease may be offered radiotherapy. In view of the negative impact of irradiation, particularly on implant-based immediate reconstruction,[3] this must therefore be discussed carefully with patients before surgery.

Additional relevant study

Clarke M et al., EBCTCG: Effects of radiotherapy and of differences in the extent of surgery for early breast cancer on local recurrence and 15-year survival: an overview of the randomised trials. *Lancet.* 2005;366:2087–106.

Conclusions

After mastectomy and axillary dissection, radiotherapy reduced the risk of recurrence and breast cancer mortality in women with node-positive disease, including 1–3 positive lymph nodes.

REFERENCES

1. Velikova G, Williams LJ, Willis S, Dixon JM, Loncaster J, Hatton M, et al. Quality of life after postmastectomy radiotherapy in patients with intermediate-risk breast cancer (SUPREMO): 2-year follow-up results of a randomised controlled trial. *Lancet Oncol.* 2018;19(11):1516–29.
2. Kunkler IH, Canney P, van Tienhoven G, Russell NS, Group MESTM. Elucidating the role of chest wall irradiation in 'intermediate-risk' breast cancer: the MRC/EORTC SUPREMO trial. *Clin Oncol.* 2008;20(1):31–4.
3. Sewart E, Turner NL, Conroy EJ, Cutress RI, Skillman J, Whisker L, et al. The impact of radiotherapy on patient-reported outcomes of immediate implant-based breast reconstruction with and without mesh. *Ann Surg.* 2022;275(5):992–1001.

CHAPTER **43**

Hypofractionated Breast Radiotherapy for 1 Week versus 3 Weeks (FAST-Forward): 5-Year Efficacy and Late Normal Tissue Effects; Results from a Multicentre, Non-Inferiority, Randomised, Phase 3 Trial

Brunt AM, Haviland JS, Wheatley DA, et al., on behalf of the FAST-Forward
Trial Management Group.
Lancet 395(10237):1613–1626, 2020

This study aimed to identify a five-fraction schedule of adjuvant radiotherapy
delivered in 1 week that is non-inferior in terms of local cancer control and is as
safe as an international standard 15-fraction regimen after primary surgery for
early breast cancer.

PAPER DESCRIPTION

- **Objective/Research Question**: To assess the non-inferiority and safety of
  five-fraction schedules of adjuvant radiotherapy delivered over a week to
  the whole breast or chest wall compared with the UK standard 15-fraction,
  3-week schedule.

- **Design**: A multicentre, nonblinded, Phase III, randomised non-inferiority
  trial, conducted between 2011 and 2014, involving 97 hospitals in the
  UK. The primary end point was ipsilateral breast tumour relapse
  (IBTR). Secondary end points included late side effects and survival
  outcomes. A non-inferiority margin of 1.6% was pre-specified in the
  protocol.

- **Sample Size**: Four thousand and ninety-six patients were included in the
  intention-to-treat analysis (1,361 to 40 Gy in 15 fractions, 1,367 to 27 Gy
  in five fractions and 1,368 to 26 Gy in five fractions).

- **Follow-Up**: Median follow-up was 71.5 months.

- **Inclusion Criteria**: Patients with invasive carcinoma of the breast (pT1–3,
  pN0–1, M0) aged ≥18 years old following breast-conserving surgery

or mastectomy. All had axillary dissection or sentinel node biopsy. Concurrent endocrine treatment and/or trastuzumab were permitted but not chemotherapy.

- **Exclusion Criteria**: A protocol amendment in February 2013 excluded the lowest risk patients (≥65 years old, pT1 pN0 M0, grade 1–2, oestrogen receptor [ER]-positive and *HER2*-negative).

- **Intervention or Treatment Received**: Each participant was allocated to one of the following groups:
  1. *Control group*: 40 Gy in 15 fractions
  2. *Test group 1*: 27 Gy in five fractions
  3. *Test group 2*: 26 Gy in five fractions

A sequential tumour bed boost dose was allowed. Nodal radiotherapy was not allowed in the main study.

- **Results**: Seventy-nine IBTRs were recorded (40 Gy = 31, 27 Gy = 27 and 26 Gy = 21). Hazard ratios (HRs) versus 40 Gy in 15 fractions were 0.86 (95% confidence interval [CI] = 0.51–1.44) for 27 Gy in five fractions, and 0.67 (95% CI = 0.38–1.16) for 26 Gy in five fractions.

  Estimated absolute differences in IBTR versus the control group were −0.3% (95% CI = −1.0 to 0.9) for 27 Gy and −0.7% (95% CI = −1.3 to 0.3) for 26 Gy. Non-inferiority was demonstrated for both five-fraction schedules compared to the 15-fraction schedule.

  Five-year prevalence of clinician-assessed moderate or marked normal tissue effects (NTEs) for the breast or chest wall was 9.9% (40 Gy), 15.4% (27 Gy) and 11.9% (26 Gy). There was a significant difference between 40 Gy and 27 Gy ($p = 0.0003$) but not with 26 Gy ($p = 0.17$), with breast shrinkage being the most prevalent. This was also demonstrated by patient and photographic assessments.

  Comparing the two five-fraction schedules, 26 Gy had significantly lower risk of any moderate or marked breast or chest wall NTEs ($p = 0.0001$) and breast shrinkage ($p = 0.0018$) compared with 27 Gy.

  Locoregional relapse, distant relapse, disease-free survival and overall survival were not statistically significant between the groups.

EXPERT COMMENTARY BY PUTERI ABDUL HARIS AND DAVID DODWELL

Paper significance

This trial builds upon existing hypofractionation trials and supports sensitivity of breast cancer cells to high fraction size. The 5-year results, demonstrating non-inferiority and safety of the 1-week schedule, are practice-changing. Compared to the 3- and 5-week schedules, the 1-week schedule has an additional advantage in terms of convenience and cost. In October 2020, the Royal College of Radiologists issued a consensus voted by the UK breast cancer radiotherapy community for five-fraction radiotherapy as the new standard of care.

The applicability and safety of the 1-week schedule for nodal irradiation remain unanswered at present, and we are awaiting the maturation of the FAST-Forward sub-study to answer this question.

Paper limitations

The size of the trial prevents reliable subgroup analyses by age, tumour characteristics and systemic treatment.

Longer-term disease outcomes and late NTEs are needed to confirm safety and efficacy.

In context of the relevant current literature

Radiotherapy after breast-conserving surgery historically has been delivered with a conventional schedule of 50–54 Gy in 25–28 fractions given over 5–6 weeks, with daily fractions of 1.8–2.0 Gy.

Hypofractionation schedules, where a larger dose is delivered per day over a shorter period of time with a modest decrease in total dose, has been an evolving strategy in delivering adjuvant radiotherapy for breast cancer. The low estimated α/β (alpha/beta) ratio (a widely used index of radiosensitivity) of breast cancer indicates sensitivity to fraction size similar to the dose-limiting normal tissue, and this radiobiological principle suggests that a hypofractionation strategy in breast cancer is potentially more effective compared to conventional fractionation.

Moderate hypofractionation has been a gold standard in the UK for treatment of breast cancer in the adjuvant setting for many years, and there have been several large randomised trials over the years to determine the effectivity and safety of this approach.

The UK Coordinating Committee for Cancer Research initiated the Standardisation of Breast Radiotherapy (START) trials to investigate the effectiveness and normal tissue toxicities of fraction sizes larger than 2.0 Gy.[1,2] The START trials demonstrated that moderate hypofractionation of a 15- or 16-fraction schedule was non-inferior to conventional fractionation in terms of breast cancer outcomes and safety.[3] This was also demonstrated by the 10-year results of the Ontario Clinical Oncology Group trial.[4] The FAST and FAST-Forward trials evolved from the START trials, utilising ultra-hypofractionated five-fraction schedules. Altogether, these studies indicated that both modest and ultra-hypofractionated schedules are as safe and effective as conventional fractionation, and they also increase cost-effectiveness and convenience for patients.

Additional relevant study

Haviland JS, et al. The UK Standardisation of Breast Radiotherapy (START) trial of radiotherapy hypofractionation for treatment of early breast cancer: 10-year follow-up results of two randomised controlled trials. *Lancet Oncol.* 2013;14:1086–94.

Conclusions

The 5-year results of the FAST-Forward trial further support the safety and efficacy of hypofractionation schedules, although we are awaiting long-term results to confirm these findings. Breast radiotherapy is expected to evolve further in the coming years based on robust radiobiological principles elucidated by randomised trials of breast radiotherapy, largely carried out in the UK.

REFERENCES

1. START Trialists' Group, Bentzen SM, Agrawal RK, et al. The UK Standardisation of Breast Radiotherapy (START) Trial A of radiotherapy hypofractionation for treatment of early breast cancer: a randomised trial. *Lancet Oncol.* 2008;9:331–41.
2. START Trialists' Group, Bentzen SM, Agrawal RK, et al. The UK Standardisation of Breast Radiotherapy (START) Trial B of radiotherapy hypofractionation for treatment of early breast cancer: a randomised trial. *Lancet.* 2008;371:1098–107.
3. Haviland JS, et al. The UK Standardisation of Breast Radiotherapy (START) trials of radiotherapy hypofractionation for treatment of early breast cancer: 10-year follow-up results of two randomised controlled trials. *Lancet Oncol.* 2013;14:1086–94.
4. Whelan T, et al. Long-term results of hypofractionated radiation therapy for breast cancer. *N Engl J Med.* 2010;362:513–20.

CHAPTER 44

Adjuvant Zoledronic Acid in Patients with Early Breast Cancer: Final Efficacy Analysis of the AZURE (BIG 01/04) Randomised Open-Label Phase 3 Trial

Coleman R, Cameron D, Dodwell D, et al., on behalf of the AZURE Investigators.
Lancet Oncol 15(9):997–1006, 2014

Breast cancer metastasises to bone in over 70% of patients with advanced disease, at which point the disease is incurable.[1] Preclinical studies provided evidence that bisphosphonates may have an effect on the primary breast tumour as well as being effective in the treatment of cancer spread to bone.[2] The main objective of the Adjuvant Zoledronic Acid to Reduce Recurrence (AZURE) study was to assess the potential anti-tumour effect (and safety) of adding the bisphosphonate zoledronic acid to standard adjuvant systemic therapy, in patients with stage II or III breast cancer. The study identified a significant disease-free survival (DFS) advantage of treatment with zoledronic acid in post-menopausal breast cancer patients, but not in premenopausal patients. Together with other data, this resulted in adjuvant zoledronic acid becoming a recommended treatment option for postmenopausal breast cancer patients.

PAPER DESCRIPTION

- **Objective/Research Question**: To assess the potential anti-tumour effect (and safety) of adding zoledronic acid to standard adjuvant systemic therapy, in patients with stage II or III breast cancer.

- **Design**: The AZURE trial was an open-label, Phase III randomised study in patients with stage II or III breast cancer. The primary outcome was DFS. Secondary outcomes included invasive disease–free survival (IDFS), overall survival (OS), skeletal morbidity and sites of recurrence.

- **Sample Size**: The study recruited 3,360 women from 174 centres in seven countries and randomised them (1:1) to receive either standard therapy or standard therapy plus intravenous zoledronic acid.

- **Inclusion Criteria**: Women with histologically confirmed, invasive breast cancer with either axillary lymph node metastasis (N1) or a T3/T4 primary tumour (American Joint Committee on Cancer [AJCC] Stage II/III).

Stratification factors included: Number of involved axillary lymph nodes, clinical tumour stage, oestrogen receptor (ER) status, type and timing of systemic therapy, menopausal status and statin use. *HER2* testing was not widely used when this study was performed and was only available in ~50% of patients.

- **Exclusion Criteria**: Patients were excluded if they had stage IV disease or a history of cancer within the preceding 5 years. Patients were excluded if they had significant renal impairment. During the trial, osteonecrosis of the jaw (ONJ) became a recognised toxicity of bisphosphonates, and the exclusion criteria were amended to exclude patients with planned jaw surgery or clinically significant, active dental problems.[3]

- **Intervention or Treatment Received**: Dosing of zoledronic acid was 4 mg intravenously every 3–4 weeks for six cycles, then every 3 months for a further eight doses, followed by five cycles 6-monthly to complete 5 years of treatment (19 doses).[4] Daily calcium and vitamin D supplements were recommended for all study patients.

- **Results**: One thousand six hundred and seventy-nine patients were recruited to the standard arm, and 1,681 to receive zoledronic acid plus standard treatment. In total, 95.5% of the patients recruited received chemotherapy, of whom 98% were planned to include an anthracycline and 24% a taxane.

  Analysis of the whole AZURE population (median follow-up of 84 months)[4] revealed no significant improvement in DFS upon adding zoledronic acid to standard systemic therapy (hazard ratio, DFS [HR_{DFS}] = 0.98, 95% confidence interval [CI] = 0.85–1.13, $p = 0.79$), in OS (HR_{OS} = 0.93, 95% CI = 0.82–1.05, $p = 0.22$) or in IDFS (HR_{IDFS} = 0.93, 95% CI = 0.81–1.08, $p = 0.37$). However, a planned analysis of the postmenopausal subgroup found that IDFS in the zoledronic acid group (78.2%) was significantly longer than in the control group (71%; adjusted HR_{IDFS} = 0.75, 95% CI = 0.59–0.96, $p = 0.02$),[5] which is a significant benefit in outcome in the zoledronic acid group.

  Further analysis at 10 years: The 10-year analysis (median follow-up = 117 months, interquartile range [IQR] = 70.4–120.4) showed that, whilst the data continued to demonstrate no significant benefit for the overall population, with IDFS and DFS being similar in both arms (HR_{IDFS} = 0.91, 95% CI = 0.82–1.02, $p = 0.116$; HR_{DFS} = 0.94, 95% CI = 0.84–1.06, $p = 0.340$), the benefit in postmenopausal women was maintained (HR_{IDFS} = 0.78, 95% CI = 0.64–0.94; HR_{DFS} = 0.82, 95% CI = 0.67–1.00, $p = 0.026$).[6]

Although osteonecrosis of the jaw was a significant side effect, it was observed to occur at a low level (cumulative incidence of 1.8% at 10 years), all within the zoledronic acid group.[3]

The annual rate of relapse over a 10-year follow-up period was ~3%.[7] Seventy-two percent of patients relapsed at distant sites, 18% at locoregional sites and 10% at both locoregional and distant sites synchronously. First recurrence in bone occurred in 14% of patients and was the most common site of relapse, with 69% of all patients in the control arm developing spread to bone. Bone metastasis occurred more frequently in ER-positive patients, whereas recurrence overall (especially at visceral sites) was more likely to occur in ER-negative patients. Zoledronic acid treatment reduced bone metastasis in both groups but increased the proportion of patients with extraskeletal metastases, particularly in women who were premenopausal.[7]

EXPERT COMMENTARY BY STEVEN WOOD, EMMA GREEN AND JANET BROWN

Paper significance

Coupled with the meta-analysis discussed below, the AZURE study has significantly contributed to saving lives and healthcare costs (for the UK alone, the potential to save more than 1,000 lives annually with greater than £50 million National Health Service [NHS] savings). It has been practice-changing, contributing to key guidance nationally and internationally with recommendations for adjuvant bisphosphonate use in the UK from the National Institute for Health and Care Excellence (NICE) in 2017 and 2018[8] and European guidance in 2020.[9] A further advantage is that patients who have been on adjuvant bisphosphonates and agents which cause bone loss, such as adjuvant aromatase inhibitors, may have significant protection against bone loss with a reduced rate of fractures.[10]

Paper limitations

Use of bisphosphonates has transformed the treatment of cancer spread to bone from breast cancer in the postmenopausal setting. Although it is unlikely to change the findings of the AZURE trial, it should be noted that the study was done before a range of modern treatments were available, including adjuvant immunotherapy for triple-negative breast cancer, adjuvant CDK4/6 inhibitors for ER-positive patients and a range of anti-HER2 therapies. Also, adjuvant bisphosphonates remain ineffective in premenopausal women, and an effective alternative is urgently needed for these patients. In addition, bisphosphonates, although inexpensive, are not without toxicities.

In context of the relevant current literature

Meta-analysis

The beneficial effects of adjuvant bisphosphonate treatment in postmeno-pausal women in the AZURE study were confirmed in a large meta-analysis of 18,766 women.[10] This analysis covered a range of trials, with both oral and intravenous bisphosphonates, and included trial durations of 2–5 years of bisphosphonate treatment.[11] The mean scheduled treatment duration was 3.4 years, and median follow-up was 5.6 years. The optimal duration of treatment remains unknown.

Overall, including all menopausal groups, the data demonstrated only border-line significance for benefit of bisphosphonates in breast cancer mortality, recurrence and distant recurrence, but a clear reduction in bone recurrence (relative risk [RR] = 0.83, 95% CI = 0.73–0.94, $2p$ = 0.004). However, for 11,767 post-menopausal women, bisphosphonates yielded significant reductions in mortality (RR = 0.82, 95% CI = 0.73–0.93, $2p$ = 0.002), disease recurrence (RR = 0.86, 95% CI = 0.78–0.94, $2p$ = 0.002) and bone recurrence (RR = 0.72, 95% CI = 0.60–0.86, $2p$ = 0.0002), with reduction in bone fractures (RR = 0.85, 95% CI = 0.75–0.97, $2p$ = 0.02). These data equated to an 18% reduction in cancer mortality and 28% reduction in bone recurrence at 10 years. There were no apparent effects on outcome in premenopausal women.[11]

In addition, several publications arising from analysis of samples taken from AZURE patients have looked into prognostic biomarkers for risk of future bone metastasis and predictive markers for response to treatment in high-risk early breast cancer. This may, in future, lead to stratified treatment recommendations to personalise treatment for prevention of bone metastasis.[13,14]

In addition to bisphosphonates, the anti-RANK-ligand antibody-based therapeutic denosumab has been proposed as a potential treatment in breast cancer spread to bone. However, in the Adjuvant Denosumab in Early Breast Cancer (D-CARE) study, comparing denosumab to placebo control, no significant difference in bone metastasis–free survival was observed between the two arms (HR = 0.97, 95% CI = 0.82–1.14, p = 0.70).[15]

Conclusions

Adjuvant bisphosphonates have provided a much-needed approach to preventing breast cancer relapse in postmenopausal patients with early breast cancer, with potential to save thousands of lives worldwide every year. Unfortunately, we still lack such treatments for premenopausal women.

REFERENCES

1. Kennecke H, et al. Metastatic behavior of breast cancer subtypes. *J Clin Oncol.* 2010;28(20):3271–7.
2. Holen I, Coleman RE. Anti-tumour activity of bisphosphonates in preclinical models of breast cancer. *Breast Cancer Res.* 2010;12(6):214.
3. Rathbone EJ, et al. Osteonecrosis of the jaw and oral health-related quality of life after adjuvant zoledronic acid: an adjuvant zoledronic acid to reduce recurrence trial subprotocol (BIG01/04). *J Clin Oncol.* 2013;31(21): 2685–91.
4. Coleman RE, et al. Breast-cancer adjuvant therapy with zoledronic acid. *N Engl J Med.* 2011;365(15):1396–405.
5. Coleman R, et al. Adjuvant zoledronic acid in patients with early breast cancer: final efficacy analysis of the AZURE (BIG 01/04) randomised open-label phase 3 trial. *Lancet Oncol.* 2014;15(9):997–1006.
6. Coleman RE, et al. Benefits and risks of adjuvant treatment with zoledronic acid in stage II/III breast cancer. 10 years follow-up of the AZURE randomized clinical trial (BIG 01/04). *J Bone Oncol.* 2018;13: 123–35.
7. D'Oronzo S, et al. Natural history of stage II/III breast cancer, bone metastasis and the impact of adjuvant zoledronate on distribution of recurrences. *J Bone Oncol.* 2021;28:100367.
8. Early breast cancer (preventing recurrence and improving survival): adjuvant bisphosphonates. July 2017 NICE Evidence summary [ES15]. Early and locally advanced breast cancer NICE Guideline NG101. July 2018. Section 1.9 contains recommendations and rationale. Full details in Evidence review G: adjuvant bisphosphonates
9. Coleman R, et al. Bone health in cancer: ESMO Clinical Practice Guidelines. *Ann Oncol.* 2020;31(12): 1650–63.
10. Anagha PP, Sen S. The efficacy of bisphosphonates in preventing aromatase inhibitor induced bone loss for postmenopausal women with early breast cancer: a systematic review and meta-analysis. *J Oncol.* 2014;2014: 625060.
11. Early Breast Cancer Trialists' Collaborative, G., Adjuvant bisphosphonate treatment in early breast cancer: meta-analyses of individual patient data from randomised trials. *Lancet.* 2015;386(10001): 1353–61.
12. Coleman R, et al. Effect of MAF amplification on treatment outcomes with adjuvant zoledronic acid in early breast cancer: a secondary analysis of the international, open-label, randomised, controlled, phase 3 AZURE (BIG 01/04) trial. *Lancet Oncol.* 2017;18(11): 1543–52.
13. Brown JE,Westbrook JA, Wood SL. Dedicator of cytokinesis 4: a potential prognostic and predictive biomarker within the metastatic spread of breast cancer to bone. *Cancer Inform.* 2019;18: 1176935119866842.
14. Westbrook JA, et al. CAPG and GIPC1: breast cancer biomarkers for bone metastasis development and treatment. *J Natl Cancer Inst.* 2016;108(4).
15. Coleman R, et al. Adjuvant denosumab in early breast cancer (D-CARE): an international, multicentre, randomised, controlled, phase 3 trial. *Lancet Oncol.* 2020;21(1): 60–72.

CHAPTER 45

Long-Term Effects of Anastrozole on Bone Mineral Density: 7-Year Results from the ATAC Trial

Eastell R, Adams J, Clack G, Howell A, Cuzick J, Mackey J, et al.
Annals Oncol 22(4):857–862, 2011

In postmenopausal women with breast cancer, large clinical trials have shown that aromatase inhibitors (AIs), including anastrozole (the Arimidex, Tamoxifen, Alone or in Combination [ATAC] study[1]), letrozole (the Breast International Group [BIG] 1-98 study[2]) and exemestane (the Intergroup Exemestane Study [IES][3]), demonstrated benefits in disease-free survival (DFS) and other positive outcomes compared to tamoxifen alone. Specifically, at a 5-year median follow-up, ATAC demonstrated significantly prolonged DFS and time to recurrence amongst postmenopausal women taking anastrozole, compared with those who took only tamoxifen. As a result of this and other similar trials, AIs have become the standard of care. The ATAC trial itself focussed on survival metrics as its primary outcome, but bone health impacts of the trial were also reported to 5 years. AIs have long-term adverse effects on bone, related to their profound suppression of circulating estrogen;[4] they increase bone loss, decrease bone mineral density (BMD) and increase fracture risk.[5] This ATAC trial follow-on study extended our understanding of the longer-term impacts of endocrine therapy after the 5 years of adjuvant treatment finishes.[1]

PAPER DESCRIPTION

- **Objective/Research Question**: The objective of the study was to assess the long-term effects of treatment with anastrozole or tamoxifen on bone health, using ATAC trial data collected out to 7 years follow-up beyond the duration of endocrine therapy treatment.

- **Design**: The ATAC trial was a randomised, double-blind, multicentre study investigating the efficacy and tolerability of adjuvant AIs (using anastrozole), tamoxifen or combination therapy for postmenopausal women with hormone receptor–positive early breast cancer. The combination arm was discontinued after the 33-month median follow-up analysis identified a lack of additional benefit compared to tamoxifen alone.

DOI: 10.1201/b23352-45

This paper describes a prospectively designed sub-study, within the ATAC trial, to assess the long-term effects of AIs and tamoxifen on BMD using a posttreatment follow-up extension study. This was a randomised, double-blind, multicentre study comparing the change in BMD during an off-treatment follow-up period of 2 years, using the end-of-treatment 5-year bone dual-energy X-ray absorptiometry (DXA) scan as baseline.

- **Sample Size**: Seventy-one participants were included in the posttreatment follow-up extension bone sub-study (n = 32 anastrozole, n = 38 tamoxifen at 6-year bone scan; n = 27 anastrozole and n = 27 tamoxifen at 7-year bone scan).

- **Inclusion Criteria**: Participants from the monotherapy arms of the bone sub-study (treatment with 1 mg anastrozole or with 20 mg tamoxifen) who remained recurrence-free, were not osteoporotic at 5 years at evaluable 5-year bone scans for both lumbar and total hip, gave written informed consent to further follow-up and did not possess any of the criteria for withdrawal.

- **Exclusion Criteria**: Participants with osteoporosis (T-score <–2.5 at the lumbar spine or total hip) or those taking bisphosphonates. Those with osteopenia (T-score –1 to –2.5) were included at the investigators' discretion.

- **Intervention or Treatment Received**: A bone densitometry (DXA) scan at treatment completion (5 years) represented baseline BMD. Additional BMD assessments were carried out at 6 years and 7 years, and compared with the 5-year baseline DXA scan.

- **Results**: Amongst anastrozole-treated participants, there was a statistically significant increase in median lumbar spine BMD at years 6 and 7 (at year 6 = +2.35%, interquartile range [IQR] = –5.34 to 8.19, P = 0.04; at year 7 = +4.02%, IQR = –6.04 to 14.01, P = 0.0004). Median total hip BMD stabilised during the off-treatment follow-up period, although this was not statistically significant (at year 6 = +0.71%, IQR = –9.42 to 4.63, P = 0.3; at year 7 = +0.5%, IQR = –8.74 to 4.27, P = 0.8).

  Amongst tamoxifen-treated participants, there was a decrease in median lumbar spine BMD across years 6 and 7 that was not statistically significant (at year 6 = –0.79%, IQR = –10.61 to 4.35, P = 0.2; at year 7 = –0.3%, IQR = –7.43 to 10.22, P = 0.9). Overall median total hip BMD showed a statistically significant decrease during this time (at year 6 = –2.09%, IQR = –4.34 to 5.70, P = 0.0003; at year 7 = –2.52%, IQR = –9.5 to 8.02, P = 0.0002).

The recovery in lumbar spine BMD and absence of further loss at the hip were consistent with the reduction in the annual rate of fracture observed after treatment cessation in the main ATAC trial.

EXPERT COMMENTARY BY SOPHIE TROTTER AND JANET BROWN

Paper significance

This sub-study found that, despite greater bone loss with anastrozole over tamoxifen during the 5-year treatment period, participants treated with anastrozole saw partial recovery of their BMD at the lumbar spine and no further loss in BMD at the hip in the posttreatment period, whereas participants treated with tamoxifen saw no significant change in BMD at the lumbar spine with further loss in BMD at the hip. Thus, in postmenopausal patients, while anastrozole carries a greater associated fracture risk in comparison with tamoxifen, this plateaus after treatment. This paper has provided a significant contribution to awareness of the need for clinicians to consider bone health during and after AI therapy and to take appropriate bone protection measures.

Paper limitations

Limitations necessitate that these results are interpreted with caution.

Firstly, a relatively low number of participants were included in this bone substudy ($n = 71$), and follow-up was relatively short (2 years post treatment, despite survival far exceeding this).

Secondly, while demographics were reported as balanced across treatment groups and representative of the overall ATAC trial population, there was limited information available, with reference instead to previously published demographic information for the overall ATAC trial. Similarly, there are no frailty and comorbidity data available here. These are particularly relevant when considering the necessity of excluding participants with known osteoporosis, potentially influencing how representative this study population may be.

Thirdly, while the ATAC trial studied the effect of anastrozole and tamoxifen on BMD during and following a 5-year treatment period, longer durations of endocrine therapy are used, particularly with higher risk tumours, and it is unclear whether the posttreatment findings here still apply with prolonged adjuvant endocrine therapy (7–10 years).

In context of the relevant current literature

Cross-study comparisons and major trials of anastrozole, letrozole and exemestane identified that the risks of bone demineralisation, osteoporosis and fracture are seen across this class.[6,7] The IBIS-II prevention trial,[8] which compared anastrozole with placebo in postmenopausal women at high risk of developing breast cancer, also included a bone sub-study of 1,410 postmenopausal women. This preventative study found, similarly to ATAC, a degree of BMD loss during the active treatment period with anastrozole (years 1 to 5) in comparison with placebo which, 2 years after stopping treatment, improved at the lumbar spine with no further reduction at the hip. IBIS-II additionally trialled administration of bisphosphonates (risedronate) to osteopenic and osteoporotic women during the treatment period and found an improvement in BMD at the lumbar spine but not at the total hip.

Bisphosphonates reduce this risk in premenopausal[9] and postmenopausal[4] women with oestrogen receptor–positive breast cancer on endocrine therapy. A meta-analysis[10] identified that among bone-modifying agents (risedronate, zoledronate and denosumab), zoledronate was associated with the greatest increase in BMD, risedronate was associated with lower fracture risk and denosumab was associated with increased BMD and reduced fracture risk. Moreover, the Early Breast Cancer Trialists' Collaborative Group (EBCTCG) meta-analysis[11] found evidence for a benefit amongst all postmenopausal women taking bisphosphonates against bone recurrence, fracture rates, breast cancer mortality and overall survival.

These studies have led to the development of bone health guidelines[12] by ESMO (European Society for Medical Oncology) advocating for aggressive risk reduction with frequent monitoring and early intervention. Clinical practice should now include a high index of suspicion for AI-induced bone loss with appropriate use of calcium and vitamin D supplementation, bisphosphonates or alternative bone-targeted agents such as denosumab. However, in the UK, many postmenopausal women with high-risk early breast cancer receive adjuvant bisphosphonates to reduce the risk of metastasis (see Chapter 44), which may negate the need for routine DXA scanning for such patients who are also on AIs.

Conclusions

Postmenopausal women with early breast cancer may be on AI therapy for many years, and it is important to optimise their quality of life. AI therapy is associated with several long-term side effects, including bone loss; careful management is needed to avoid this and the associated osteoporosis and fracture risk. This paper has highlighted these issues and the measures which need to be adopted to manage them.

REFERENCES

1. Howell A, Cuzick J, Baum M, Buzdar A, Dowsett M, Forbes JF, et al. Results of the ATAC (Arimidex, Tamoxifen, Alone or in Combination) trial after completion of 5 years' adjuvant treatment for breast cancer. *Lancet*. 2005;365:60–62.

2. Thürlimann B, Keshaviah A, Coates A, et al. A Comparison of letrozole and tamoxifen in postmenopausal women with early breast cancer. *New Engl J Med*. 2005;353:2747–57. doi:10.1056/NEJMoa052258

3. Coombes RC, Hall E, Gibson LJ, et al. A randomized trial of exemestane after two to three years of tamoxifen therapy in postmenopausal women with primary breast cancer. *New Engl J Med*. 2004;350:1081–92. doi:10.1056/NEJMoa040331

4. Confavreux CB, Fontana A, Guastalla JP, et al. Estrogen-dependent increase in bone turnover and bone loss in postmenopausal women with breast cancer treated with anastrozole. Prevention with bisphosphonates. *Bone*. 2007;41:346–52. doi: 10.1016/j.bone.2007.06.004

5. Hadji P. Aromatase inhibitor-associated bone loss in breast cancer patients is distinct from postmenopausal osteoporosis. *Critical Reviews in Oncology/Hematology*. 2009;69:73–82. doi:10.1016/j.critrevonc.2008.07.013

6. McCloskey E, Hannon R, Lakner G, et al. The letrozole (L), exemestane (E), and anastrozole (A) pharmacodynamics (LEAP) trial: A direct comparison of bone biochemical measurements between aromatase inhibitors (AIs) in healthy postmenopausal women. *J Clin Oncol*. 2006;24.

7. De Placido S, Gallo C, De Laurentiis M, et al. Adjuvant anastrozole versus exemestane versus letrozole, upfront or after 2 years of tamoxifen, in endocrine-sensitive breast cancer (FATA-GIM3): a randomised, phase 3 trial. *Lancet Oncol*. 2018;19:474–85. doi:10.1016/S1470-2045(18)30116-5

8. Sestak I, Blake G, Patel R, et al. Off-treatment bone mineral density changes in postmenopausal women receiving anastrozole for 5 years: 7-year results from the IBIS-II prevention trial. *Br J Cancer*. 2021;124:1373–8.

9. Gnant MFX, Mlineritsch B, Luschin-Ebengreuth G, et al. Zoledronic acid prevents cancer treatment-induced bone loss in premenopausal women receiving adjuvant endocrine therapy for hormone-responsive breast cancer: a report from the Austrian Breast and Colorectal Cancer Study Group. *J Clin Oncol*. 2007;25:820–8. doi:10.1200/JCO.2005.02.7102

10. Miyashita H, Satoi S, Kuno T, et al. Bone modifying agents for bone loss in patients with aromatase inhibitor as adjuvant treatment for breast cancer; insights from a network meta-analysis. *Breast Cancer Res Treat*. 2020;181:279–89. doi:10.1007/s10549-020-05640-3

11. (EBCTCG) EBCTCG. Adjuvant bisphosphonate treatment in early breast cancer: meta-analyses of individual patient data from randomised trials. *Lancet*. 2015;386:1353–61.

12. Cardoso F, Kyriakides S, Ohno S, et al. Early breast cancer: ESMO Clinical Practice Guidelines for diagnosis, treatment and follow-up†. *Ann Oncol*. 2019;30:1194–220. doi: 10.1093/annonc/mdz173.

CHAPTER 46

Locoregional Treatment versus No Treatment of the Primary Tumour in Metastatic Breast Cancer: An Open-Label Randomised Controlled Trial

Badwe R, Hawaldar R, Nair N, Kaushik R, Parmar V, Siddique S, et al.
Lancet Oncol 16:1380–1388, 2015

Surgery to remove the primary breast cancer in women presenting with *de novo* metastatic disease has been a controversial issue for many years. Theoretically, some argued that removal of the source of tumour cells and cytokines would reduce metastatic progression. Numerous observational studies had usually reported survival benefit. However, selection bias, with women with low metastatic burdens and better disease biology being offered surgery, meant that these results were unreliable. It was long believed that a randomised trial in this setting would be impossible due to lack of patient and clinician equipoise. The Tata Memorial Centre trial was the first randomised trial to rigorously evaluate the survival benefit of surgery in *de novo* stage IV breast cancer. It found no survival benefit and a small benefit to local control. It has since been followed by several other randomised trials including the US-based Eastern Cooperative Oncology Group–American College of Radiology Imaging Network (ECOG-ACRIN) E2108 trial, the Turkish Trial and most recently the Japanese Clinical Oncology Group Trial. With the exception of the Turkish Trial (which had unbalanced groups in favour of surgery), all have found no survival benefit to surgery.

PAPER DESCRIPTION

- **Objective/Research Question**: This study was undertaken to compare the effect of locoregional treatment (LRT) to no LRT on overall survival (OS) in women with *de novo* metastatic breast cancer (MBC).

- **Design**: Open-label, randomised controlled trial (RCT).

- **Sample Size**: Three hundred and fifty patients with MBC.

- **Inclusion Criteria**:
  - Histopathological confirmation of MBC
  - Have not received any cancer-directed treatment

DOI: 10.1201/b23352-46

- Age ≤65 years
- Patients with resectable hormone receptor (HR)-positive tumours upfront and unresectable tumours with partial or complete response to chemotherapy
- Estimated life expectancy of at least 1 year during registration and at least 6 months during randomisation

- **Exclusion Criteria**:
  - Multiple liver metastases with grossly deranged liver function test, and involvement of more than two visceral organs, because of shorter life expectancy
  - Post-chemotherapy and before randomisation: stable disease
  - Ulceration, fungation or bleeding at the local site mandating palliative LRT

- **Intervention Received**: LRT in the form of surgery to the primary in the breast (mastectomy or breast conservation surgery) and axilla (axillary lymph node dissection) followed by radiotherapy (RT).

- **Results**: From 7 February 2005 to 18 January 2013, 716 patients presented at Tata Memorial Centre with *de novo* MBC, of whom 350 were randomised and included in the study (14 responders post primary endocrine treatment and 336 post first-line chemotherapy).

    Of the 350 randomised patients, 173 patients were allocated to the LRT arm and 177 to the no-LRT arm. Baseline demographics and disease characteristics were well balanced between arms, including baseline patient characteristics, tumour characteristics and systemic treatment. At a median follow-up of 23 months (interquartile range [IQR] = 12.2–38.7), the results were analysed with an intention-to-treat analysis.

    The authors reported that eight (5%) of 173 patients in the LRT group did not undergo LRT. Eighteen (10%) of 177 patients in the no-LRT group underwent surgical removal of the primary tumour for palliation of symptoms upon progression at a median of 4.1 months (IQR = 3–15) after randomisation.

    The authors reported that there was no difference in OS with or without LRT (median survival = 19.2 months, 95% CI = 15.98–22.46 vs. 20.5 months, 95% CI = 16.96–23.98; hazard ratio [HR] = 1.04, 95% CI = 0.81–1.34, p = 0.79).

    Two-year OS was 41.9% (95% CI = 33.9–49.7) in the LRT group and 43.0% (95% CI = 35.2–50.8) in the no-LRT group. The findings from subgroup analyses of OS were consistent with the overall result.

    On multivariate analysis, OS was independently associated with expression of the oestrogen receptor (ER) or progesterone receptor (PR) (HR = 0.37, 95% CI = 0.28–0.48, p < 0.0001) and fewer distant metastatic sites at initial presentation (HR = 0.61, 95% CI = 0.45–0.83, p = 0.0020).

The authors reported a significant improvement in locoregional progression-free survival (LR-PFS) in the LRT group compared to the no-LRT group (median not attained vs. 18.2 months, 95% CI = 15.1–21.3; HR = 0.16, 95% CI = 0.10–0.26, $p < 0.0001$). On the contrary, there was a significant detriment reported in the distant disease–free survival (DDFS) in the LRT group compared to the no-LRT group (median = 11.3 months, 95% CI = 7.7–14.84 vs. 19.8 months, 95% CI = 10.26–29.0; HR = 1.42, 95% CI = 1.08–1.85, $p = 0.012$).

Health-related quality of life (HR-QoL) was only assessed in a subset of patients in this trial and was analysed and reported separately.[1]

EXPERT COMMENTARY BY URVASHI JAIN, ASHUTOSH KOTHARI AND RAJENDRA BADWE

Paper significance

This was the first level-1 evidence in the form of an RCT with the largest patient series published at a very crucial time that assessed the role of LRT and discouraged its routine use in *de novo* MBC with conclusive findings. Preclinical data in animal studies have suggested that surgical removal of the primary tumour could potentially promote growth of disease at distant sites.[2–5] Although the conventional wisdom has been to treat MBC as a systemic disease, with treatment to the primary being reserved for palliative reasons only, there was no robust evidence until this time that guided or supported treatment decisions in these patients. With the advent of newer systemic treatments and their promising effect on distant metastatic sites with evolving evidence, a clinician could be tempted to treat the primary disease with curative intent. Moreover, several retrospective studies along with a meta-analysis of these studies reported a significant benefit with LRT on OS in this group of patients.[6] However, these were fraught with selection bias and could not account for potential confounding factors to reach a definitive conclusion to change practice. This was a practice-changing landmark trial in this regard, as there was a conflicting body of evidence reported before this.

This is the first study to report the impact of removal of primary on distant metastases in humans and the importance of events at the time of surgery in breast cancer. These data align with those from animal experiments and should offer major insights into the biology of breast cancer and its interaction with treatment, as well as open a window of opportunity to modulate tumour behaviour at the time of delivery of treatment.

Study limitations

Since this was a single-centre study conducted in India, one could argue that this study is not representative of the world population. However, this was conducted at one of the high-volume cancer centres in Asia and was followed by four other

RCTs: one in North America (ECOG-ACRIN E2108), one in Austria (Austrian Breast Cancer Study Group [ABCSG]-28 POSYTIVE), one in Turkey (MF07-01) and one in Japan (Japan Clinical Oncology Group [JCOG] 1017, published in abstract form in 2023 at American Society of Clinical Oncology [ASCO]), with three of the published trials and a meta-analysis of the four published RCTs showing similar results.[7–11]

Thirty-one percent (107/350) of patients had *HER2* receptor–positive disease, and most of these patients (92% = 98/107) did not receive *HER2*-targeted therapy due to financial constraints at the time. This could be critiqued as suboptimal systemic treatment. The authors argue that because of random allocation, these factors are unlikely to affect the outcome of this study. The results from three other RCTs support this argument, as they published similar results with *HER2*-directed treatment in this group of patients.[7,8]

HR-QoL was deemed as one of the secondary outcome measures of this study which was only assessed in a subset of the patients and analysed and reported separately.[1] One could argue that this pertinent outcome could skew the conclusive results. However, the two other RCTs did not report any quality-of-life (QoL) advantage with LRT or no LRT.[7,8] In fact, the ECOG-ACRIN E2108 trial did show a detriment in QoL at 18 months in the LRT group.[7]

The random allocation of responders to chemotherapy as the first-line treatment could limit the applicability of these results in patients who receive endocrine treatment or *HER2*-directed therapy along with chemotherapy as their first-line systemic treatments. However, there is no reason to believe that there is an interaction between these treatments and the effect of locoregional treatment of the primary tumour. The ECOG-ACRIN E2108 trial supports this reasoning by publishing similar results accounting for these differences in first-line systemic therapy options.[7]

In context of the relevant current literature

To get an overall perspective on this subject, it is essential to review the other RCTs that produced similar results and closely compare the Turkish trial that reported conflicting results.

The key difference between the four RCTs is in their design: The Indian (Tata) and North American (ECOG-ACRIN E2108) trials randomised responders following first-line systemic therapy, whereas the Turkish (MF07-01) and Austrian (ABCSG-28 POSYTIVE) trials randomised patients with *de novo* metastatic disease upfront without systemic treatment.[7-9]

The Austrian trial was halted prematurely due to poor accrual (90 instead of the planned 254 patients), thus making it underpowered to detect the differences between the two groups. Although it did not reach statistical significance, it showed an improved trend for OS in the no-LRT arm.

The ECOG-ACRIN E2108 trial also made amendments to the original design plan due to the slow accrual rate to maintain the power of the study to detect differences. It was more flexible with primary systemic treatment options, offering endocrine treatment and *HER2*-directed treatment as appropriate, which is reflected in an OS rate of approximately 65% in both arms at 3 years as compared to about 40% at 2 years in the Indian trial. However, the difference in OS within a resource-rich healthcare system with optimal systemic treatments and early presentation of disease in the developed countries did not translate into an OS difference between the two arms.

Of note, the Turkish trial, which did report an advantage in OS at 5 years, did not demonstrate this advantage at 2 years, showcasing results consistent with all the other RCTs at 2 years.[9] There are several caveats in the Turkish MF07-01 trial which may have influenced the results favouring the LRT group, resulting in an OS advantage at 5 years. There were no stratification criteria applied, which resulted in a significant imbalance between the two groups: significantly higher ER-positive patients in the LRT group (86% vs. 73%), patients with higher solitary bone metastases in the LRT group (23% vs. 15%) and a significantly lower proportion of triple-negative patients in the LRT group (7% vs. 18%). This demonstrates that the LRT group predominantly consisted of patients with a lower volume of metastatic disease and good biology which may have resulted in favourable outcomes in this group. The subset analyses did show favourable outcomes in HR-positive disease, younger women and women with bone metastases only, particularly solitary bone metastasis (HR = 0.47, 95% CI = 0.23–0.98), but this was unplanned and post hoc.

A recent systematic review and meta-analysis of the four published RCTs with 970 patients reports no advantage in OS in the LRT group in the pooled analysis (HR = 0.97, 95% CI = 0.72–1.29).[11] These results are consistent on multiple sensitivity analyses for OS and leave-one-out sensitivity analyses for OS. The results did not vary on subgroup analysis based on either receptor status or bone versus visceral disease. Since then, the Japanese (JCOG) trial has reported its findings in abstract form (at ASCO 2023), reinforcing these findings.

Conclusions

Based on this trial, and evidence published so far, the routine use of LRT is not justified; it should be discouraged in patients with *de novo* MBC and reserved for situations that necessitate palliation. With advances in systemic and local therapy, oligometastatic disease with a low-volume burden of metastases and favourable biology needs to be dealt with as a separate entity, awaiting the results of evolving research in this field.

REFERENCES

1. Badwe RA, Parmar V, Hawaldar R, et al. Surgical removal of primary tumor in metastatic breast cancer: Impact on health-related quality of life (HR-QOL) in a randomized controlled trial (RCT). *Proc Am Soc Clin Oncol.* 2014;32(suppl 5S):abstr 1124.
2. Gunduz N, Fisher B, Saffer EA. Effect of surgical removal on the growth and kinetics of residual tumor. *Cancer Res.* 1979;39:3861–65.
3. Braunschweiger PG, Schiffer LM, Betancourt S. Tumour cell proliferation and sequential chemotherapy after primary tumour resection in C3H/HeJ mammary tumours. *Breast Cancer Res Treat.* 1982;2:323–29.
4. Fisher B, Gunduz N, Coyle J, Rudock C, Saffer E. Presence of a growth-stimulating factor in serum following primary tumor removal in mice. *Cancer Res.* 1989;49:1996–2001.
5. Demicheli R, Retsky MW, Swartzendruber DE, Bonadonna G. Proposal for a new model of breast cancer metastatic development. *Ann Oncol.* 1997;8:1075–80.
6. Harris E, Barry M, Kell MR. Meta-analysis to determine if surgical resection of the primary tumour in the setting of stage IV breast cancer impacts on survival. *Ann Surg Oncol.* 2013;20:2828–34.
7. Khan SA, Zhao F, Solin LJ, et al. A randomized phase III trial of systemic therapy plus early local therapy versus systemic therapy alone in women with *de novo* stage IV breast cancer: a trial of the ECOG-ACRIN Research Group (E2108). *J Clin Oncol.* 2020;38.
8. Fitzal F, Bjelic-Radisic V, Knauer M, et al. Impact of breast surgery in primary metastasized breast cancer: outcomes of the prospective randomized phase III ABCSG-28 POSYTIVE trial. *Ann Surg.* 2019;269:1163e9. doi: 10.1097/SLA.0000000000002771
9. Soran A, Ozmen V, Ozbas S, et al. Randomized trial comparing resection of primary tumor with No surgery in stage IV breast cancer at presentation: protocol MF07-01. *Ann Surg Oncol.* 2018;25:3141e9. doi: 10.1245/s10434-018-6494-6
10. Shien T, Nakamura K, Shibata T, et al. A randomized controlled trial comparing primary tumour resection plus systemic therapy with systemic therapy alone in metastatic breast cancer (PRIM-BC): Japan Clinical Oncology Group Study JCOG1017. *Jpn J Clin Oncol.* 2012;42:970–3.
11. Reinhorn D, Mutai R, Yerushalmi R, et al. Locoregional therapy in *de novo* metastatic breast cancer: systemic review and meta-analysis. *Breast.* 2021;58:173–81.
12. Gupta S, Chaubal R, Gardi N, et al. Abstract P3-05-01: Molecular effects of surgical resection on primary breast tumor. *Cancer Res.* 2020;80(4_Supplement):P3–05–01. doi: 10.1158/1538-7445.SABCS19-P3-05-01
13. Badwe RA, Parmar V, Nair N, et al. Effect of peritumoral infiltration of local anaesthetic before surgery on survival in early breast cancer. *JCO.* 2023;41:3318–28. doi: 10.1200/JCO.22.01966

CHAPTER 47

Treatment of Breast Cancer during Pregnancy: An Observational Study

Loibl S, Han SN, Minckwitz GV, Bontenbal M, Ring A, Giermek J, et al.
Lancet Oncol 13:887–896, 2012

PAPER DESCRIPTION

- **Objective/Research Question**: To determine whether breast cancer treatment during pregnancy is safe for mother and child, and if pregnant patients should therefore be treated as similarly as possible to non-pregnant patients with breast cancer.

- **Design**: International, multicentre, retro- and prospective observational cohort study.

- **Sample Size**: Four hundred and forty-seven participants.

- **Inclusion Criteria**: All women diagnosed with breast cancer during pregnancy were included in the study irrespective of pregnancy outcome, breast cancer stage and type of treatment received.

- **Exclusion Criteria**: Participants were excluded if data about disease and outcomes were not received.

- **Intervention or Treatment Received**: Participants received routine care, with some treated as per a German Breast Group treatment algorithm. Chemotherapy was administered to 205 women during pregnancy and 192 women after delivery or interruption. Breast conservation surgery was performed in 179 women. No patients received immunotherapy, endocrine therapy or radiotherapy during pregnancy.

- **Results**: Median gestational age at breast cancer diagnosis was 24 weeks (range = 5–40). Women with stage T4 disease were more likely to receive chemotherapy during pregnancy compared to after delivery ($p = 0.005$). Taxane-free chemotherapy regimens were more common in women who started chemotherapy during pregnancy compared to after delivery.

DOI: 10.1201/b23352-47

Women with distant metastases were more likely to have a first-trimester discontinuation of pregnancy (miscarriage or termination). There was no difference in preterm delivery rates in patients with or without distant metastases, nor those who received chemotherapy during or after pregnancy. Lower birth weight (adjusted by gestational age) and higher incidence of adverse neonatal events were observed in infants exposed to chemotherapy in utero. Two neonatal deaths occurred, both following chemotherapy exposure in pregnancy which was reportedly unrelated. No differences in the incidence of fetal growth restriction or Apgar scores were seen following chemotherapy exposure during pregnancy. Obstetric complications were more commonly reported in women with early breast cancer who were treated with chemotherapy during pregnancy. Disease-free and overall survival varied by tumour stage and nodal status, but **was not statistically significant in relation to** timing of antenatal chemotherapy compared to postpartum chemotherapy.

EXPERT COMMENTARY BY LYDIA NEWMAN, CHRIS COYLE, AVI AGRAWAL AND EDWARD R. ST JOHN

Paper significance

Although breast cancer in pregnancy is rare, it is one of the most common cancers to present antenatally. The management of breast cancer in pregnancy is complex, requiring difficult decision making regarding whether to continue the pregnancy, possible complications of treatment during pregnancy and timing of delivery. This landmark registry study provides data on both maternal and neonatal short-term outcomes from a large cohort of women with breast cancer in pregnancy. The study reports an increased risk of obstetric and neonatal complications in women who received chemotherapy during pregnancy, but emphasises the need to balance this with the potentially greater harm to neonates associated with iatrogenic preterm delivery.

Paper limitations

It is inevitable that this paper is observational, and therefore inferences about the superiority of one management strategy relative to another cannot be made with certainty, but this is one of the highest quality studies of breast cancer in pregnancy and has been very influential. There were significant differences in tumour characteristics between patients receiving chemotherapy in pregnancy compared to postpartum, although the authors have adjusted for this in some analyses. When early outcomes were reported in this study, first-trimester discontinuation of pregnancy was not differentiated by miscarriage or termination of pregnancy, and it was not reported if any women received chemotherapy during the first trimester. It is therefore not possible to discern whether breast cancer treatment during pregnancy was associated with a risk of miscarriage or congenital anomaly in the cohort. Furthermore, neonates were only followed-up for a short period which does not exclude potential longer-term harm associated with chemotherapy treatment during pregnancy.

In context of the relevant current literature

The interim findings of the UK Obstetric Surveillance System (UKOSS) Breast Cancer in Pregnancy study reported an estimated incidence of primary breast cancer diagnosed in pregnancy of 5.3 per 100,000 maternities in the UK.[1] The true incidence of breast cancer associated with pregnancy is unclear and may be rising due to breast cancer risk increasing with age and women increasingly opting to delay pregnancy until later in life.

Breast cancer associated with pregnancy presents risks to the mother, including delayed diagnosis and undertreatment. More recent results (2019) from a single institution found that pregnancy-associated breast cancer (PABC) patients had high rates of induction of labour and preterm births.[2] A recent meta-analysis (2020) reported that breast cancer diagnosed during pregnancy and/or the postpartum period is associated with a poor prognosis in overall survival and disease-free survival.[3] A nationwide Dutch study revealed that those with PABC had a more aggressive histopathologic profile compared to matched breast cancer patients.[4] However, it has been argued that the term 'PABC' should no longer be used, instead separating those patients whose breast cancer occurs during pregnancy (PrBC) and those whose cancer occurs during the postpartum period (PPBC). The literature gives a mixed view of whether PrBC confers a worse prognosis than breast cancer not diagnosed during pregnancy. Conversely, PPBC is associated with worse survival rates and a >2 times increased risk of metastases compared to either those diagnosed during pregnancy or those who have never been pregnant.[5]

The developing fetus is at risk of iatrogenic harm due to the adverse effects of oncology treatments and elective preterm delivery. When breast cancer is diagnosed in early pregnancy, termination may be considered after individualised counselling. There is no robust evidence that miscarriage risk is increased in women treated for breast cancer during pregnancy. Chemotherapy treatment is usually commenced after the first trimester to mitigate teratogenicity risks to the fetus. It is reported that anthracycline-based chemotherapy may be administered during the second and third trimesters, with seemingly few short-term implications. Although limited data exist, taxanes may also be given with few adverse events reported.[6] The consequences of preterm deliveries prior to 37 weeks on short- and long-term neonatal outcomes are well established and should be avoided where possible. Careful timing of chemotherapy to ensure a 2–3-week recovery period prior to delivery is advised to reduce the risks of immunosuppression at birth. There is limited evidence regarding the long-term implications on oncology treatments during pregnancy on the offspring. Shielding should be used for those undergoing mammography, whilst certain imaging modalities such as computerised tomography (CT) should be avoided to reduce radiation exposure risk to the fetus. UK guidelines support the use of tailored surgery and chemotherapy during pregnancy, and advise delaying routine radiotherapy as well as hormone and monoclonal antibody therapies until after delivery.[7]

Pregnancy after breast cancer

Meta-analyses have been performed focussing on pregnancy outcomes after breast cancer treatment. A synthesis of 16 studies demonstrated that women who had received systemic therapy after surgery had an overall pooled estimate of 14% of becoming pregnant, whilst 12% suffered a miscarriage. The pregnancy rate after breast cancer treatment for survivors was on average 40% lower than the general population's pregnancy rate.[8] These findings were similar in another meta-analysis, demonstrating that breast cancer survivors were significantly less likely to have a subsequent pregnancy compared with the general population.[9] Low birth weight, preterm birth and small-for-gestational-age babies were more common in breast cancer survivors, particularly in those with previous chemotherapy exposure, compared with the general population.[9] However, there was no significant risk of fetal congenital abnormalities. It is therefore important that women are informed about the effects of breast cancer treatment and are provided with sufficient fertility-related information, access to fertility preservation and psychosocial support before commencing treatment. Those with a subsequent pregnancy had better disease-free and overall survival compared to patients with breast cancer without subsequent pregnancy; therefore, breast cancer survivors should not be unduly counselled against pregnancy.[9] The POSITIVE trial shows that for young women with ER-positive breast cancer, a temporary interruption of endocrine treatment to attempt pregnancy does not confer a greater short-term risk of recurrence, when compared to the control group without interruption of treatment.[10]

Conclusions

Understanding the consequence of pregnancy in association with breast cancer is important for both the mother and fetus. Termination of pregnancy or iatrogenic preterm delivery is not routinely necessary to commence systemic breast cancer treatment and achieve good maternal cancer prognosis. As there are relatively few research studies addressing the topic of breast cancer and pregnancy, there are still uncertainties around the management, treatment and long-term safety for the mother and baby which lead to variation in clinical practice. Further research is needed in order to achieve optimal long-term maternal and fetal outcomes following pregnancy-associated breast cancer. The UK Royal College of Obstetricians and Gynaecologists have produced some excellent guidelines for those wishing to learn more about best practice.[7]

REFERENCES

1. O'Connor M, Kurinczuk JJ, Knight M. UKOSS Annual Report 2018. Oxford: National Perinatal Epidemiology Unit 2018. *Available online at:* https://www.npeu.ox.ac.uk/ukoss/publications-ukoss/annual-reports (accessed 20/08/2023).
2. Gomez-Hidalgo NR, Mendizabal E, Joigneau L, Pintado P, De Leon-Luis J. Breast cancer during pregnancy: results of maternal and perinatal outcomes in a single institution and systematic review of the literature. *J Obstet Gynaecol.* 2019;39(1):27–35.
3. Shao, C., Yu, Z., Xiao, J., et al. Prognosis of pregnancy-associated breast cancer: a meta-analysis. *BMC Cancer.* 2020;20:746.
4. Suelmann BBM, van Dooijeweert C, van der Wall E, Linn S, van Diest PJ. Pregnancy-associated breast cancer: nationwide Dutch study confirms a discriminatory aggressive histopathologic profile. *Breast Cancer Res Treat.* 2021;186(3):699–704.
5. Amant F, Lefrère H, Borges VF, Cardonick E, Lambertini M, Loibl S, Peccatori F, Partridge A, Schedin P. The definition of pregnancy-associated breast cancer is outdated and should no longer be used. *Lancet Oncol.* 2021;22(6):753–4.
6. Mir O, Berveiller P, Goffinet F, Treluyer JM, Serreau R, Goldwasser F, et al. Taxanes for breast cancer during pregnancy: a systematic review. *Ann Oncol.* 2010;21(2):425–6.
7. Royal College of Obstetricians and Gynaecologists. Pregnancy and Breast Cancer (Green top guideline No. 12). 2011. Available online at: https://rcog.org.uk/guidance/browse-all-guidance/green-top-guidelines/pregnancy-and-breast-cancer-green-top-guideline-no-12/ *(accessed 20/08/2023).*
8. Gerstl B, Sullivan E, Ives A, Saunders C, Wand H, Anazodo A. Pregnancy Outcomes After a Breast Cancer Diagnosis: A Systematic Review and Meta-analysis. *Clin Breast Cancer.* 2018;18(1):e79–e88.
9. Lambertini M, Blondeaux E, Bruzzone M, Perachino M, Anderson RA, de Azambuja E, et al. Pregnancy after breast cancer: a systematic review and meta-analysis. *J Clin Oncol.* 2021;39(29):3293–305.
10. Partridge AH, Niman SM, Ruggeri M, Peccatori FA, Azim HA Jr, Colleoni M, et al. International Breast Cancer Study Group; POSITIVE Trial Collaborators. Interrupting endocrine therapy to attempt pregnancy after breast cancer. *N Engl J Med.* 2023;388(18):1645–56.

Germline BRCA Mutation and Outcome in Young-Onset Breast Cancer (POSH): A Prospective Cohort Study

Copson ER, Maishman TC, Tapper WJ, Cutress RI, Greville-Heygate S, Altman DG, et al.

Lancet Oncol 19(2):169–180, 2018

Young-onset breast cancer (YOBC) is defined as breast cancer (BC) diagnosed in women under the age of 40 years.[1] YOBC accounts for 5% of all female BCs and is associated with higher stage disease on presentation, higher rates of local recurrence and distant disease and poor survival.[2] A higher number of YOBC patients carry inherited pathogenic *BRCA1* or *BRCA2* variants (*gBRCA1/2*) compared to older patients diagnosed with BC. The *BRCA* genes are tumour suppressor genes involved in DNA repair by homologous recombination. They have an autosomal dominant pattern of inheritance.[3] Pathogenic mutations in the *BRCA* genes result in ineffective DNA repair, leading to chromosomal instability. They are characterised by high penetrance, with a lifetime BC risk of up to 70%, and are associated with aggressive histopathological characteristics, such as triple-negative breast cancer (TNBC).[4] However, there is no clear evidence on the impact of *gBRCA* mutations on the prognosis of patients with BC. The Prospective Study of Outcomes in Sporadic versus Hereditary Breast Cancer (POSH) study investigated the association between *gBRCA1/2* pathogenic variants and clinical outcomes in patients with YOBC.

PAPER DESCRIPTION

- **Objective**: To evaluate the association between *gBRCA1/2* mutations and clinical outcomes in YOBC.

- **Design**: The POSH study was a UK multicentre prospective cohort study that recruited patients from the years 2000 to 2008.

  Clinical, pathological and treatment data were collected from medical records, and family history was obtained via a questionnaire at study entry. The risk of carrying a *BRCA* mutation was estimated using the BOADICEA algorithm. The oestrogen receptor (ER), progesterone receptor (PR) and *HER2*-receptor status of the primary tumours was obtained from local pathology reports. Tissue microarrays were stained for hormone receptors to supplement missing data.

DOI: 10.1201/b23352-48

Whole blood was collected at recruitment for DNA analysis, and next-generation sequencing was performed using a targeted gene panel that included *BRCA1/2* and *TP53* genes. All pathogenic variants were confirmed by Sanger sequencing. Patients with pathogenic *BRCA* variants were categorised as *BRCA*-positive, and all other patients as *BRCA*-negative.

The primary and secondary outcomes were overall survival (OS) and distant disease–free survival (DDFS), respectively. OS was defined as the time from first diagnosis to death from any cause. DDFS was defined as the time from primary diagnosis to first distant recurrence. Subgroup analysis of TNBC patients, comparing OS between *BRCA*-positive and *BRCA*-negative patients, was performed.

- **Sample Size**: In total, 3,021 patients were recruited, of whom 2,733 were included in the analysis, of whom 338 patients were found to be *BRCA*-positive. TNBC was diagnosed in 558 patients, of whom 136 were *BRCA*-positive.

- **Inclusion Criteria**: Women aged between 18 and 40 years old, diagnosed with primary invasive BC, within 12 months of their initial histopathological diagnosis, were recruited into the study. All disease stages, histological subtypes, comorbidities and performance statuses were allowed.

- **Exclusion Criteria**: Patients were excluded if they had a previous invasive malignancy, not including non-melanomatous skin cancer. Patients with absent primary tumour data, without genotyping data, with non-invasive BC or with a constitutional *TP53* mutation were also excluded.

- **Intervention or Treatment Received**: All patients received oncological treatment according to local protocols.

- **Results**:

  1. *Whole cohort*: Overall, of the 2,733 YOBC patients included in the analysis, 12% (*n* = 338) were *BRCA*-positive. Pathogenic *BRCA1* or *BRCA2* variants were reported in 7% (*n* = 201) and 5% (*n* = 137), respectively. Clinical genetic consultation and *BRCA* testing occurred in only 14% (*n* = 388) of patients, of whom 47% (*n* = 182) had a pathogenic variant. Twenty-two percent (*n* = 75) of those found to be *BRCA*-positive did not meet the criteria for genetic testing in place at the time of study recruitment.

     The median follow-up was 8.2 years (interquartile range [IQR] = 6.0–9.9), with losses to follow-up accounting for 3% of the participants (*n* = 91). There was no significant difference in OS between *BRCA*-positive and *BRCA*-negative patients on univariable (hazard ratio [HR] = 0.99, 95% confidence interval [CI] = 0.78–1.24) or multivariable

(HR = 0.96, 95% CI = 0.76–1.22) analyses. No statistically significant difference was demonstrated in OS between *BRCA*-negative and *BRCA1*- or *BRCA2*-positive patients when compared separately. There was no evidence of association between *BRCA* status and distant DFS (HR = 0.82, 95% CI = 0.55–1.20).

BRCA-positive tumours were associated with younger age, higher histological tumour grade and an ER-negative, PR-negative and *HER2*-negative receptor profile ($p < 0.05$). *BRCA1*-positive tumours were correlated with the presence of histological tumour grade 3, ER and *HER2*-receptor negativity and an absence of lymph node metastases or lymphovascular invasion ($p < 0.05$). Contralateral BC occurred in 6% ($n = 151$) of all patients. Subgroup analysis showed that 18% ($n = 37$) of *BRCA1*-positive, 12% ($n = 17$) of *BRCA2*-positive and 4% ($n = 97$) of *BRCA*-negative patients developed contralateral BC. The median time from diagnosis to contralateral BC was 3.0 years (IQR = 1.5–4.8) in the *BRCA*-positive and 2.7 years (1.2–5.3) in the *BRCA*-negative group. Distant recurrence was reported in 28% ($n = 752$) of patients.

2. *TNBC cohort*: Pathogenic *BRCA* variants were found in 24% ($n = 136$) of TNBC patients, of whom 90% ($n = 123$) were *BRCA1*-positive. The distant recurrence rate and BC-specific mortality in the TNBC cohort were 28% ($n = 159$) and 27% ($n = 153$), respectively. OS was significantly higher at 2 years of follow-up in *BRCA*-positive compared to *BRCA*-negative patients (HR = 0.49, 95% CI = 0.35–0.99). However, there was no significant difference in OS between these groups at 5 years and 10 years ($p > 0.05$). Similarly, there was no statistically significant difference in distant DFS between *BRCA*-positive and -negative patients ($p > 0.05$). Post-hoc multivariable analysis showed that immediate-risk-reducing mastectomy was not associated with early survival benefit in *BRCA*-positive patients; however, the number of patients who underwent preventative mastectomy was small.

EXPERT COMMENTARY BY WILSON CHEAH PUI FUI, CAMELLIA RICHARDS, CONSTANTINOS SAVVA AND RAMSEY CUTRESS

Paper significance

The POSH study has brought new insights into the prognostic value of pathogenic *BRCA* variants in women with YOBC. Although there was no statistically significant difference in OS or DFS, patients with *BRCA* mutations have demonstrated improved 2-year survival compared to *BRCA*-negative patients, suggesting that *BRCA*-positive tumours may be more sensitive to chemotherapy-induced DNA damage.[5] This association may potentially confound early outcomes of TNBC patients and hence should be considered in clinical trials and prognostic models. A comparison of survival outcomes of the POSH cohort with predicted outcomes from the PREDICT tool (http://www.predict.nhs.uk), demonstrated that the short-term estimates of the PREDICT tool were less accurate for women with YOBC.[6] Inclusion of POSH data has improved the PREDICT prognostic model which is widely used by cancer physicians to inform chemotherapy decision making.[7]

The POSH cohort has also contributed to an international collaboration demonstrating the incidence of *gBRCA1/2* mutations in women with YOBC, leading to the update of the National Institute for Health and Care Excellence (NICE) genetic testing criteria for *gBRCA* mutations.[8] The POSH study has reported a higher percentage of *BRCA*-positive patients compared to historical studies, which can be attributed not only to the use of more sensitive genetic testing methods but also to the early-onset BC which is associated with genetic predisposition. In addition, the POSH study suggested that additional surgery may be delayed to a later date after primary diagnosis whilst patients recover from their oncological treatment, given the use of enhanced BC screening and the lack of early survival benefit of bilateral mastectomy in *BRCA*-positive patients with TNBC. This has challenged the tendency for BC specialists to recommend immediate bilateral mastectomy in newly diagnosed BC patients with a pathogenic *BRCA* variant.

This cohort has also evaluated the prognostic significance of body mass index, ethnicity, surgical margins and family history in women with YOBC, demonstrating that clear surgical margins, lifestyle factors (obesity) and ethnicity impact outcomes in patients with YOBC, whereas family history of BC and *BRCA* status, at least in the first few years following diagnosis, do not.[9–12] The POSH data have also contributed to genome-wide association studies, identifying novel BC susceptibility loci associated with risk, pathological subtypes and survival.[13–15]

Paper limitations

The main strength of the POSH study is the large sample size with a median follow-up of 8.2 years and few missing data. However, it has been shown that recurrences of ER-positive BCs occur steadily for up to 20 years, with 17–26% of them occurring between 5 and 20 years from initial diagnosis.[3] Furthermore, survival analysis following diagnosis suggests that the transient survival advantage in TNBC patients with *gBRCA* mutations may be reversed over a longer time period, and hence longer follow-up is required. Also, the study was not powered to detect a statistically significant difference between *BRCA*-positive and *BRCA*-negative patients with TNBC, as the design of this study pre-dated the recognition of the association between *BRCA1* mutations and TNBC.

The POSH study only recruited patients aged 40 years or younger, and these observations may not be generalisable to older women. Since publication of the study, and in part due to the results, as well as greater availability and reduced costs, genetic testing criteria have widened and become more readily available. There have also been significant advances in the management of TNBC and g*BRCA*-associated BC since the recruitment period, including the use of platinum-based chemotherapy, immunotherapy and poly (ADP-ribose) polymerase (PARP) inhibitors. Furthermore, recommendations for adjuvant treatment changed during recruitment, with taxanes recommended for node-positive disease and adjuvant trastuzumab becoming routinely available for *HER2*-positive BC only since 2006 in the UK. Observations from this cohort should therefore be interpreted with the knowledge that, whilst it might not reflect current oncological practice, it was representative of the UK YOBC population[16] and therefore provides a historic "natural history" description against which these newer interventions may be evaluated.

Other limitations include the use of multiplex ligation probe analysis only in patients who underwent clinical *BRCA* testing rather than research genotyping, which may have resulted in some structural *BRCA* variants not being identified. Notably, mutations in other BC susceptibility genes such as *PALB2*, *CHEK2* and *ATM*, which have been associated with TNBC, higher risk of contralateral disease and poorer clinical outcomes, have not been excluded from the study, which might have confounded the results.[17]

In context of the relevant current literature

Multiple published retrospective studies and systematic reviews of oncological outcomes in YOBC and *BRCA1/2* mutation carriers have reported inconsistent results.

A meta-analysis by Liu and colleagues, which included 35,972 women with BC including 3,402 *BRCA*-positive patients, showed that *BRCA*-positivity is associated with shorter survival (*BRCA1*: OS, HR = 1.2, 95% CI = 1.08–1.33; *BRCA2*: DFS, HR = 1.35, 95% CI = 1.1–1.67).[18] While OS was worse in *BRCA1*-positive patients compared to noncarriers, there were no differences in DFS and BC-specific survival in this group, which could be attributed to confounding factors such as the development of ovarian cancer and use of different treatment modalities. In *BRCA2*-positive patients, there was no difference in 5-year OS, whereas OS was significantly poorer in studies with greater than 5 years of follow-up. This could be explained by the late recurrence of ER-positive BCs, which are more frequent in *BRCA2*-positive patients, or by the increased incidence of other types of *BRCA2*-related malignancies. Liu and colleagues did demonstrate that BRCA mutations were not correlated with worse OS or BC-specific survival in patients with TNBC, a finding which was also supported by a meta-analysis by Baretta and colleagues. These meta-analyses were characterised by methodological limitations that included a lack of clear definitions of the end points, as well as use of different end point definitions by the individual studies which might have introduced bias.[19] Furthermore, Liu and colleagues did not report the individual studies from which the survival data were extracted, and adjusted HRs were used if available, meaning that confounding was not controlled for. Older systematic reviews and meta-analyses which evaluated the associations of *BRCA* mutations with survival outcomes showed conflicting results, with either statistically significant evidence[20–22] or trends of associations[23,24] between *gBRCA* mutations and worse survival. Recent studies evaluating clinical outcomes in BC patients with pathogenic *BRCA* variants have supported the results of the POSH cohort.[25–27]

Overall, the POSH study addressed the methodological limitations of the previous studies, providing strong evidence characterised by a low risk of bias, a large sample size, a complete dataset for genetic testing and confounding factors and longer follow-up.

Conclusions

YOBC is associated with the presence of pathogenic *BRCA1* or *BRCA2* variants and high BC-specific mortality. The POSH study has shown that YOBC patients with a pathogenic *BRCA* variant have similar survival rates compared to noncarriers. In patients with TNBC, *gBRCA*-positive patients may have a survival advantage over noncarriers during the first 2 years after initial diagnosis.

REFERENCES

1. Paluch-Shimon S, et al. ESO–ESMO 4th International Consensus Guidelines for Breast Cancer in Young Women (BCY4). *Ann Oncol.* 2020;31(6):674–96.
2. Han W, et al. Young age: an independent risk factor for disease-free survival in women with operable breast cancer. *BMC Cancer.* 2004;4:82.
3. Foulkes WD. Inherited susceptibility to common cancers. *N Engl J Med.* 2008;359(20): 2143–53.
4. Yoshimura A, Imoto I, Iwata H. Functions of Breast Cancer Predisposition Genes: Implications for Clinical Management. *Int J Mol Sci.* 2022;23(13).
5. Copson ER, et al. Germline—BRCA—mutation and outcome in young-onset breast cancer (POSH): a prospective cohort study. *Lancet Oncol.* 2018;19(2): 169–80.
6. Maishman T, et al. An evaluation of the prognostic model PREDICT using the POSH cohort of women aged ≤40 years at breast cancer diagnosis. *Br J Cancer.* 2015;112(6):983–91.
7. Candido dos Reis FJ, et al. An updated PREDICT breast cancer prognostication and treatment benefit prediction model with independent validation. *Breast Cancer Res.* 2017;19(1):58.
8. National Institute for Health and Care Excellence. Familial breast cancer: classification, care and managing breast cancer and related risks in people with a family history of breast cancer. in *NICE guideline [CG164]*. 2013, London; NICE.
9. Copson E, et al. Ethnicity and outcome of young breast cancer patients in the United Kingdom: the POSH study. *Br J Cancer.* 2014;110(1):230–41.

10. Copson ER, et al. Obesity and the outcome of young breast cancer patients in the UK: the POSH study. *Ann Oncol.* 2015;26(1): 101–12.
11. Eccles BK, et al. Family history and outcome of young patients with breast cancer in the UK (POSH study). *Br J Surg.* 2015;102(8): 924–35.
12. Maishman T, et al. Local recurrence and breast oncological surgery in young women with breast cancer: the POSH observational cohort study. *Ann Surg.* 2017;266(1): 165–72.
13. Khan S, et al. Meta-analysis of three genome-wide association studies identifies two loci that predict survival and treatment outcome in breast cancer. *Oncotarget.* 2018;9(3): 4249–57.
14. Zhang H, et al. Genome-wide association study identifies 32 novel breast cancer susceptibility loci from overall and subtype-specific analyses. *Nat Genet.* 2020;52(6): 572–81.
15. Rafiq S, et al. Identification of inherited genetic variations influencing prognosis in early-onset breast cancer. *Cancer Res.* 2013;73(6): 1883–91.
16. Copson E, et al. Prospective Observational Study of Breast Cancer Treatment Outcomes for UK Women Aged 18–40 Years at Diagnosis: The POSH Study. *J Natl Cancer Inst.* 2013;105(13): 978–88.
17. Mavaddat N, et al. Pathology of tumors associated with pathogenic germline variants in 9 breast cancer susceptibility genes. *JAMA Oncol.* 2022;8(3): e216744.
18. Liu M, et al. Association between BRCA mutational status and survival in patients with breast cancer: a systematic review and meta-analysis. *Breast Cancer Res Treat.* 2021;186(3): 591–605.
19. Wang Y, van den Broek AJ, Schmidt MK. Letter to the editor regarding: 'Association between BRCA mutational status and survival in patients with breast cancer: a systematic review and meta-analysis'. *Breast Cancer Res Treat.,* 2021;188(3): 821–3.
20. Lee EH, et al. Effect of BRCA1/2 mutation on short-term and long-term breast cancer survival: a systematic review and meta-analysis. *Breast Cancer Res Treat.* 2010;122(1): 11–25.
21. Zhong Q, et al. Effects of BRCA1- and BRCA2-related mutations on ovarian and breast cancer survival: a meta-analysis. *Clin Cancer Res.* 2015;21(1): 211–20.
22. Zhu Y, et al. BRCA mutations and survival in breast cancer: an updated systematic review and meta-analysis. *Oncotarget.* 2016;7(43): 70113–27.
23. van den Broek AJ, et al. Worse Breast Cancer Prognosis of BRCA1/BRCA2 Mutation Carriers: What's the Evidence? A Systematic Review with Meta-Analysis. *PLOS ONE.* 2015;10(3): e0120189.
24. Templeton AJ, et al. Interaction between hormonal receptor status, age and survival in patients with BRCA1/2 germline mutations: a systematic review and meta-regression. *PLOS ONE.* 2016;11(5): e0154789.
25. De Talhouet S, et al. Clinical outcome of breast cancer in carriers of BRCA1 and BRCA2 mutations according to molecular subtypes. *Sci Rep.* 2020;10(1):7073.
26. Mailliez A, et al. Survival outcomes of metastatic breast cancer patients by germline BRCA1/2 status in a large multicenter real-world database. *Int J Cancer.* 2023;152(5): 921–31.
27. Kurian AW, et al. Association of genetic testing results with mortality among women with breast cancer or ovarian cancer. *J Natl Cancer Inst.* 2021;114(2): 245–53.

Efficacy of Bilateral Prophylactic Mastectomy in Women with a Family History of Breast Cancer

Hartmann L, Schaid D, Woods J, Crotty T, Myers J, Arnold P, et al.
N Engl J Med 340(2):77–84, 1999

It has long been known that some women are at increased breast cancer risk as a result of their family history. The *BRCA1* and *BRCA2* genes were identified in the early 1990s, and studies began to investigate the protective effect of risk-reducing mastectomy (RRM). RRM has been used for over 50 years, well before genetic testing was made available, and several retrospective studies had been published prior to this article suggesting a protective effect. This study set out to assess breast cancer rates in women after bilateral risk-reducing mastectomy (BRRM), relative to their own untreated relatives or relative to their predicted breast cancer risk, derived from Gail model[1] estimates (an online tool which uses a woman's personal data about family history, parity and previous breast biopsy to derive a breast cancer risk estimate).

PAPER DESCRIPTION

- **Objective/Research Question**: This study was undertaken to investigate the effectiveness of BRRM as a risk-reducing strategy for women with a high or moderate increased breast cancer risk due to their family history of breast cancer.

- **Design**: Retrospective cohort study design with a predicted risk of cancer derived from the Gail model or by comparison to cancer rates in untreated relatives. Surgery took place between 1960 and 1993, an era when scientists were aware that there must be inherited potent breast cancer genes, but those genes had not yet been identified and could not be tested for. Risk assessment was therefore based on family history.

- **Sample Size**: A total of 639 women with a family history of breast cancer who had undergone a BRRM between 1960 and 1993.

- **Follow-Up**: Median length of follow-up was 14 years.

DOI: 10.1201/b23352-49

- **Inclusion Criteria**: A documented family history of breast cancer. The high-risk category included women who had two or more first-degree relatives with breast cancer, a first-degree relative with breast cancer before the age of 45 years and one other relative with breast cancer, or a family history of breast cancer plus ovarian cancer or bilateral breast cancer. The moderate-risk category included women with an affected first-degree relative, two aunts or cousins with breast cancer or family histories of breast cancer involving second- or third-degree relatives.

- **Exclusion Criteria**: Previous breast cancer in the surgically treated breast. Women without a family history of breast cancer who underwent mastectomy. Male patients were excluded.

- **Intervention or Treatment Received**: BRRM (575 subcutaneous mastectomy and 64 total mastectomy).

- **Risk Prediction**: The sisters of the high-risk women were assessed for breast cancer incidence and survival. In the moderate-risk group, a Gail model breast cancer risk calculation was performed to determine their expected breast cancer risk. The Gail model breast cancer incidence data were also used alongside Surveillance, Epidemiology, and End Results (SEER) data on breast cancer survival rates to estimate the survival rate these women should have had if they had not undergone BRRM.

- **Results**: This study investigated a cohort of 639 women with a family history of breast cancer, who underwent BRRM at the Mayo Clinic between 1960 and 1993. Among them, 425 had a moderate risk of breast cancer based on family history, while 214 women had a high risk. The median age in both groups was 42 years. The high-risk women had 403 sisters who did not undergo BRRM and for whom cancer diagnoses and survival were ascertained.

  The study findings revealed that BRRM, whether total or subcutaneous, was associated with a significant reduction in the incidence of breast cancer in both the moderate-risk and high-risk groups. Among the moderate-risk group, the predicted incidence of breast cancer according to the Gail model was 37.4, but the actual incidence was only 4. This represents an 89.5% reduction in the risk of breast cancer after RRM ($p < 0.001$), and reduction in the risk of death was 100% (no deaths in the RRM cohort, and 10 deaths predicted using the Gail model and SEER survival data). In the high-risk group, the expected number of breast cancers among the cohort ranged from 30.6 to 37.4. However, the actual number of breast cancers was only three, resulting in a risk reduction of 90%–94%. Two of the women from the high-risk group developed ovarian cancer.

  Medical records, including cancer occurrence data, were available for all participants. After a median follow-up of 14 years, only seven cases of breast cancers were observed, all of which occurred after subcutaneous bilateral mastectomy. The study included 575 cases of subcutaneous mastectomy and 64 cases of total mastectomy. Among the seven women who developed breast cancer, the median time from mastectomy to diagnosis was 6 years. Breast cancers were confined to the chest wall in six out of seven cases, indicating that the mastectomy effectively prevented spread of cancer beyond the chest wall. One woman from the high-risk group presented with bone metastases. Two of the seven women died of breast cancer, while the remaining five were alive and disease-free after local treatment of their chest wall disease.

The study reviewed the pathological specimens obtained from BRRM. Tissue from 603 women were available for review, and most specimens (74.5%) were categorised as normal. Proliferative changes without atypia were observed in 23.9% of cases, while atypical hyperplasia was present in 1.5% of cases. Invasive carcinoma was found in only 0.1% of specimens, and none were categorised as carcinoma *in situ*.

Regarding follow-up, 95% of the women were alive at the time of analysis, with a median follow-up of 14 years. The study had a high follow-up rate, with complete questionnaire and chart information available for 93% of the women.

EXPERT COMMENTARY BY HAMZA IKRAM AND LYNDA WYLD

Paper significance

This study had a significant impact on the potential risk management benefits of BRRM in high-risk women, reducing both the incidence of breast cancer and the mortality rate. It influenced clinical practice by informing guidelines, risk assessment and further research in the field of breast cancer risk management and prevention. Subsequent data, including meta-analyses, have confirmed their findings, and more recently, data on women specifically identified as gene carriers have been published. There is also more sophistication in the identification of the age- and gene mutation–specific benefits of BRRM, with understanding of the differential protective effects of *BRCA1* versus *BRCA2* and the upper age limits for survival benefit to be seen. The effectiveness of BRRM in women without cancer is now well established. For women who have already had cancer, there is ongoing clinical uncertainty about the benefits of contralateral RRM, with a more nuanced approach being required, taking into account the prognosis of their initial cancer, their age and their gene mutation.

Paper limitations

There were several limitations in this study. This was retrospective, so the data were collected from historic records and patient recall. This introduces the possibility of recall bias and incomplete or inaccurate information. In addition, the study relied on medical record information for all women, but there were cases where women or their next of kin declined to fill out the questionnaire, which may have resulted in missing data.

The study had a long duration, spanning from 1960 to 1993. During this time, there may have been changes in surgical techniques, advances in breast reconstruction and improvements in breast cancer screening and treatment. These factors could have influenced the outcomes observed in the study.

Another limitation is the lack of a proper control group. The study did not include a comparison group of women who did not undergo prophylactic mastectomy. The Gail model was used to estimate breast cancer risk and has been found to both overestimate and underestimate breast cancer risk. Therefore, it is challenging to determine the true efficacy of the procedure in preventing breast cancer and reducing mortality compared to other management strategies, such as surveillance, bilateral salpingo-oophorectomy or chemoprevention. Furthermore, the study did not provide detailed information on the specific criteria used to determine the risk level for patients. The criteria for high- and moderate-risk classification were briefly mentioned, but the specific details and thresholds were not provided. The study also did not specifically address the efficacy of RRM in women with *BRCA1/2* mutations, as these genes had not been identified and routine testing was not available.

In addition, the study did not address the psychosocial implications and quality-of-life outcomes associated with RRM. The decision to undergo RRM is a complex one that involves considerations beyond medical outcomes, such as body image, sexuality and psychological well-being. Subsequent studies have explored these issues in more detail (nicely reviewed in the Cochrane Review of 2018[2]), but at the time, quality-of-life research was not widely performed.

Lastly, the study had a relatively short follow-up period, with a median follow-up duration of 14 years. Breast cancer can have a long latency period, and longer-term follow-up would be necessary to fully evaluate the effectiveness of RRM in preventing breast cancer and reducing mortality.

In context of the relevant current literature

A further study by the same lead author assessed the efficacy of bilateral prophylactic mastectomy in reducing breast cancer risk in women with *BRCA1* and *BRCA2* gene mutations. The researchers obtained samples from 176 high-risk women who had undergone BPM and analysed them for *BRCA1* and *BRCA2* mutations. The study identified 26 women with alterations in *BRCA1* or *BRCA2*. None of these women developed breast cancer after a median follow-up of 13.4 years. The study acknowledges the limitations of the testing strategies, which may fail to detect certain types of *BRCA1* and *BRCA2* mutations.[3]

An excellent systematic review and meta-analysis of BRRM was published by the Cochrane Review in 2005 and most recently updated in 2018.[2] This confirmed the effectiveness of BRRM in reducing breast cancer incidence and mortality in high-risk women, particularly those with known *BRCA* mutations, based on data from 15,000 women.

UK National Institute for Health and Care Excellence (NICE) guidelines recommend a BRRM as a risk-reducing strategy option for discussion with women at high breast cancer risk.[4] This should be managed by a multidisciplinary team, and women should undergo genetic counselling in a specialist cancer genetic clinic before deciding. Preoperative counselling should cover the psychosocial and sexual consequences of the procedure, as well as the possibility of breast cancer being diagnosed histologically following mastectomy. Furthermore, women should have the opportunity to discuss breast reconstruction options with a surgical team specialising in breast reconstructive skills. Women considering this should be offered access to support groups.[4]

Conclusions

This study was one of the first to show that BRRM reduced breast cancer incidence and improved survival in women at increased breast cancer risk. Whilst it had some methodological flaws, the outcomes shown have been corroborated by numerous subsequent studies which have added more details and stratification factors for decision making.

REFERENCES

1. Gail MH, Brinton LA, Byar DP, Corle DK, Green SB, Schairer C, Mulvihill JJ. Projecting individualized probabilities of developing breast cancer for white females who are being examined annually. *J Natl Cancer Inst*. 1989;81(24): 1879–86.
2. Carbine NE, et al. Risk-reducing mastectomy for the prevention of primary breast cancer. *Cochrane Database Syst Rev*. 2018;4:CD002748.
3. Hartmann LC, et al. Efficacy of bilateral prophylactic mastectomy in BRCA1 and BRCA2 gene mutation carriers. *J Natl Cancer Inst*. 2001;93(21): 1633–7.
4. (NICE), N.I.o.H.a.C.E. Familial breast cancer: classification, care and managing breast cancer and related risks in people with a family history of breast cancer. 2019:p. 1.7.20–1.7.29. http://www.nice.org.uk/guidance/cg164

Wire- and Magnetic-Seed-Guided Localization of Impalpable Breast Lesions: iBRA-NET Localisation Study (Arm 1)

Dave RV, Barrett E, Morgan J, et al., on behalf of the iBRA-NET Localisation Study Collaborative.
Br J Surg 109:274–282, 2022

Wire guidance is the historical standard of care for localisation of impalpable breast lesions. However, limitations including wire migration and the need for day-of-surgery placement led to the emergence of implantable seeds for localisation.

PAPER DESCRIPTION

- **Objective/Research Question**: Effectiveness and safety of magnetic seed (Magseed®) localisation for impalpable breast lesions in comparison to wire localisation.

- **Design**: A multicentre, prospective, cohort study in the UK between August 2018 and August 2020 across 35 units. Units recruited into only one or both arms of the study according to local practice.

- **Sample Size**: Using the reported wire failure rate of 0.6% from the literature (99.4% identification rate), and a single-tailed 95% confidence interval difference of less than 0.9%, with 80% power, the power calculation resulted in a planned sample size of 1,000 patients per group. One thousand and three patients had magnetic seed localisation, 1,296 underwent wire localisation and four patients had both seed and wire localisation.

- **Inclusion Criteria**: All women undergoing breast-conserving surgery who required preoperative localisation were eligible, although only patients having unifocal, unilateral lesion localisation were included for primary end point analysis.

- **Exclusion Criteria**: (Magnetic seed group only) Patients who had an iron oxide injection in the previous 6 months, a pacemaker or an electronic chest wall device.

DOI: 10.1201/b23352-50

- **Intervention or Treatment Received**: Magnetic seed localisation for impalpable breast lesions. The magnetic seed is made of **steel and iron oxide** and is detected using a magnetometer device which can detect **a magnetic signature from the seed** in close proximity to the probe head.

  Units offering magnetic seed localisation needed to have adopted the technique as part of routine care. For quality assurance, a minimum caseload was set for each group to ensure adequate radiological and surgical experience prior to study enrolment.

  Wire-guided localisations were performed on the morning of surgery in all patients, but magnetic seed placement (localisations) could be performed in advance.

- **Results**: Two thousand one hundred and sixteen patients (1,170 wire-guided and 946 magnetic seed–guided) who underwent unifocal, unilateral lesion localisation formed the population for the primary end point analysis. The groups were well matched for baseline clinicopathological variables.
  - **Primary outcomes**: Identification of the index lesion occurred in 99.8% (905 of 907 patients, unknown in 39 patients) of magnetic seed–guided excisions and 99.1% (1,150 of 1,161 patients, unknown in nine patients) of wire-guided excisions, a small but statistically significant difference ($p = 0.048$, Fisher's exact test) favouring seed localisation.
  - **Secondary outcomes**: No significant differences in closest or involved margins, re-excision rates (12.3% vs. 13.2%, $p = 0.574$), rates of routine shaves taken during surgery, procedure duration or specimen weight (adjusted for lesion size) were found.

    Significant findings included failed localisation requiring a second localisation method being more common with wire localisation (1.98% vs. 1.64%, $p = 0.032$), and magnetic seeds being less likely to be dislodged from the lesion during surgery compared with wire (0.4% vs. 1.4%, $p = 0.039$). Magnetic seed–guided surgeries were started earlier in the day, as the seed could be placed days before surgery rather than on the day of surgery.

    There were no differences in perioperative surgical complications, reoperation rates or day-of-surgery cancellations.

EXPERT COMMENTARY BY IRAM HASSAN, SAMANTHA CHEN, MASOOMA ZAIDI, PETER A BARRY AND EDWARD R. ST JOHN

Paper significance

This is the largest localisation study to date comparing wire- and magnetic seed–guided localisation for nonpalpable breast lesions. The results demonstrate that magnetic seed is a safe and viable localiser technique for impalpable breast lesions.

The two modalities were equivalent in terms of positive margins, re-excision rate, adjusted specimen weight and procedure duration. There were no differences in complications, reoperation rate and cancellations on the day of surgery. However, magnetic seed localisation was superior in facilitating identification of the index lesion, and it was less likely to require a second method of localisation or be dislodged from the lesion during surgery. As magnetic seeds can be placed prior to the morning of surgery, enabling decoupling of localisation and surgery, they allowed an earlier start time of surgery compared with wire localisation and thus more flexibility for scheduling.

A strength of this study is its prospective multicentre design involving over 2,000 patients. A randomised controlled trial comparing wire and magnetic seed localisation is unlikely to be feasible, as many units in the UK no longer perform wire localisation.

Paper limitations

Whilst the clinical significance of the primary end point demonstrating superiority of seed localisation is marginal at best, and sensitivity analysis imputing missing cases reduces statistical significance ($p = 0.0677$), the study certainly demonstrates the equivalence of magnetic seed to wire localisation for lesion localisation and removal. Localisation accuracy was not examined, only successful surgical removal of the target breast lesion, as defined on final pathology.

The study had potential for selection bias, as choice of localisation method was dependent on unit policy, and hence influenced by surgeons and radiologists. An additional source of bias was that not all units performed both localisation methods, and the study did not detail the number of units performing one or both localisation methods. Centres performing magnetic seed localisation may have had a higher volume of cases and greater radiology and surgical expertise than units performing wire guidance alone.

There was no standardisation of wire localisation (but there was a suggested protocol for magnetic seed localisation) or surgical technique, such as the routine use of intraoperative specimen X-ray to guide additional margin shaves, which are potential sources of bias.

Despite this, the results likely reflect real-world practice across different centres in the UK. As the study occurred during the initial years of magnetic seed implementation, there is potential for an ongoing learning curve, although it has been suggested that the learning curve is minimal.[1,2]

The study was not powered to examine more complex breast localisation, such as multiple lesions or bracketing of larger lesions, and level-2 oncoplastic procedures were excluded. The study did not examine patient or clinician satisfaction or cost analysis between wire- and magnetic seed–guided localisation, which has been reported in other prospective studies.[2]

In context of the relevant current literature

Over the last two decades, several localisation techniques including radio-guided occult lesion localisation (ROLL), radioactive seed localisation, carbon-track marking[3] and intraoperative ultrasonography[4] have emerged as alternatives to standard wire-guided localisation for surgical excision of impalpable breast lesions.

Recently, a variety of non-radioactive seed-based localisation devices have been introduced with the principal aim of guiding surgeons in targeting nonpalpable breast lesions.

In contrast to day-of-surgery wire placement, these seeds can be placed weeks or months before the operation, with subsequent improvement in radiology scheduling, theatre utilisation, patient comfort and experience. These devices differ in their mechanism of detection during surgical localisation, and current literature lacks comparative data.

Outcomes of magnetic seed localisation have been reported in mostly single-institution case series or cohort studies comprising small numbers of patients. Such studies often lacked a control group, were underpowered, were retrospective or did not have well-defined outcome measures. This has led to heterogeneity in results, with some studies reporting a reduction in re-excision rates and specimen weights,[5] while others found no difference in re-excision rates[6,7] or found smaller specimen weights but similar rates of positive margins.[1,2]

A systematic review and pooled analysis of 1,559 magnetic seed (Magseed)-guided procedures across 16 studies demonstrated successful placement in 94.42% of cases and successful localisation in 99.86%, although most studies did not provide a clear definition of either.[8]

A large single-centre study compared magnetic seed ($n = 561$) with conventional wire placement ($n = 825$) and radioactive seed localisation ($n = 449$). Magseed was reported as a safe and effective alternative to the others, with statistically comparable localisation and negative resection margins whilst overcoming radiation safety issues and increasing efficiency.[7]

Patient-related outcome data are limited, although lower preoperative patient anxiety with magnetic seed when compared with wire has been reported.[2,8]

Prospective multicentre audits based on the methodology of the iBRA-NET Magseed landmark study have been replicated to evaluate other novel localisation devices—namely, the Hologic LOCalizer device, the SCOUT Radar Localisation device and Sirius–Pintuition—in comparison to conventional wire guides procedures, with results expected to be published in due course.

Ongoing large, observational, international, prospective cohort studies include EUBREAST's MELODY (Methods for Localization of Different Types of Breast Lesions) study, which aims to prospectively evaluate localisation methods in current use to report oncological safety and patient-reported outcomes.[9] These results are expected to add to the evidence for seed-based localisation and contribute to the ongoing shift away from wire-based localisation.

Magnetic seeds are also used in localising lymph nodes to facilitate accurate axillary de-escalation in targeted axillary dissection.[10]

The future requirements of localisation devices include providing increasingly accurate localisation, smaller devices to enable easier placement and devices designed to prevent migration and facilitate bracketing, as well as reducing magnetic resonance imaging (MRI) artefacts and enabling use in both the breast and axilla (seed- and/or dye-based techniques). As these devices come to market, it is important that they are similarly evaluated to ensure that any advantages and disadvantages of the techniques and technologies are identified, so that any benefits can be translated to patients, clinicians and healthcare providers.

Conclusions

This study demonstrates that magnetic seed localisation (Magseed) is safe and effective at identification of index lesions for impalpable breast lesions compared to traditional wire-based techniques.

Further studies on complex breast localisation such as multiple lesions and bracketing, patient and clinical satisfaction and cost analysis comparing seed and wire localisation are required to determine if efficiencies gained in the patient care pathway offset costs of the devices evaluated.

REFERENCES

1. Redfern RE, Shermis RB. Initial experience using Magseed for breast lesion localization compared with wire-guided localization: analysis of volume and margin clearance rates. *Ann Surg Oncol*. 2022;29(6):3776–83.
2. Micha AE, Sinnett V, Downey K, Allen S, Bishop B, Hector LR, et al. Patient and clinician satisfaction and clinical outcomes of Magseed compared with wire-guided localisation for impalpable breast lesions. *Breast Cancer*. 2021;28(1):196–205.
3. Rose A, Collins JP, Neerhut P, Bishop CV, Mann GB. Carbon localisation of impalpable breast lesions. *Breast*. 2003;12(4):264–9.

4. Haloua MH, Volders JH, Krekel NMA, Lopes Cardozo AMF, De Roos WK, De Widt-Levert LM, et al. Intraoperative Ultrasound Guidance in Breast-Conserving Surgery Improves Cosmetic Outcomes and Patient Satisfaction: Results of a Multicenter Randomized Controlled Trial (COBALT). *Ann Surg Oncol.* 2016;23(1):30–7.
5. Lake B, Wilson M, Thomas G, Williams S, Usman T. P006: The triple effect of the Magseed for localisation of impalpable breast cancer: Significant reduction in re-excision rate, cost saving by reducing further surgery and high patient satisfaction. *Eur J Surg Oncol.* 2020;46(6):e12.
6. Zacharioudakis K, Down S, Bholah Z, Lee S, Khan T, Maxwell AJ, et al. Is the future magnetic? Magseed localisation for non-palpable breast cancer. A multi-centre non randomised control study. *Eur J Surg Oncol.* 2019;45(11):2016–21.
7. Liang DH, Black D, Yi M, Luo CK, Singh P, Sahin A, et al. Clinical outcomes using magnetic seeds as a non-wire, non-radioactive alternative for localization of non-palpable breast lesions. *Ann Surg Oncol.* 2022;29(6):3822–8.
8. Gera R, Tayeh S, Al-Reefy S, Mokbel K. Evolving Role of Magseed in Wireless Localization of Breast Lesions: Systematic Review and Pooled Analysis of 1,559 Procedures. *Anticancer Res.* 2020;40(4):1809–15.
9. Banys-Paluchowski M, Kühn T, Masannat Y, Rubio I, De Boniface J, Ditsch N, et al. Localization Techniques for Non-Palpable Breast Lesions: Current Status, Knowledge Gaps, and Rationale for the MELODY Study (EUBREAST-4/iBRA-NET, NCT 05559411). *Cancers.* 2023; 15(4):1173.
10. Barry PA, Harborough K, Sinnett V, Heeney A, St John ER, Gagliardi T, et al. Clinical utility of axillary nodal markers in breast cancer. *Eur J Surg Oncol.* 2023;49(4):709–15.

Index

Note: Page numbers in *italics* and **bold** refer to figures and tables respectively.

4AC (four cycles of Adriamycin and cyclophosphamide) regimens, 160–162
5-fluorouracil (5-FU), 159, 166
21-gene assay Oncotype Dx, 120, 123–126
70-gene signature, 117–121

A

ACOSOG Z0011 trial, 71, 73–76, 80
ACOSOG Z1071 trial, 81–85
Adjuvant Denosumab in Early Breast Cancer (D-CARE) study, 240
Adjuvant endocrine therapy, 142, 144, 150, 156, 174, 180, 183–191, 217–218, 245
Adjuvant! Online, 117–118, 120, 125, 132
Adjuvant radiotherapy, 97, 137, 143, 149, 165, 227, 233, 235
Adjuvant systemic therapy, 62, 74–75
Adjuvant tamoxifen, 132, 149, 171, 173, 177–181
Adjuvant trastuzumab, 193, 196–198, 213–214, 265
Adjuvant Zoledronic Acid to Reduce Recurrence (AZURE), 237–240
Alcohol consumption, 3, 9
and cancer incidence, 7–10
ALND, *see* Axillary lymph node dissection
AMAROS (After Mapping of the Axilla: Radiotherapy or Surgery), 71, 77, 79
American Society for Radiation Oncology (ASTRO), 59
American Society of Clinical Oncology (ASCO), 143
Anastrozole, 187–191, 244–245
on bone mineral density, 243–246
dose, 187
plus tamoxifen, 187–191
Anthracyclines, 205

Anthracycline–taxane chemotherapy, 196
Antibody–drug conjugate (ADC), 211
Anti-*HER2*
antibody, 211
therapy, 53, 195, 239
APHINITY trial, 197
Arimidex, Tamoxifen, Alone or in Combination (ATAC) trial, 191, 245
Aromatase inhibitors (AIs), 180, 183, 187, 243
Association of Breast Surgery (ABS), 97
AstraZeneca, 190
ATK1 gene, 113
ATLAS (Adjuvant Tamoxifen: Longer against Shorter) trial, 132, 176–181
ATM gene, 265
ATNEC trial, 84
ATTom (Adjuvant Tamoxifen—To Offer More?) trial, 132, 180
Atypical ductal hyperplasia, 14
Austrian Breast Cancer Study Group (ABCSG) XII, 186
Axilla, 79
Axillary clearance, 67–71
Axillary de-escalation, 71
Axillary lymph nodes, 52, 82
metastasis, 237
Axillary lymph node dissection (ALND), 52, 73–75, 79, 82
Axillary node clearance (ANC), 117, 123
Axillary radiotherapy, 67–71, 75, 77, 79–80
Axillary recurrence-free survival, 78
Axillary surgery, 77–80, 118
AZURE, *see* Adjuvant Zoledronic Acid to Reduce Recurrence

B

Basal-like breast cancer, 110
BCS, *see* Breast-conserving surgery

BCT, *see* Breast-conserving therapy
Bilateral risk-reducing mastectomy
        (BRRM), 269–273
Biopsy-proven node-positive (cN1)
        breast cancer, 81
Bisphosphonates, 239, 246
Block randomisation, 187
BOADICEA algorithm, 261
Body mass index (BMI), 3, 8, 96
Bone demineralisation, 245
Bone fractures, 13
Bone mineral density (BMD), 243
Bonferroni analysis, 32
BRCA1
    gene, 203
    mutation, 40–41, 113, 203, 208
BRCA1, proteins, 199
BRCA1/2 gene, 262
BRCA2
    gene, 203
    mutation, 41, 113, 203, 208
BRCA2, proteins, 199
BRCA genes, 261
BRCA-positive tumours, 263
Breast
    biopsy, 269
    density, 102
    radiotherapy, 52
    reduction, 93
    removal, 52
Breast cancer: *see also Specific entries*
    classes, 111
    heterogenicity, 108
    hormone receptors, 171–174
    metastasises to bone, 237
    molecular analyses, 112
    mortality, 21, 172, 230–231
    risk, 1–3, 139
        and menopausal hormone therapy
            (MHT), 1–4
        risk factor for, 3, 9
    screening
        benefits and harms, 25–29
        with Digital Breast Tomosynthesis
            (DBT), 36
        detection rates, 34
        digital mammography, 31–36
        film mammography, 31–36
        image interpretation, 32–33
        mortality benefits of, 25
        staging, 48
        subtypes, 110–114
        surgery, 103
Breast cancer occuring during pregnancy
        (PrBC), 257
Breast-conserving surgery (BCS), 45, 61–65,
        75, 78, 87–89, 91, 102–103, 117, 123,
        130, 148, 153
    management, 223
    with or without irradiation, 217–219
    radiotherapy after, 221–223, 235
Breast-conserving therapy (BCT), 53, 57, 62
Breast Imaging Reporting and Data System
        (BI-RADS) scoring system, 33, 102
Breast International Group (BIG) 1-98
        trial, 191
BREAST-Q, 97
British Association of Plastic,
        Reconstructive and Aesthetic
        Surgeons (BAPRAS), 97

C

CAF (cyclophosphamide, Adriamycin and
        fluorouracil) regimen, 160
Cancer predisposition genes (CPGs), 202
Capecitabine, 165, 203, 206, 208, 214
Capecitabine for Residual Cancer as
        Adjuvant Therapy (CREATE X)
        trial, 165–169
Carbon-track marking, 278
Cardiotoxicity, 196
CEF (cyclophosphamide, epirubicin and
        fluorouracil) regimen, 160
Cell-mediated cytotoxicity, 193
CHEK2, 265
Chemo-endocrine therapy, 124
Chemopreventative therapy, 15
Chemotherapy
    benefits of, 119, 124
    immune checkpoint inhibitors (ICPIs), **209**
    neoadjuvant chemotherapy, 189, 227
    platinum-based chemotherapy, 167, 265
    platinum-based neoadjuvant
        chemotherapy, 205
    for postmenopausal women, 124

pregnancy, during, 255
premenopausal women, 124–125
side effects, 125–126
timing, 201
Cigarette consumption, 8
Claustrophobia, 41
Clinical Evaluation of Pertuzumab and
    Trastuzumab (CLEOPATRA)
    trial, 197
CMF (cyclophosphamide, methotrexate
    and 5-fluorouracil) chemotherapy,
    159–163
Cochrane Central Register of Controlled
    Trials (CENTRAL), 91
Cochrane Group, 27
Collaborative Group on Hormonal Factors
    in Breast Cancer (CGHFBC), 1–3, 9
Comparative Effectiveness of MRI in Breast
    Cancer (COMICE) trial, 45–49
Comparison of Operative *versus*
    Monitoring and Endocrine Therapy
    (COMET) trial, 150, 153
CompassHER2 RD (Comprehensive Use
    of Pathologic Response Assessment
    to Optimize Therapy in HER2-
    Positive Breast Cancer Residual
    Disease), 214–215
Complementary DNA (cDNA)
    microarray, 108
Computerised tomography (CT), 258
Contralateral invasive breast cancer, 199
Contralateral prophylactic mastectomy
    (CPM), 64
Contralateral tumours, 149
Contrast-enhanced magnetic resonance
    imaging (CE MRI), 39–43
Copy number (CN) profiling, 136
Cosmesis, 91
Cox regression models, 8, 154, 194
Cox's proportional hazards, 188
Cytotoxic chemotherapy, 114

D

Danish trial, 63
Data Monitoring Ethics Committee
    (DMEC), 46
DCIS, *see* Ductal carcinoma *in situ*

DCIS tumour pairs, 137
De-epithelialisation, 102
Deep vein thrombosis (DVT), 14
Denosumab, 246
Deprivation, 8
Digital breast tomosynthesis, 23
Digital Mammographic Imaging Screening
    Trial (DMIST), 31, 34–36
Digital mammography, 31–36
    Digital mammograms, 33, 142–143
    in DCIS, 155
Disease-free survival (DFS), 68, 78, 166,
    185, 187, 199, 237, 243
Distal metastasis-free survival (DMFS), 117
Distant disease–free survival (DDFS),
    68–69, 201, 262
Distant recurrence, 199
Distant relapse-free survival (DRFS), 124
DNA, 111
    methylation, 113
    microarrays, 107–110
    mutations, 143
    repair mechanisms, 199–204
Double-blind placebo-controlled trial, 15
Dual-agent mapping, 82, 85
Dual-energy X-ray absorptiometry
    (DXA), 244
Ductal carcinoma *in situ* (DCIS), 35, 46, 59,
    130, 135–139, 141–144
    endocrine therapy and radiotherapy, 149
    high grade, 142–143
    ipsilateral recurrence, 142
    prognostic index, 153–157
    tamoxifen and radiotherapy in, 147–150
Ductal hyperplasia, 148
Duke Hospital cohort, 136
Dutch DCIS cohort study, 136
Dutch Dense Tissue and Early Breast
    Neoplasm Screening (DENSE)
    trial, 42

E

Early Breast Cancer Trialists' Collaborative
    Group (EBCTCG), 161
    meta-analysis, 54, 179, 246
Eastern Cancer Registration and
    Information Centre (ECRIC), 129

Eastern Cooperative Oncology Group
    (ECOG), 82, 166, 206
Eastern Cooperative Oncology
    Group–American College of
    Radiology Imaging Network
    (ECOG-ACRIN), 249
  E2108 trial, 253
Edinburgh Randomized Trial of Breast
    Cancer Screening, 27
Embase, 91
EMBRACA trial, 203
Endocrine therapy, 125, 150, 165, 246
Endometrial cancer, 180
Endopredict, 120
Epigenetic changes (DNA
    methylation), 111
Epithelial abnormalities, 143
Epithelial-like group, 107
ERBB2-overexpressing group, 107
EUBREAST's MELODY, 279
European Organisation for Research and
    Treatment of Cancer (EORTC)
    trial, 54, 80
  10801 trial, 63, 227
European Society for Medical Oncology
    (ESMO), 80, 186, 213
Exemestane, 185, 243, 245
ExteNET trial, 215

F

False-negative rate (FNR), 81
Familial risk (FaMRIsc), 29
Film mammography, 31–36
FinXX trial, 168
First Early Breast Cancer Trialists'
    Collaborative Group (EBCTCG)
    meta-analysis, 223
Fisher's alternative hypothesis, 53
Fluorescent *in situ* hybridisation
    (FISH), 114
Fluorouracil, 165
Food and Drug Administration
    (FDA), 15
Formalin-fixed paraffin-embedded
    (FFPE), 135
Fractures, 245
Full-thickness excision, 102

G

Gail model, 269
GATA3, 111
gBRCA mutations, 261
GEICAM/2003-10 trial, 168
Gene expression patterns, 107–110
Genetic assays, 113
Genetic profiling of tumours, 54
Genomic analysis, 135–139
Genomic clonality, 136
Glandular density, 101–102
Glandular re-approximation, 102
GRADEpro tool, 94
Grading of Recommendations Assessment,
    Development and Evaluation
    (GRADE), 91
GRETA (Group for REconstructive and
    Therapeutic Advancements) group,
    93–94

H

Haematoxylin and eosin (H&E) staining, 74
Halstedian paradigm, 52
Halsted radical mastectomy, 69
Hazard ratios (HRs), 194
Health Insurance Plan (HIP) trial, 25
Health-related quality of life
    (HR-QoL), 251
HER2, 132
  protein, 193
  targeted treatment, 183
  testing, 114
HER2+, 108
  breast cancer, 110–111
HER2-negative, 110
  breast cancer, 123, 205
  cancer, 186
  disease, 165
  tumours, 214
HERA trial, 214
HERceptin Adjuvant (HERA) study, 193
Hologic LOCalizer device, 279
Hormonal bone effects (HOBE), 186
Hormone positivity, 188
Hormone receptor, 148
  –negative patients, 190
  –positive breast cancer, 218

Hormone replacement therapy (HRT), 138, 189; *see also* Menopausal hormone therapy
Human epidermal growth factor 2 *(HER2)* receptors, 114, 120
Human immunodeficiency virus (HIV) infection, 206
Hypertension, 184
Hypofractionated breast radiotherapy, 233–236

I

IBIS-II DCIS trial, 139
IBIS-II prevention trial, 246
iBRANET Magseed landmark, 278
Imaging discordancy, 49
Immediate implant-based breast reconstruction (IBBR), safety outcomes, 95–98
Immune checkpoint inhibitors (ICPIs), 205, **209**
Immunodeficiency, 206
Immunotherapy, 205, 265
Implant-based immediate reconstruction, 231
Implant breast reconstruction (IBR), 88–89
Implant breast reconstruction evaluation (iBRA), 97
Implant loss rates, 96
Institute Gustaf Roussy (IGR) trial, 63
Intention-to-treat analysis, 200, 205
International Clinical Trials Registry Platform, 91
Intraoperative ultrasonography, 278
Invasive breast tumour recurrence (IBTR), 156
Invasive disease–free survival (IDFS), 123, 211, 237
Invasive lobular carcinoma (ILC), 48
Ipsilateral axillary lymph nodes, 78
Ipsilateral breast tumour, 150 recurrence (IBTR), 51–52, 58, 226
Ipsilateral invasive breast cancer, 136, 199 recurrence, 137

K

Kaplan–Meier survival scores, 154, 194
KATHERINE trial, 197, 211–215
KEYNOTE-522 trial, 205, 207–208
Ki67, 132

L

Left ventricular ejection fraction (LVEF), 194, 212
Letrozole, 243, 245
Level-1 OPBCS, 102
Level-2 oncoplastic techniques, 103–104
Li–Fraumeni syndrome, 40
Liver function tests, 212
Lobular carcinoma, 47, 148
Lobular carcinoma *in situ* (LCIS), 14, 130, 139
Localisation for impalpable breast lesions, 275–279
Local recurrence (LR), 57–60
Locoregional invasive disease, 199
Locoregional lymph nodes, 161
Locoregional treatment (LRT), 249
LR, *see* Local recurrence
Luminal A and B breast cancer, 110
Luminal A tumours, 108–109
Luminal breast cancers, 114
Luminal ER-positive tumours, 112
Lumpectomy, 51, 74, 222
Lumpectomy plus tamoxifen, 219
Lymphatico-venous communications, 52
Lymphoedema, 79
Lymphoedema, 67–71, 78

M

Magnetic resonance imaging (MRI), 29, 45, 279
in DCIS, 155
Magnetic Resonance Imaging for Breast Screening (MARIBS), 39–43
Magnetic seed localisation, 276, 279
Malmö Breast Tomosynthesis Screening Trial, 26
MammaPrint, 118–121, 125–126, 162
Mammary Prevention 3 (MAP.3) trial, 16
Marmot Review, 25

Mastectomy, 51–55, 61, 67–71, 75, 88, 103, 117
survival rate, 61
Mastopexy techniques, 93
Medial-lateral oblique (MLO) mammogram, 20
MEDLINE, 91
Menopausal hormone therapy (MHT), 1–4, 8
alcohol intake and cancer incidence, 7–10
and breast cancer risk, 1–4
Mesh-assisted techniques, 96
Metastatic breast cancer (MBC), 123, 249
Methylation, 112
MHT, *see* Menopausal hormone therapy
MicroRNA expression, 110, 113
Million Women Study (MWS), 3–4, 7
MINDACT trial, 120, 126, 163
Molecular architecture of breast cancer, 111–114
Mortality, 19
Multigene expression tumour-profiling tests, 125
Musculoskeletal symptoms, 184
Mutational Significance in Cancer (MuSiC), 112
Myelodysplastic syndromes, 201
Myocardium, 162

N

NAC undermining, 102
National Cancer Institute Common Terminology Criteria for Adverse Events (NCICTCAE), 166
National Cancer Institute (NCI) trial, 63
National Genomic Test Directory, 202
National Health Service Breast Screening Programme (NHS BSP), 4, 26–27, 34, 149
National Institute for Health and Care Excellence (NICE) guidelines, 15, 80, 132, 149, 186, 191, 195, 202, 213, 239, 264, 273
National Institutes of Health (NIH), 63
National Mastectomy and Breast Reconstruction Audit (NMBRA), 96

National Surgical Adjuvant Breast and Bowel Project (NSABP), 13, 69, 153
B-04 trial, 67–68, 73, 77, 79
B-06, 53–54
B-06 trial, 61, 63, 221
B-17 trial, 153
B-24 trial, 147, 150
B-32 trial, 83
B-35, 139
Negative margins, 58
Neoadjuvant chemotherapy (NACT), 81–85, 165, 189, 211, 227
NeoSphere trial, 197
Night shift work, 10
Nipple–areolar complex (NAC), 102
Nipple deviation, 102
Node localisation, 83
Node-negative breast cancer, 110
Node-negative disease, *68*, 68–69
Node-positive disease, *68*, 68–69, 81, 223
Node-positive patients, 230
Non-Hodgkin lymphoma, 8
Non-pathological complete response (non-pCR), 169
Normal breast–like group, 107
Nottingham Prognostic Index (NPI), 110, 120, 125, 131
NSABP Breast Cancer Prevention Trial (NSABP P-1), 15–16
Nuclear factor I (NFI), 143

O

Oestrogen, 1, 3, 10, 13
Oestrogen-only MHT, 4
Oestrogen–progestogen MHT, 4
Oestrogen receptor (ER), 138, 149, 191, 222, 261
-negative breast cancer, 205
-positive, 171
-positive breast cancer, 177–181, 246
-positive patients, 165
status, 238
Olaparib, 199–204
OlympiAD trial, 203
OlympiA study, 199, 201
Oncoplastic breast-conserving surgery (OPBCS), 87, 91–94, 101–104
Oncoplastic Breast Consortium, 93

Oncoplastic classification system, 102
Oncoplastic techniques, 102
Oncotype Dx, 120, 125, 143–144, 162
OPBCS, *see* Oncoplastic breast-conserving
    surgery
OptimICE-pCR trial, 208
Oral contraceptives, 8
Osteonecrosis of the jaw (ONJ), 238
Osteoporosis, 184, 245
OTOASOR trial, 80
Ovarian function suppression, 125
Ovarian oestrogen suppression, 185
Ovarian suppression, 184–185
Overall survival (OS), 68–69, 78, 262

P

P53, 143
Paget's disease, 49, 62
  of nipple, 148
PALB2 gene, 265
PAM50 gene expression assay, 110
Pathogenic gene mutation, 39
Pathological complete responses (pCRs),
    165, 205
Pathological features and DCIS,
    141–144
Patient-reported outcome measures
    (PROMs), 92
Pectoral fascia, 52
Pembrolizumab, 205–209
Pertuzumab, 197
  plus trastuzumab, 197
Physical activity, 8
PIK3CA, 111–112, 143
Planned non-inferiority test, 79
Plastic surgery, 93
Platinum-based chemotherapy,
    167, 265
Platinum-based neoadjuvant
    chemotherapy, 205
Pneumonitis, 201
Polychemotherapy, 81, 159–163
Poly (ADP-ribose) polymerase (PARP)
    inhibitors, 163, 199–204, 265
POSH (Prospective Outcomes in
    Sporadic *versus* Hereditary Breast
    Cancer), 131
Positive margins, 58

POSNOC trial, 75
Postmastectomy radiotherapy, 229–232
Postmenopausal women
  chemotherapy for, 124
  Mammary Prevention 3 (MAP.3) trial
    in, 16
  tamoxifen in, 191
PREDICT, 110, 120, 129–132, 264
Prediction Analysis of Microarray 50
    (PAM50), 109
PREDICT Plus, 125
Pregnancy, breast cancer treatment during,
    255–258
Pregnancy after breast cancer, 258
Pregnancy-associated breast cancer (PABC)
    patients, 257
PreludeDx assays, 144
Premenopausal oestrogen receptor
    (ER)-positive breast cancer,
    183–186
Premenopausal women, endocrine therapy
    for, 174
Pre-pectoral reconstruction, 97
PRIME II trial, 217–219
Progesterone receptor (PR), 172
  -negative breast cancer, 205
  -positive disease, 200
Progestogen, 2
Programmed cell death ligand (PDL)
    pathway, 64
Programmed death ligand-1 (PDL1),
    114, 205
  receptor, 205
Prosigna®, 120, 125
  gene expression assay, 110
  test, 110
Prospective Study of Outcomes in Sporadic
    versus Hereditary Breast Cancer
    (POSH) study, 261–266
Protein expression, 110
Pulmonary embolism (PE), 14, 173, 180

Q

Quadrantectomy, 222
Quality of life (QoL), 91, 93–94,
    229–232, 252
Quantitative RT-PCR (qRT-PCR) assay
    test, 109–110

R

Radical mastectomy, 52–54
Radioactive isotope tracer, 78
Radioactive seed localisation, 278
Radio-guided occult lesion localisation
    (ROLL), 278
Radiotherapy (RT), 63
    after breast-conserving surgery, 235
    BCS and, 153
    benefits, 150
    ipsilateral breast tumour recurrence
        (IBTR), 51–52
    whole-breast radiotherapy (WBRT),
        225–228
Raloxifene, 16
Randomisation, 20, 63, 78, 118, *187*,
    187–188, 211
Randomised controlled trials (RCTs), 94, 97
Receiver operating characteristic (ROC)
    analysis, 32
Recurrence score (RS), 123
Regional radiotherapy utilisation, 78
Relapse-free survival, 68
Relative risks (RRs), 8
    of breast cancer mortality, 26
Renal cell carcinoma, 8
Residual invasive HER2-positive breast
    cancer, 211–215
Risedronate, 246
Risk of Bias in Non-Randomised Studies of
    Interventions [ROBINS-I] tool, 91
Risk-reducing mastectomy (RRM), 41,
    269–272
RNA, 111
RxPONDER, 126

S

SCOUT Radar Localisation device, 279
Screening mammography, 31
Second primary invasive cancer, 199
Seed-based localisation, 279
Selective ER modulators (SERMs), 15
Selective Use of Postoperative
    Radiotherapy after Mastectomy
    (SUPREMO) trial, 231
SENTINA (SENTinel NeoAdjuvant)
    multicentre cohort study, 83, *84*

Sentinel lymph node biopsy (SLNB), 71, 73,
    77, 81, 117, 123
Sentinel lymph node dissection (SLND), 73
Sentinel lymph node (SLN) metastase, 73
Sentinel node biopsy, 77, 79, 83
    Sentinel node procedure, 78
Shoulder mobility, 78
Significance analysis of microarrays
    (SAM), 108
Single-agent mapping technique, 83
Single-cell DNA sequencing
    (scDNA-seq), 137
Single-nucleotide polymorphism (SNP)
    arrays, 112, 136
Sirius–Pintuition wire guides, 279
Skin incision, 102
Skin undermining, 102
Sloane project, 136, 143
Smoking, 96
Society of Surgical Oncology (SSO), 59, 143
Standardisation of Breast Radiotherapy
    (START) trials, 227, 235–236
Staging tumour, 47
Stress, 41
Stromal changes, 143
Study of Tamoxifen and Raloxifene
    (STAR) trial, 16
Sublocalisation of tumour, 62
Suppression of Ovarian Function Trial
    (SOFT), 125, 183–186
Surgical de-escalation, 61
Surgical margins in breast conservation
    therapy and local recurrence (LR),
    57–60
Surgical quality control, 78
Surveillance, epidemiology, and end
    results (SEER)
    data, 270
    registry, 132
Swedish National Board of Health and
    Welfare, 19
Swedish Two-County Trial, 19–23, 26
Systemic adjuvant therapies, 223

T

TAILORx (Trial Assigning Individualized
    Options for Treatment [Rx]) trial,
    120, 126, 163

Tamoxifen, 13–16, 148–149, 177–181, 183–191, 222, 243–244
dose, 187
effectiveness, 15
and lumpectomy, 219
in postmenopausal women, 191
side effects, 180
therapy, 171–174
Tamoxifen and Exemestane Trial (TEXT), 125, 183–186
Targeted axillary dissection (TAD), 81
Targeted sequencing, 136
Taxanes, 165–166, 205
anthracycline regimens, 161
-based chemotherapy, 212
T-DM1 (ado-trastuzumab emtansine; Kadcyla), 211–215
Therapeutic mammaplasty (TM), 87–89, 93, 102
Third-field radiation, 74
Thrombocytopenia, 212
Thromboembolic disease, 173
Thromboembolic events, 16
Thyroid cancer, 8
TM, see Therapeutic mammaplasty
Tobacco consumption, 9
Tomosynthesis Mammographic Imaging Screening Trial (TMIST), 36
TP53, 111
Transcription polymerase chain reaction (RT-PCR), 108
Translational Arimidex, Tamoxifen, Alone or in Combination (transATAC), 125
Trastuzumab, 193–198, 212
Trastuzumab emtansine, 211–215
Trial Assigning Individualized Options for Treatment (TAILORx), 126
Triple-negative breast cancer (TNBC), 165, 205, 207, 261
Triple-negative disease, 114
Triple-negative type breast cancer, 111

Tumour bed boost, 227
Tumour-free resection margins, 51
Tumour location, 101
Two-County Trial, see Swedish Two-County Trial

U

UK National Quality Criteria for Breast Reconstruction, 96
Ultra-hypofractionated five-fraction schedules, 235
Uterine cancer, 173

V

Van Nuys Prognostic Index (VNPI), **70**, 153–157, **154**
Volume displacement techniques, 93

W

WBRT, see Whole-breast radiotherapy
Whole-breast irradiation, 74, 225–228
Whole-breast radiotherapy (WBRT), 58, 225–228
Whole-exome sequencing (WES), 136
Wide local excision (WLE), 51–52, 137
Wire- and magnetic-seed-guided localization, 275–279
Women's Health Initiative (WHI) trial, 3

X

X-rays, 277

Y

Young-onset breast cancer (YOBC), 261–266

Z

Z0011 trials, see ACOSOG Z0011 trial
Zoledronate, 246
Zoledronic acid, 237–238

Printed in the United States
by Baker & Taylor Publisher Services

Printed in the United States
by Baker & Taylor Publisher Services